Saunders'

Q&A
REVIEW
for the

PHYSICAL
THERAPY
BOARD
EXAMINATION

Saunders'

Q&A
REVIEW
for the
PHYSICAL
THERAPY
BOARD
EXAMINATION

Edited by

Brad Fortinberry, PT, DPT, SCS

President
Fortinberry Physical Therapy
Physical Therapist
St. Luke Home Health
McComb, Mississippi

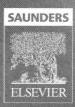

SAUNDERS

ELSEVIER

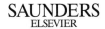

SAUNDERS
ELSEVIER

3251 Riverport Lane
St. Louis, Missouri 63043

SAUNDERS' Q&A REVIEW FOR THE PHYSICAL THERAPY
BOARD EXAMINATION   ISBN: 978-1-4160-4979-1
Copyright © 2011 by Saunders, an imprint of Elsevier Inc.

Notice

Knowledge and best practice in this field are constantly changing. As new research and experience broaden our understanding, changes in research methods, professional practices, or medical treatment may become necessary.

Practitioners and researchers must always rely on their own experience and knowledge in evaluating and using any information, methods, compounds, or experiments described herein. In using such information or methods they should be mindful of their own safety and the safety of others, including parties for whom they have a professional responsibility.

With respect to any drug or pharmaceutical products identified, readers are advised to check the most current information provided (i) on procedures featured or (ii) by the manufacturer of each product to be administered, to verify the recommended dose or formula, the method and duration of administration, and contraindications. It is the responsibility of practitioners, relying on their own experience and knowledge of their patients, to make diagnoses, to determine dosages and the best treatment for each individual patient, and to take all appropriate safety precautions.

To the fullest extent of the law, neither the Publisher nor the authors, contributors, or editors, assume any liability for any injury and/or damage to persons or property as a matter of products liability, negligence or otherwise, or from any use or operation of any methods, products, instructions, or ideas contained in the material herein.

978-1-4160-4979-1

Fortinberry, Brad, 1974-
   Saunders' Q & A review for the physical therapy board examination /
Brad Fortinberry.
      p. ; cm.
   Includes index.
   ISBN 978-1-4160-4979-1 (pbk. : alk. paper) 1. Physical
therapy--Examinations--Study guides. I. Title. II. Title: Q & A review
for the physical therapy board examination. III. Title: Q and A review
for the physical therapy board examination.
   [DNLM: 1. Physical Therapy Modalities--Examination Questions. WB
18.2 F742s 2011]
   RM706.F67 2011
   615.8'2076--dc22
                                                                    2009051980

Vice President and Publisher: Linda Duncan
Executive Editor: Kathy Falk
Senior Developmental Editor: Christie M. Hart
Publishing Services Manager: Hemamalini Rajendrababu
Project Manager: Jagannathan Varadarajan
Book Designer: Jessica Williams

Printed in The United States of America

Last digit is the print number: 9   8   7   6   5   4   3   2   1

Dedication

Without the love and support of my wife, Melissa, and the sacrifices of my children, Austin and Hayden, this project would have never been possible.

Also, thanks to my parents, Bebo and Brenda, for a great beginning to a rewarding career.

Contributors

NANCY ADACHI, PT, BS
Clinical Specialist and Coordinator of Clinical Education
Kaiser Permanente;
Department of Physical Medicine and Rehabilitation
University of California;
Part-time Faculty UCLA Orofacial Pain
Lecturer Kaiser Permanente Orthopedic Residency Program
Lecturer UCLA Orofacial Pain and Dental School
Los Angeles, California

LEESHA AUGUSTINE, PT, DPT
Lead Inpatient Physical Therapist
Children's Hospital of Orange County
Orange, California

ROSS BIEDERMAN, DPM
Professor
Department of Physical Therapy
Chapman University
Orange, California

TERESA BRIEDWELL, PT, DPT
Clinical Assistant Professor/Director of Admissions
Department of Physical Therapy
University of Missouri;
Clinic Director
Renaissance Therapy Rehabilitation and Fitness
Columbia, Missouri

LUCY K. CHUNG, PharmD
Adjunct Professor
School of Recreation, Health, and Tourism
George Mason University
Manassas, Virginia

PETER GERBINO, MD
Orthopedic Surgeon
Monterey Joint Replacement and Sports Medicine
Monterey, California

VICTORIA GRAHAM, PT, DPT, OCS, NCS
Assistant Professor
Department of Physical Therapy Education
College of Allied Health Professions
Western University of Health Sciences
Pomona, California

JULIE GUTHRIE, PT, DPT, OCS
Adjunct Faculty
Department of Physical Therapy
Mount St. Mary's College
Los Angeles, California;
Physical Therapist
Davis and Derosa Physical Therapy
El Segundo, California

MARTHA R. HINMAN, PT, EdD, CEEAA
Professor
Department of Physical Therapy
Hardin-Simmons University
Abilene, Texas

REVAY MEAD, PT, DPT
Inpatient Physical Therapist
Loma Linda University Children's Hospital
Loma Linda, California;
Inpatient Physical Therapist
Children's Hospital of Orange Country
Orange, California

WILLIAM H. O'GRADY, PT, DPT, MA, OCS, FAAOMPT, DAAPM
Former CEO
Olympic Sports and Spine Rehabilitation
Lakewood, Washington;
Past Chief Examiner
AAOMPT;
Adjunct Faculty
Physical Therapy Program
University of Nevada
Las Vegas, Nevada

RICHARD B. SOUZA, PhD, PT, ATC, CSCS
Assistant Professor
Department of Physical Therapy and Rehabilitation Science
University of California, San Francisco
San Francisco, California

DERRICK SUEKI, DPT, GCPT, OCS
Adjunct Orthopedic Faculty
Department of Physical Therapy
Mount St. Mary's College
Los Angeles, California;
Clinical Mentor
Orthopedic Residency Program
Division of Biokinesiology and Physical Therapy
University of Southern California
Los Angeles, California;
Owner
Knight Physical Therapy, Inc.
Garden Grove, California

WOLFGANG H. VOGEL, PhD
Professor Emeritus of Pharmacology
Formerly Professor and Acting Chairman
Department of Pharmacology
Jefferson Medical College of Thomas Jefferson University
Philadelphia, Pennsylvania

ROBERT WELLMON, PT, PhD, NCS
Associate Professor
Institute for Physical Therapy Education
Widener University
Chester, Pennsylvania

Preface

The purpose of any exam preparation study guide is to help you find the area of weakness in your knowledge base. You should already have a vague idea of which topic in physical therapy has challenged you in the past. It is not important that you memorize answers to the questions included in this book, only that you understand how to prepare and pass the exam. Careful study of this book and its associated CD-ROM will allow you to tackle these different areas.

This book does not attempt to take the place of the vast array of knowledge gained in course work and clinical rotations, nor should this preparation tool be used to cram for hours before taking the exam. Instead this text and accompanying CD-ROM should be used to simulate actual exam scenarios and find faults in your knowledge base. For this reason, we have divided this book into 6 sections:

1. Clinical Application of Foundational Sciences
2. Examination
3. Foundations for Evaluation, Differential Diagnosis and Prognosis
4. Interventions
5. Equipment and Devices
6. Safety and Professional

Each section has a wide variety of scenarios, diagnoses, patient populations practice settings, and types of questions designed to help you prepare for the national examination. References were selected primarily from sources and textbooks familiar to physical therapy programs across the country.

Examination Preparation

Remember, it is not important that you get the questions right when practicing but that you understand how to prepare yourself for the exam and your career as a physical therapist. You should consider several factors in preparing for the exam. First and foremost you should consider the actual material on the test. Your knowledge in the varied subject areas of physical therapy will be tested. Although cramming for this sort of comprehensive exam is usually futile, you may prefer to study in that fashion. Previous coursework, clinical studies, peer-group study sessions, and observation of experienced physical therapists over the years is what prepares you for this type of national exam.

The practice exams should be administered in the same environment as the actual national exam. Rooms should be quiet and at a comfortable temperature. Limit interruptions for the duration of your simulated examination. The

CD-ROM included in this book is an excellent source for practice exams. It will randomly select 250 questions to create a practice test. Each practice test will have roughly the same percentage of questions in each of the six sections as the actual exam. If you are using the actual text for your practice, block off enough time, and treat the text as if it were an actual computerized test.

In the final weeks prior to the exam, concentrate study on those areas in which you have found yourself to be weak. Cramming huge amounts of facts only increases your level of anxiety. Establish a routine of sleeping, eating, and exercise before the exam. If your routine is the same day in and day out, your anxiety level will be decreased at exam time.

Familiarize yourself with the testing center. It may be a good idea to map your route to the testing center in the days before the exam. This would give you time to find alternate routes for road construction or poor weather. Also check with the testing center for specific rules such as: Will there be a lunch break? Can I bring lunch in to the testing center? Will lockers be provided? Will scratch paper be provided?

Taking the Exam
RELAX!!! The exam allows ample time for completion, so do not get nervous about time in the first portions. The exam is computerized, so read all directions and familiarize yourself with all controls before beginning. Read each question carefully and slowly. Each question or stem will be followed by four choices. There will be one correct answer and three distracters or incorrect answers to each question. Remember that you are required to choose the correct or best answer for each question. There may seem to be more than one correct answer, but look for the most correct one for the question provided.

Bring appropriate supplies to the exam, such as pencils and erasers. Consider ear plugs if you are distracted by noise. Ask the exam center if they will provide such items in advance.

Most computerized exams offer a tutorial of the computerized controls used in the exam. Even if you feel you are very computer literate, it is still advisable to take this opportunity to familiarize yourself with the specific controls for the test. The tutorials do not usually count into your actual exam time.

Be cognizant of what exactly the question is asking. Some of the distracters are designed to lead you into an incorrect answer. Reread the stem along with each choice if necessary before deciding upon an answer. Determine what part of the therapy process the question is referring. For example, is the question asking you about examination, intervention, plan, or goals? Also pay attention to words related to timing of a particular action, like initial, first, next, or last step.

Answer all questions even if you have no idea of the correct answer. Unmarked and incorrect questions equally count against the tested student. Narrow the distracters to the best of your ability and guess at the answer if necessary. If applicable, skip the question and come back if you have time. Sometimes questions early in the exam can seem unfamiliar to you, but a question later can jog your memory and help you answer earlier questions.

It is certainly normal to feel a little nervous before taking the exam. Control your emotions and breathing rate before you begin the actual test. If allowable, take a break during the exam just to clear your head and refocus your thoughts.

After the Exam

Allow some time to decompress after you leave the testing area. Most people are mentally exhausted after such an expansive test. Consider a good meal and some relaxation time for the evening after the exam. Also, plan something fun for the next day to take your mind off of the test.

It is imperative that you do not discuss the specifics after completing the exam. The organization that manages the national exam, the Federation of State Boards of Physical Therapy (FSBPT), is very explicit in their desire to stop students from discussing questions after the test. If you are found to have circulated actual test items, you could face disciplinary action from the FSBPT such as voiding of your test score and an inability to retake the exam.

We wish you the best of luck as you prepare for the exam. This is an important step to launch a long and successful career as a physical therapist.

Brad Fortinberry, PT, DPT, SCS

Contents

CHAPTER 1

Clinical Application of Foundational Sciences

1. The sinoatrial node is located in what chamber of the heart?
   a. Left atrium
   b. Right atrium
   c. Left ventricle
   d. Right ventricle

2. Where in the tissues does nutrient exchange take place?
   a. Capillaries
   b. Interstitial spaces
   c. Arterioles
   d. Venules

3. During which phase of the cardiac cycle is ventricular volume the lowest?
   a. Atrial systole
   b. Isovolumetric ventricular contraction
   c. At the onset of rapid ventricular ejection
   d. Isovolumetric ventricular relaxation

4. The heart contains a variety of different types of muscle fibers, each with a different frequency of spontaneous contraction. Which of the following has the shortest period (highest frequency) of spontaneous contraction?
   a. Purkinje fibers
   b. SA node
   c. AV node
   d. Myocardium

5. Stimulation of CN X will cause which of the following effects?
   a. Atrial fibrillation
   b. Sinus bradycardia
   c. Cardiac rigor
   d. Ventricular fibrillation

6. The volume of air moved going from full forced expiration to full forced inspiration is known as
   a. Inspiratory capacity
   b. Vital capacity
   c. Total lung capacity
   d. Inspiratory reserve volume

7. During periods of intense physical activity, many physiologic adaptations occur, especially in the circulatory system. Which of the following occurs during increased physical exertion?
   a. Increased ventricular refilling, secondary to increased venomotor tone
   b. Decreased cardiac output
   c. Decreased stroke volume
   d. Increased cardiac cycle time

8. Which of the following is indicative of left heart failure?
   a. Pitting pedal edema
   b. Neck vein distention
   c. Orthopnea
   d. Ascites

9. A patient asks the therapist to explain the function of his medication verapamil (a calcium antagonist). Which of the following points should be conveyed in the therapist's explanation?
   a. Verapamil causes decreased contractility of the heart and vasodilation of the coronary arteries.
   b. Verapamil causes decreased contractility of the heart and vasoconstriction of the coronary arteries.
   c. Verapamil causes increased contractility of the heart and vasodilation of the coronary arteries.
   d. Verapamil causes increased contractility of the heart and vasoconstriction of the coronary arteries.

10. The protocol for a cardiac patient states that the patient should not exceed 5 metabolic equivalents (METs) with any activity at this stage of recovery. Which of the following activities would be inappropriate for the patient?
    a. Cycling 11 mph
    b. Walking 4 mph
    c. Driving a car
    d. Weeding a garden

11. During the opening of a patient's mouth, a palpable and audible click is discovered in the left temporomandibular joint. The physician informs the therapist that the patient has an anteriorly dislocated disk. This click most likely signifies that
    a. The condyle is sliding anteriorly to obtain normal relationship with the disk
    b. The condyle is sliding posteriorly to obtain normal relationship with the disk
    c. The condyle is sliding anteriorly and losing normal relationship with the disk
    d. The condyle is sliding posteriorly and losing normal relationship with the disk

12. In what position should the therapist place the upper extremity to palpate the supraspinatus tendon?
    a. Full abduction, full flexion, and full external rotation
    b. Full abduction, full flexion, and full internal rotation
    c. Full adduction, full external rotation, and full extension
    d. Full adduction, full internal rotation, and full extension

13. A 13-year-old girl has fractured the left patella during a volleyball game. The physician determines that the superior pole is the location of the fracture. Which of the following should be avoided in early rehabilitation?
    a. Full knee extension
    b. 45 degrees of knee flexion
    c. 90 degrees of knee flexion
    d. 15 degrees of knee flexion

14. During conference with the physical therapist, a respiratory therapist indicates that the patient has a low expiratory reserve volume. What does this mean?
    a. The volume of air remaining in the lungs after a full expiration is low.
    b. The volume of air in a breath during normal breathing is low.
    c. The volume of air forcefully expired after a forceful inspiration is low.
    d. The amount of air expired after a resting expiration is low.

15. During an evaluation a 74-year-old woman informs you that she is "taking a heart pill." The patient does not have her medication with her but states that the medication "slows down my heart rate." Which of the following is the most probable medication?
    a. Epinephrine
    b. Digitalis
    c. Quinidine
    d. Norepinephrine

16. A patient is referred to physical therapy with a secondary diagnosis of hypertension. The physician has ordered relaxation training. The therapist first chooses to instruct the patient in the technique of diaphragmatic breathing. Which of the choices below is the correct set of instructions?
    a. Slow the breathing rate to 8 to 12 breaths per minute, increase movement of the upper chest, and decrease movement in the abdominal region.
    b. Slow the breathing rate to 12 to 16 breaths per minute, increase movement of the abdominal region, and decrease movement in the upper chest.
    c. Slow the breathing rate to 8 to 12 breaths per minute, increase movement of the abdominal region, and decrease movement in the upper chest.
    d. Slow the breathing rate to 12 to 16 breaths per minute, increase movement of the upper chest, and decrease movement in the abdominal region.

17. Which of the following statements about cardiovascular response to exercise in trained and/or sedentary patients is false?
    a. If exercise intensities are equal, the sedentary patient's heart rate will increase faster than the trained patient's heart rate.
    b. Cardiovascular response to increased workload will increase at the same rate for sedentary patients as it will for trained patients.
    c. Trained patients will have a larger stroke volume during exercise.
    d. The sedentary patient will reach anaerobic threshold faster than the trained patient if workloads are equal.

18. A therapist is asked to examine a patient in the intensive care unit. The patient is comatose but breathing independently. During the assessment of range of motion in the right upper extremity, the therapist notices that the patient is breathing unusually. The pattern is an increase in breathing rate and depth followed by brief pauses in breathing. The therapist should notify the appropriate personnel that the patient is exhibiting which of the following patterns?
    a. Biot's respiration
    b. Cheyne-Stokes respiration
    c. Kussmaul respiration
    d. Paroxysmal nocturnal dyspnea

19. Which of the following statements is not a common physiologic change of aging?
    a. Blood pressure taken at rest and during exercise increases.
    b. Maximal oxygen uptake decreases.
    c. Residual volume decreases.
    d. Bone mass decreases.

20. A patient with cardiac arrhythmia is referred to physical therapy services for cardiac rehabilitation. The therapist is aware that the heart receives nerve impulses that begin in the sinoatrial node of the heart and then proceed to the
    a. Atrioventricular node, then to the Purkinje fibers, and then to the bundle branches
    b. Purkinje fibers, then to the bundle branches, and then to the atrioventricular node
    c. Atrioventricular node, then to the bundle branches, and then to the Purkinje fibers
    d. Bundle branches, then to the atrioventricular node, and then to the Purkinje fibers

21. A 65-year-old man is scheduled to begin a wellness program. He has no cardiovascular disease, major systemic illness, or musculoskeletal abnormality. However, he is deconditioned because of an extremely sedentary lifestyle. Resting heart rate is 90 beats/minute, and resting blood pressure is 145/92 mm Hg. Which of the choices below describes the most correct intensity, frequency, and duration at which the patient should begin exercise?
    a. 75% Vo$_2$ max; 30 min/day; 3 days/wk
    b. 40% Vo$_2$ max; 30 min/day; 5 days/wk
    c. 40% Vo$_2$ max; 10 minutes twice daily; 5 days/wk
    d. 75% Vo$_2$ max; 10 minutes twice daily; 3 days/wk

22. A 17-year-old athlete has just received a posterior cruciate ligament reconstruction. The therapist is attempting to explain some of the characteristics of the posterior cruciate ligament. Which of the following is incorrect information?
    a. The posterior cruciate ligament prevents posterior translation of the tibia on the femur.
    b. Posterior bands of the posterior cruciate ligament are their tightest in full knee extension.
    c. The posterior cruciate ligament is attached to the lateral meniscus and not to the medial meniscus.
    d. The posterior cruciate ligament helps with medial rotation of the tibia during full knee extension with open chain activities.

23. A patient starting to use antihypertensive medications must be observed when getting up or leaving a warm therapeutic pool in order to avoid an episode of
    a. Bradycardia
    b. Orthostatic hypotension
    c. Dysrhythmias
    d. Skeletal muscle weakness

24. A patient whose exercise-induced heart rate is less than the heart rate was before exercise is most likely starting therapy with
    a. Anticholinergic drugs
    b. Alpha blockers
    c. Beta blockers
    d. Antianginals

25. A patient inhales a beta agonist to relieve his asthma. After its use, you may notice
    a. An increase in heart rate
    b. A few moments of incoordination
    c. Flushing with red face
    d. A decrease in blood pressure

26. A patient is using a statin drug. Which of the following drug-induced signs or symptoms should be reported to the treating physician?
    a. Muscle pain
    b. Irregular heart beat
    c. Persistent diarrhea
    d. Intermittent confusion

27. Statin drugs lower cholesterol by
    a. Preventing cholesterol absorption
    b. Binding to cholesterol in the intestines
    c. Inhibiting HMG-CoA reductase
    d. Inhibiting lipoprotein lipase

28. A patient is being treated with an antiarrhythmic drug. The drug might cause all of the following adverse reactions except
    a. Dizziness and fainting
    b. Stevens Johnson syndrome
    c. Irregular heart beats
    d. Joint and muscle pain

29. An asthmatic patient is to be exercised in a rather cool environment. It is recommended that the patient use the inhaler
    a. About 1 hr before the exercise
    b. About 20 minutes before exercise
    c. Just at the beginning of exercise
    d. At the first onset of breathing problems during exercise

30. A patient using a beta blocker is exercised and might experience all of the following except
    a. Some breathing difficulties
    b. Muscle cramps and pain
    c. A smaller than expected increase in heart rate
    d. Some drowsiness

31. A beta blocker reduces blood pressure by all of the following actions except
   a. A reduction in cardiac output
   b. A reduction in central sympathetic outflow
   c. Inhibition of renin release
   d. A reduction in peripheral resistance

32. A patient on calcium channel blocker therapy might complain during therapy sessions about all of the following except
   a. Lightheadedness and dizziness
   b. Muscle pain and joint stiffness
   c. Tremors
   d. Edema

33. A patient under the influence of local anesthetic therapy might experience all of the following except
   a. Some sensory impairment
   b. Increased blood pressure
   c. Tremors
   d. Motor deficits

34. A patient with angina pectoris experiences some pain during exercise therapy and uses three tablets of sublingual nitroglycerin, but the pain does not subside. You should
   a. Ask the patient to stretch out quietly and breathe deeply
   b. Tell patient to continue the medication until the pain stops
   c. Call 911 since this could signal a true heart attack
   d. Administer two tablets of a non-narcotic analgesic to help reduce the pain

35. Your patient is a 48-year-old male who reports to physical therapy with complaints of left shoulder and neck pain. Symptoms began insidiously 3 weeks ago and have been increasing in frequency and duration since that time. He notices the symptoms with lifting heavy objects and shoveling dirt for a garden that he is building. Walking fast elicits symptoms. Symptoms abate after several minutes of rest. He is in relatively good health with the exception of high blood pressure and shortness of breath. What system is most likely affected?
   a. Cardiovascular
   b. Pulmonary
   c. Musculoskeletal
   d. Hepatic

36. Your patient is a 38-year-old male who is a patient that you have been treating for left shoulder pain. He was in a motor vehicle accident since you last treated him 2 days ago. He was the driver and was rear-ended. He hit his left side on the door handle and has been having sharp pain in his ribs. X-rays the day of the accident revealed fractured ribs (ribs 6 and 7 on the left). He has been having difficulty breathing and has been very short of breath. Sharp pain is noted on the left with breathing and coughing. He has also noticed some blood in his sputum. What system is mostly likely the source of the patient's symptoms?
   a. Musculoskeletal
   b. Pulmonary
   c. Cardiovascular
   d. Hepatic

37. Aspirin and clopidogrel (Plavix) fall into which class of antithrombics?
   a. Thrombolytics
   b. Platelet aggregator inhibitors
   c. Anticoagulants
   d. Fibrinolytics

38. Which of the following drugs should angina patients always carry with/on them in case of an angina attack?
   a. Nitroglycerin patch
   b. An ACE inhibitor
   c. Digoxin
   d. Sublingual nitroglycerin

39. The part of the respiratory system that is most effected by asthma is/are the
   a. Bronchioles
   b. Trachea
   c. Nasal cavity
   d. Bronchi

40. Some of the classes of drugs used to treat angina include
   a. Nitrates
   b. HMG-CoA reductase inhibitors
   c. Alpha-blockers
   d. Diuretics

41. Beta-blockers that are useful in the treatment of hypertension
   a. Work by competitively inhibiting beta receptors, thereby decreasing heart rate
   b. Are always selective for $beta_1$-receptors
   c. Do not cause bronchoconstriction in patients with asthma
   d. Should not be combined with any other type of antihypertensive

42. Which of the following medications should be used to treat an acute asthma attack?
    a. An oral steroid such as prednisone
    b. A long-acting beta-agonist such as salmeterol
    c. An inhaled steroid such as fluticasone
    d. A short-acting beta-agonist such as albuterol

43. In children with osteogenesis imperfecta, fractures heal
    a. Within the normal healing time
    b. More quickly than normal
    c. More slowly than normal
    d. Only with assistance of medication

44. Components of lower extremity alignment that contribute to toe in include
    a. Femoral retroversion
    b. Femoral anteversion
    c. Calcaneovalgus feet
    d. External tibial torsion

45. Osteochondritis dissecans occurs most commonly in the
    a. Capitellum
    b. Humeral condyle
    c. Medial femoral condyle
    d. Lateral femoral condyle

46. The joint most frequently involved in pauciarticular juvenile rheumatoid arthritis is the
    a. Cervical spine
    b. Lumbar spine
    c. Knee
    d. Wrist

47. The most common onset type of juvenile rheumatoid arthritis is
    a. Systemic
    b. Juvenile ankylosing spondylitis
    c. Polyarticular
    d. Pauciarticular

48. Considering an injury to the medial collateral ligament (MCL) of the knee, when does the inflammatory phase of healing begin?
    a. First days after injury
    b. 2 to 3 weeks after injury
    c. 4 to 6 weeks after injury
    d. 6 to 8 weeks after injury

49. Which of the following types of exercise is most likely to intensify delayed onset muscle soreness (DOMS)?
    a. Concentric exercise is most likely to intensify DOMS.
    b. Eccentric exercise is most likely to intensify DOMS.
    c. Isometric exercise is most likely to intensify DOMS.
    d. DOMS will remain constant no matter the type of exercise.

50. What is the correct order of the stages of bone healing after a fracture?
    a. Inflammatory phase, hard callous phase, soft callous phase, remodeling phase
    b. Inflammatory phase, soft callous phase, hard callous phase, remodeling phase
    c. Remodeling phase, soft callous phase, hard callous phase, inflammatory phase
    d. Remodeling phase, hard callous phase, soft callous phase, inflammatory phase

51. Which type of connective tissue includes the superficial sheath of body tissue under the skin, muscle, and nerve sheaths, and the framework of internal organs?
    a. Dense regular connective tissue
    b. Dense irregular connective tissue
    c. Loose irregular connective tissue
    d. Loose regular connective tissue

52. Which patient population is most likely to have osteophyte formation that leads to rotator cuff damage?
    a. 16-year-old baseball player
    b. 34-year-old factory worker
    c. 45-year-old tennis player
    d. 75-year-old sedentary individual

53. You are seeing a patient who has just received a steroid injection into a joint. You should
    a. Treat this joint vigorously
    b. Treat this joint gently
    c. Not touch this joint at all
    d. Postpone the session for at least 1 week

54. A patient with osteoporosis might be treated with all of the following drugs except
    a. Bisphosphonates
    b. Calcitonin
    c. Calcium with vitamin D
    d. Thyroid hormones

55. A patient has been told to use Advil for rheumatoid arthritis. You notice that the patient uses acetaminophen because a friend uses it, and it is cheaper. You can tell the patient that acetaminophen
    a. Can be used since it is the same as Advil
    b. Is different from Advil but has the same therapeutic action
    c. Is actually more effective than Advil
    d. Does not work in rheumatoid arthritis

56. Skeletal muscle relaxants
    a. May interfere with walking in patients who use their spasticity to control balance
    b. Selectively paralyze certain muscle groups
    c. Should be stopped quickly after long-term use when problems have been resolved
    d. Have never been proven effective

57. While doing a worksite assessment in the hospital business office, a physical therapist found several employees complaining of neck and shoulder pain. It was determined that making a simple change in the set-up of the computer stations could reduce symptoms. The change to the computer monitor that would MOST affect neck and shoulder discomfort is
    a. Lowering the monitor to the desk surface
    b. Moving the computer monitor closer to the employee's face
    c. Tilting the monitor forward
    d. Putting a nonglare screen on the monitor

58. The cuboid bone is located just posterior to the
    a. Base of the first metatarsal
    b. Head of the first metatarsal
    c. Medial cuneiform bone
    d. Tuberosity of the fifth metatarsal

59. The metacarpophalangeal joints are classified as what type of joint?
    a. Plane
    b. Hinge
    c. Condyloid
    d. Saddle

60. Which muscle would move the abducted (90 degree) arm anteriorly?
    a. Sternocostal head of the pectoralis major
    b. Clavicular head of the pectoralis major
    c. Inferior fibers of the serratus anterior
    d. Pectoralis minor

61. Which one of the following structures does NOT pass through the foramen magnum of the occipital bone?
    a. Spinal cord
    b. Meninges
    c. Cranial nerve XII
    d. Vertebral artery

62. Contraction of which muscle produces extension of the head?
    a. Spinalis cervicis
    b. Longus capitis
    c. Longus colli
    d. Sternocleidomastoid

63. The nucleus pulposus is thickest in which region of the spine?
    a. Lumbar spine
    b. Inferior half of the thoracic spine
    c. Superior half of the thoracic spine
    d. Cervical spine

64. The speed of muscle contraction is a function of which of the following factors?
    a. Resting length of the muscle fiber
    b. Cross-sectional diameter of the muscle
    c. Creatine phosphate of the muscle
    d. Glycolytic capacity of the muscle

65. Which of the following describes the proper normal anatomy of the proximal carpal row, from lateral to medial?
    a. Capitate, lunate, triquetrum, pisiform
    b. Lunate, trapezium, capitate, hamate
    c. Scaphoid, lunate, triquetrum, pisiform
    d. Scaphoid, hamate, lunate, capitate

66. A therapist is testing key muscles on a patient who recently suffered a spinal cord injury. The current test assesses the strength of the long toe extensors. Which nerve segment primarily innervates this key muscle group?
    a. L2
    b. L3
    c. L4
    d. L5

67. A physician notes a vertebral fracture in the x-ray of a patient involved in a car accident. The fractured vertebra has a bifid spinous process. Which of the following vertebrae is the most likely to be involved?
    a. Fourth lumbar vertebra
    b. Fifth cervical vertebra
    c. Twelfth thoracic vertebra
    d. First sacral vertebra

68. If the line of gravity is posterior to the hip joint in standing, on what does the body first rely to keep the trunk from moving into excessive lumbar extension?
    a. Iliopsoas muscle activity
    b. Abdominal muscle activity
    c. Anterior pelvic ligaments and the hip joint capsule
    d. Posterior pelvic ligaments and the hip joint capsule

69. What is the closed-packed position of the shoulder?
    a. Internal rotation and abduction
    b. External rotation and abduction
    c. Internal rotation and adduction
    d. External rotation and adduction

70. A patient with a diagnosis of a rotator cuff tear has just begun active range of motion. The therapist is strengthening the rotator cuff muscles to increase joint stability and oppose the superior shear of the deltoid. Which of the rotator cuff muscles participate least in opposing the superior sheer force of the deltoid?
    a. Infraspinatus
    b. Subscapularis
    c. Teres minor
    d. Supraspinatus

71. What portion of the adult knee meniscus is vascularized?
    a. The outer edges are vascularized.
    b. The inner edges are vascularized.
    c. The entire meniscus is vascular.
    d. The entire meniscus is avascular.

72. At what age does a human have the greatest amount of fluid in the intervertebral disc?
    a. 1 year
    b. 4 years
    c. 7 years
    d. 10 years

73. Which of the following is not an example of a synarthrodial joint in the body?
   a. Coronal suture
   b. The fibrous joint between the shaft of the tibia and fibula
   c. Symphysis pubis
   d. Metacarpophalangeal

74. A football player presents to an outpatient clinic with complaints of pain in the right knee after an injury suffered the night before. The physician determines that the anterior cruciate ligament (ACL) is torn. Which of the following is most commonly associated with an injury causing damage to the ACL only?
   a. Varus blow to the knee with the foot planted and an audible pop
   b. Foot planted, medial tibial rotation, and an audible pop
   c. Valgus blow to the knee with the foot planted and no audible pop
   d. Foot planted, lateral tibial rotation, and no audible pop

75. A 27-year-old woman is referred to a physical therapy clinic with a diagnosis of torticollis. The right sternocleidomastoid is involved. What is the most likely position of the patient's cervical spine?
   a. Right lateral cervical flexion and left cervical rotation
   b. Right cervical rotation and right lateral cervical flexion
   c. Left cervical rotation and left lateral cervical flexion
   d. Left lateral cervical flexion and right cervical rotation

76. Observing a patient in a standing position, the therapist notes that an angulation deformity of the right knee causes it to be located medially in relation to the left hip and left foot. This condition is commonly referred to as
   a. Genu varum
   b. Genu valgum
   c. Pes cavus
   d. None of the above

77. Which of the following is the most vulnerable position for dislocation of the hip?
   a. 30 degrees hip extension, 30 degrees hip adduction, and minimal internal rotation
   b. 30 degrees hip flexion, 30 degrees hip adduction, and minimal external rotation
   c. 30 degrees hip flexion, 30 degrees hip abduction, and minimal external rotation
   d. 30 degrees hip extension, 30 degrees hip abduction, and minimal external rotation

78. Which of the following articulate with the second cuneiform?
    a. Navicular
    b. Talus
    c. First metatarsal
    d. Cuboid

79. The terms below refer to properties of water that make hydrotherapy valuable to a variety of patient populations. Match the following terms with the statement that best relates to each term.
    1. Viscosity
    2. Buoyancy
    3. Relative density
    4. Hydrostatic pressure
    A. This property can assist in the prevention of blood pooling in the lower extremities of a patient in the pool above waist level.
    B. This property makes it harder to walk faster through water.
    C. A person with a higher amount of body fat can float more easily than a lean person because of this property.
    D. This property makes it easier to move a body part to the surface of the water and harder to move a part away from the surface.
    a. 1-B, 2-C, 3-D, 4-A
    b. 1-B, 2-D, 3-C, 4-A
    c. 1-C, 2-B, 3-A, 4-D
    d. 1-A, 2-C, 3-B, 4-D

80. A physician ordered a splint for a patient who should keep the thumb of the involved hand in abduction. A new graduate is treating the patient and is confused about the difference between thumb flexion, extension, abduction, and adduction. Which of the following lists is correct?
    a. Extension is performed in a plane parallel to the palm of the hand, and abduction is performed in a plane perpendicular to the palm of the hand.
    b. Flexion is performed in a plane perpendicular to the palm of the hand, and adduction is performed in a plane parallel to the palm of the hand.
    c. Extension is performed in a plane perpendicular to the palm of the hand, and adduction is performed in a plane parallel to the palm of the hand.
    d. In referring to positions of the thumb, flexion and adduction are used synonymously, and extension and abduction are used synonymously.

81. A physical therapist receives an order from the physician to treat a patient using iontophoresis. The order indicates that the purpose of the treatment is to attempt to dissolve a calcium deposit in the area of the Achilles' tendon. When preparing the patient for treatment, the therapist connects the medicated electrode to the negative pole. Which of the following medications is the therapist most likely preparing to administer?
    a. Dexamethasone
    b. Magnesium sulfate
    c. Hydrocortisone
    d. Acetic acid

82. A therapist is assisting a patient in gaining lateral stability of the knee joint. The therapist is using strengthening exercises to strengthen muscle groups that will increase active restraint on the lateral side of the joint. Which of the following offers the least amount of active lateral restraint?
    a. Gastrocnemius
    b. Popliteus
    c. Biceps femoris
    d. Iliotibial band

83. A patient is in an outpatient facility because of an injury sustained to the right knee joint. Only the structures within the synovial cavity were compromised during the injury. Knowing this information only, the therapist is not concerned with injury to which of the following structures?
    a. Patellofemoral joint
    b. Anterior cruciate ligament
    c. Medial meniscus
    d. Femoral condyles

84. A patient is being examined by a physical therapist because of bilateral knee pain. The therapist is attempting to rule out ankle or foot dysfunction as the source of the pain. Which of the following observations is not true in examining a patient without foot or ankle problems in the standing position?
    a. The talus is situated somewhat medially to the midline of the foot.
    b. In quiet standing, the muscles surrounding the ankle joint remain silent.
    c. The first and second metatarsal heads bear more weight than the fourth and fifth metatarsal heads.
    d. The talus transmits weight to the rest of the bones of the foot.

85. A physical therapist is examining a female distance runner who complains of intermittent medial ankle pain. In static standing, the therapist palpates excessive lateral deviation of the head of the talus. From this information, in what position is the subtalar joint during palpation?
    a. Supination
    b. Pronation
    c. Neutral
    d. Unable to determine from the information given

86. Which of the following is not part of the triangular fibrocartilage complex of the wrist?
    a. Dorsal radioulnar ligament
    b. Ulnar collateral ligament
    c. Radial collateral ligament
    d. Ulnar articular cartilage

87. A physical therapist is attempting to explain the importance of slow stretching to an athlete training to compete in a marathon. The therapist explains that quick stretching often causes the muscle to _____, which is a response initiated by the _____, which are located in the muscle fibers.
    a. Relax, Golgi tendon organs
    b. Contract, Golgi tendon organs
    c. Relax, muscle spindles
    d. Contract, muscle spindles

88. What is the normal low-end range for interincisal opening with a TMD patient?
    a. 50 mm
    b. 30 mm
    c. 40 mm
    d. 60 mm

89. What is dental trismus?
    a. Capsulitis of the TMJ
    b. Osteoarthritis of the TMJ
    c. Muscle spasm of the TMJ
    d. The trigger point of the TMJ

90. Temporomandibular anterior disc displacement without reduction occurs between the
    a. Disc and the lower joint compartment
    b. Disc and the ementia articularis
    c. Disc and the lateral pterygoid muscle
    d. Disc and the upper joint compartment

91. What are the signs and symptoms of a temporomandibular anterior displaced disc with reduction?
    a. Crepitation with loss of opening
    b. Clicking with opening
    c. No clicking with loss of opening
    d. Temporomandibular joint tenderness and loss of opening

92. What is the normal TMJ arthrokinematics for lateral movements?
    a. Bilateral translation
    b. Bilateral rotation
    c. Contralateral rotation and ipsilateral translation
    d. Ipsilateral rotation and contralateral translation

93. What is the normal TMJ arthrokinematics for protrusion?
    a. Bilateral anterior translation
    b. Bilateral posterior translation
    c. Ipsilateral rotation with contralateral translation
    d. Bilateral rotation

94. What is the normal TMJ arthrokinematics for wide opening?
    a. Bilateral translation
    b. Combination of rotation occurs first 26 mm then anterior translation
    c. Combination of anterior translation occurs first 26 mm then anterior rotation
    d. Bilateral rotation

95. Positioning of a patient in right side-lying can create pressure on the
    a. Right ischial tuberosity
    b. Left greater trochanter
    c. Right lateral malleolus
    d. Occiput

96. Ideal postural alignment is influenced by appropriate muscle balance. What combinations of muscle imbalance would likely contribute to increased anterior pelvic tilt?
    a. Short hamstrings and elongated hip flexors
    b. Strong anterior abdominals and strong hip flexors
    c. Short hip flexors and lengthened anterior abdominals
    d. Strong anterior abdominals and strong hip extensors

97. A patient presents with anterior knee pain, which of the following cannot be the source of that pain?
    a. Synovium
    b. Capsule
    c. Patella cartilage
    d. Patella bone

98. Anterior cruciate ligament tears do not heal as well as medial collateral ligament tears because
    a. The ACL is under greater tension
    b. Synovial fluid inhibits ACL healing
    c. The MCL is broad and flat allowing better healing
    d. There is more motion in the ACL

99. Patellofemoral joint reactive forces are highest with
    a. Running
    b. Straight leg raises
    c. Prolonged sitting
    d. Plyometrics

100. Rotator cuff tear
    a. Is rare under the age of 40
    b. Is usually painful
    c. Progresses from the bursal side toward the articular side
    d. Requires surgical repair

101. Foot drop following total hip arthroplasty most likely indicates
    a. Stroke
    b. Disc herniation
    c. Sciatic laceration
    d. Traction neurapraxia

102. Sever's apophysitis
    a. Frequently occurs with Achilles tendinitis
    b. Is a result of leg length inequality
    c. Is not an inflammatory condition
    d. Responds to ultrasound treatment

103. Pes planus
    a. Is a painful condition
    b. Is common in patients with hyperlaxity
    c. Requires orthotics treatment
    d. Results in anterior knee pain if not corrected

104. A patient was referred for physical therapy after removal of a long arm cast extending to the forearm. She lacks full passive elbow extension. What may be causing this problem?
    a. Active insufficiency of the biceps
    b. Tightness in posterior humeroulnar joint capsule
    c. Passive insufficiency of the pronator teres
    d. Passive insufficiency of the triceps

105. A 10 degrees hip flexion contracture produces _____ torque at the hip that increases muscle demand on the _____.
   a. Extension, quadriceps
   b. Flexion, biceps femoris
   c. Abduction, adductor magnus
   d. Flexion, iliopsoas

106. The physical therapist is analyzing a patient's gait with descending stairs. During left single limb stance, the patient demonstrates a right pelvic drop with left trunk lean. The physical therapy hypothesis is
   a. Weak right gluteus medius with left trunk lean to move center of mass towards stronger side
   b. Weak left gluteus medius with left trunk lean to move center of mass towards weaker side
   c. Weak left quadratus lumborum producing left trunk lean
   d. Weak right gluteus medius with left trunk lean to move center of mass towards stronger side

107. Left lateral trunk flexion is limited primarily by
   a. The thoracic spine because of sagittal facet alignment
   b. The rib cage because of multiple attachments
   c. The lumbar spine because of horizontal plane facet orientation
   d. The left quadratus lumborum

108. Which is true about the hip joint?
   a. The hip joint's closed pack position is extension with full external rotation.
   b. The hip joint's loose pack position is 30 degrees of abduction, 70 degrees of flexion with lateral rotation.
   c. With its capsular pattern of restriction, medial rotation is most restricted in the hip joint.
   d. With its capsular pattern of restriction, flexion is most restricted in the hip joint.

109. A physical therapist is conducting a screen for visual field deficits by having the client look straight ahead and presenting a stimulus at the outer margins of the person's visual fields. The examination technique checks cranial nerve(s) _____ function.
   a. II
   b. III, IV, VI
   c. V
   d. VIII

110. The next patient on your schedule is a 69-year-old Asian woman with a diagnosis of "T8 fracture." What condition are you most concerned with for this patient?
    a. Neck pain
    b. Myopathy
    c. Dizziness
    d. Osteoporosis

111. Which of the following are not appropriate interventions for a patient with osteoporosis and a T8 compressions fracture?
    a. Balance exercises
    b. Postural exercises
    c. Proprioceptive training
    d. Ultrasound

112. A patient is suffering from chronic back pain as a result of a recent automobile accident. He is currently taking an opioid medication for relief of this pain. Which of the following medications is an opioid?
    a. Ibuprofen
    b. Aspirin
    c. Codeine
    d. Acetaminophen

113. An athlete has been complaining of muscle spasms. Her physician decided to treat her with a medication called cyclobenzaprine, which is a muscle relaxant. She is unfamiliar with this medication and asks if you can tell her anything about it. Which of the following is a correct statement?
    a. There are no such medications as muscle relaxants.
    b. Muscle relaxants are the same thing as anti-inflammatory medications.
    c. Drowsiness, blurred vision, and dry mouth are some of the side effects of muscle relaxants.
    d. You cannot overdose on muscle relaxants.

114. All NSAIDs inhibit _____ in some manner or another.
    a. Bradykinin
    b. Cyclooxygenase (COX)
    c. Prostaglandins
    d. Lipoxygenase

115. Which NSAID has been used because of its lower incidence of GI complications?
    a. Naproxen
    b. Aspirin
    c. Ketoprofen
    d. Celecoxib

116. Your patient had a laceration anterior to the medial malleolus that required stitches. He is now in your office complaining of pain along the medial border of the foot. Which nerve is most likely involved?
   a. Sural nerve
   b. Deep fibular
   c. Tibial nerve
   d. Saphenous nerve

117. Which named peripheral nerve is responsible for pain sensation from the pericardium, mediastinal pleura, diaphragmatic pleura, and diaphragmatic peritoneum?
   a. Vagus nerve
   b. Phrenic nerve
   c. Greater thoracic splanchnic nerve
   d. Tenth intercostal nerve

118. The neural canal is smallest and circular in shape in the _____ region of the vertebral canal.
   a. Cervical
   b. Thoracic
   c. Lumbar
   d. Sacral

119. Ascending tracts in the white matter of the spinal cord carry _____information.
   a. Sensory
   b. Motor
   c. Both sensory and motor
   d. Autonomic

120. Which of the following cranial nerves does NOT contain parasympathetic fibers?
   a. Oculomotor
   b. Facial
   c. Trigeminal
   d. Vagus

121. A number of significant clinical conditions involve abnormalities of neurotransmitter release or reception at the myoneural junction. The neurotransmitter associated with the motor endplate is
   a. Norepinephrine
   b. Dopamine
   c. Acetylcholine
   d. Myasthenia gravis

122. Which is an inhibitory neurotransmitter in the central nervous system?
   a. GABA
   b. Epinephrine
   c. Glutamate
   d. Norepinephrine

123. On examination of a cross-section of the spinal cord of a cadaver, the examiner notes plaques. This finding is most characteristic of
   a. Parkinson's disease
   b. Myasthenia gravis
   c. Multiple sclerosis
   d. Dementia

124. The therapist is ordered to evaluate a patient in the intensive care unit. The patient appears to be in a coma and is totally unresponsive to noxious, visual, and auditory stimuli. What rating on the Rancho Los Amigos Cognitive Functioning Scale is most appropriate?
   a. I
   b. III
   c. IV
   d. VIV

125. Which of the following is not an acceptable long-term goal for a patient with a complete C7 spinal cord injury?
   a. Independence with dressing
   b. Driving an automobile
   c. Balance a wheelchair for 30 seconds using a "wheelie"
   d. Independence with performing a manual cough

126. Which of the following neural fibers are the largest and fastest?
   a. C fibers
   b. A beta fibers
   c. A delta fibers
   d. B fibers

127. A posterior lateral herniation of the lumbar disc between vertebrae L4 and L5 most likely results in damage to which nerve root?
   a. L4
   b. L5
   c. L4 and L5
   d. L5 and S1

128. A therapist is examining a patient in the intensive care unit. The therapist notes no eye opening, no verbal response, and no motor response. On the Glasgow coma scale, what is the patient's score?
   a. 0
   b. 3
   c. 5
   d. 9

129. During the examination of an infant, the therapist observes that with passive flexion of the head the infant actively flexes the arms and actively extends the legs. Which of the following reflexes is being observed?
   a. Protective extension
   b. Optical righting
   c. Symmetrical tonic neck
   d. Labyrinthine head righting

130. A patient asks the therapist whether she should be concerned that her 4-month-old infant cannot roll from his back to his stomach. The most appropriate response to the parent is:
   a. "This is probably nothing to be concerned about because, although it varies, infants can usually perform this task by 10 months of age."
   b. "This is probably nothing to be concerned about because, although it varies, infants can usually perform this task by 5 months of age."
   c. "Your infant probably needs further examination by a specialist because, although it varies, infants can usually perform this task at 2 months of age."
   d. "Your infant probably needs further examination by a specialist because, although it varies, infants can usually perform this task at birth."

131. A patient has traumatically dislocated the tibia directly posteriorly during an automobile accident. Which of the following structures is the least likely to be injured?
   a. Tibial nerve
   b. Popliteal artery
   c. Common peroneal nerve
   d. Anterior cruciate ligament

132. A patient is referred to physical therapy with complaints of sensation loss over the area of the radius of the right upper extremity, extending from the elbow joint distally to the wrist. Therapy sessions are focused on assisting the patient in regaining normal sensation. Which of the following nerves is responsible for sensation in this region?
   a. Medial antebrachial cutaneous
   b. Lateral antebrachial cutaneous
   c. Musculocutaneous
   d. Both B and C

133. While examining a patient who suffered a complete spinal cord lesion, the therapist notes the following strength grades with manual muscle testing: wrist extensors = 3+/5, elbow extensors = 2+/5, and intrinsic muscles of the hand = 0/5. What is the highest possible level of this lesion?
    a. C3
    b. C4
    c. C5
    d. C7

134. A physical therapist must have a clear understanding of the normal development of the human body to treat effectively and efficiently. Which of the following principles of treatment is incorrect?
    a. Early motor activity is influenced primarily by reflexes.
    b. Motor control develops from proximal to distal and from head to toe.
    c. Increasing motor ability is independent of motor learning.
    d. Early motor activity is influenced by spontaneous activity.

135. Which of the following statements about developmental motor control is incorrect?
    a. Isotonic control develops before isometric control.
    b. Gross motor control develops before fine motor control.
    c. Eccentric movement develops before concentric movement.
    d. Trunk control develops before distal extremity control.

136. Which of the following statements is true in comparing infants with Down's syndrome to infants with no known abnormalities?
    a. Motor milestones are reached at the same time with both groups.
    b. Postural reactions are developed in the same time frame with both groups.
    c. Postural reactions and motor milestones are developed slower in patients who have Down's syndrome, but with the same association as with normal infants.
    d. Postural reactions and motor milestones are not developed with the same association with patients who have Down's syndrome as with normal infants.

137. The spastic type of cerebral palsy usually results from involvement of the
    a. Corpus callosum
    b. Basal ganglia
    c. Motor cortex
    d. Cerebellum

138. A complete rupture of a cord of the brachial plexus is best described using the term
   a. Neurotmesis
   b. Neuropraxia
   c. Axonotmesis
   d. Axonopraxia

139. Which of the following statements is true regarding myelodysplasia?
   a. Myelodysplasia is defined as defective development limited to the anterior horn cells of the spinal cord.
   b. Embryologically, myelodysplastic lesions can be related to either abnormal nervous system neurolation or canalization.
   c. Myelodysplasia is often associated with genetic abnormalities; however, there is no association with teratogens.
   d. Myelodysplasia refers to defects in the lower spinal cord only.

140. Which of the following statements is true regarding progressive neurologic dysfunction?
   a. Progressive neurologic dysfunction is common during periods of rapid growth but does not occur once skeletal maturity is reached.
   b. Deterioration of the gait pattern is one of the last symptoms to be detected.
   c. Symptoms include loss of sensation and/or strength, pain along a dermatome or incision, spasticity onset or worsens, and changes in bowel or bladder sphincter control.
   d. Development of scoliosis will always be rapid.

141. Fine synergistic control of neck flexors and extensors in the upright position typically appears in the
   a. Second month
   b. Third month
   c. Fourth month
   d. Fifth month

142. Ballistic movements of arms and legs are characterized by
   a. Reciprocal activation of antagonist muscles.
   b. Coactivation of antagonist muscles.
   c. Need for proprioceptive feedback during movement.
   d. Visual guidance during movement.

143. In typically developing children, successful head turning in a prone position with an erect head is characterized by
    a. Hip extension, medial rotation, and abduction
    b. Cervical spine extension and rotation with weight bearing on the upper abdomen
    c. Shoulder flexion and abduction with weight bearing on elbows
    d. Caudal weight shift with load bearing on lateral thighs and lower abdomen

144. Development in children with cerebral palsy is characterized by
    a. Failure to develop reciprocal patterns of muscle activation
    b. The appearance of fidgety movements as defined by Prechtl and colleagues at about 9 weeks of age
    c. The appearance of chorea at about 6 months of age
    d. Failure to develop binocularity of vision

145. Circling arm movements, finger spreading, and a poor repertoire of general movements are characteristic of
    a. Down syndrome
    b. Muscular dystrophy
    c. Spastic cerebral palsy
    d. Dyskinetic cerebral palsy

146. The movement repertoire of the human newborn includes
    a. Projection of the arm toward stationary objects, kicking, and mouth-to-hand behaviors
    b. Projection of the arm toward stationary objects, reaching with grasping, and neonatal stepping behaviors
    c. Projection of the arm toward moving objects, reaching and grasping, and light-avoidance behaviors
    d. Projection of the arm toward moving objects, mouth-to-hand, and kicking behaviors

147. Once a new motor skill is obtained, further development entails
    a. Performance with more use of sensory feedback
    b. Constricting the degrees of freedom used when performing the skill
    c. Perfecting postural control and transitions between postures
    d. Developing a single way of performing the skill

148. Which is the strongest predictor of skill in walking for children with typical development?
    a. Age
    b. Duration of time since walking began
    c. Weight
    d. Extent of walking practice

149. It is typical of a 3-year-old child to
    a. Manage buttoning well
    b. Alternate feet when ascending stairs
    c. Be unafraid of falling
    d. Show no dysmetria during block stacking

150. A patient with Parkinson's disease on levodopa/carbidopa therapy might experience during therapy all of the following except
    a. The "off" phase
    b. Dizziness
    c. Involuntary movements
    d. Marked bradycardia

151. A patient whose seizures are controlled with an anticonvulsant should be treated in a room or an area that
    a. Is devoid of bright flickering lights and repetitive, loud noises
    b. Has no electronic equipment near the patient
    c. Is warm and somewhat humid
    d. Is not frequented by many people

152. You might want to inform a patient on lithium therapy to contact the physician or call the physician directly if this patient shows
    a. Ataxia and a fine tremor
    b. Increased blood pressure and dyspnea
    c. Excessive salivation and tearing
    d. Constipation and trouble voiding

153. Your patient is on antipsychotic drug therapy. During your therapy sessions you might notice a number of movement abnormalities. The most severe one is
    a. Tardive dyskinesia
    b. Tremor
    c. Akathisia
    d. Dystonia

154. Which of the following adverse reactions experienced during antiviral drug treatment might be encountered most frequently during therapy?
    a. Elevated blood pressure
    b. Aggressive and inappropriate behavior
    c. Neuralgia and myopathies
    d. Sedation and incoordination

155. Which of the following adverse reactions might be encountered during therapy sessions by a patient receiving anxiolytic drugs?
    a. Psychomotor impairment
    b. Erratic heart rates
    c. Frequent interruptions due to diarrhea
    d. Excessive sweating

156. A patient starting cholinergic agonist therapy for myasthenia gravis might have to interrupt the therapy session repeatedly because of
    a. Abdominal cramps and diarrhea
    b. Intermittent tachycardia
    c. Joint stiffness and muscle cramps
    d. Extremely dry mouth

157. Among other reasons, mental activity and motor control is the result of excitatory and inhibitory neurotransmitter actions in the CNS. The most important inhibitory neurotransmitter is
    a. Glutamate
    b. GABA
    c. Norepinephrine
    d. Acetylcholine

158. A patient has a tumor in the parietal lobe. The physical therapist anticipates problems with
    a. Muscle strength
    b. Perception of spatial relationships
    c. Sensation and motor function
    d. Vision

159. What are the components of upper motor neuron syndrome?
    a. Fasciculations, spasticity, hyperreflexia
    b. Spasticity, rigidity, hyporeflexia
    c. Spasticity, positive Babinski sign, rigidity
    d. Spasticity, hyperreflexia, positive Babinski sign

160. After completing a developmental assessment on a seven month old, which of the following reflexes wound not be integrated?
    a. Galant Reflex
    b. Moro Reflex
    c. Landau reflex
    d. Symmetrical tonic neck reflex

161. Nerve regeneration occurs at a pace of _____ per month
    a. 5 mm
    b. 1 inch
    c. 1 cm
    d. 2.5 inches

162. A physical therapist working in an early intervention program is providing intervention to an infant diagnosed with Erb's palsy. This condition most often involves what nerve roots?
    a. C2-C3
    b. C3-C4
    c. C5-C6
    d. C8-T1

163. A patient with an Erb's palsy will have paralysis of all of the following muscles except the
    a. Flexor carpi ulnaris
    b. Rhomboids
    c. Brachialis
    d. Teres minor

164. The physical therapist is beginning the examination of a patient in an outpatient cardiac rehabilitation facility. A chart review shows that this patient has active atrial fibrillation with a controlled ventricular rate. What is the most appropriate intervention for this patient?
    a. Low intensity aerobic exercise
    b. High intensity aerobic exercise
    c. High intensity lower extremity exercise only.
    d. Low intensity lower extremity exercise only.

165. Which of the following is incorrect advice to give to a patient with a diagnosis of congestive heart failure who complains of shortness of breath and "smothering" while attempting to sleep?
    a. Sleep with the head on 2 to 3 pillows
    b. Sleep without any pillows
    c. Sleep in a recliner during exacerbations
    d. During exacerbations come to a standing position for short-term relief

166. A physical therapist is treating a patient with significant burns over the limbs and upper trunk. Which of the following statements is false about some of the changes initially experienced after the burn?
    a. This patient initially experienced an increase in the number of white blood cells.
    b. This patient initially experienced an increase in the number of red blood cells.
    c. This patient initially experienced an increase in the number of free fatty acids.
    d. This patient initially experienced a decrease in fibrinogen.

167.   The most common cause of burn injury in infants is
    a.   Accidental flame burn from a smoking adult
    b.   Car accidents with immolation.
    c.   Scald injury, either intentional or accidental by neglect
    d.   House fires, in which all family members are injured

168.   What are the four stages, in time order, of wound healing after surgery?
    a.   Coagulation, inflammatory phase, granulation phase, and scar
        formation and maturation
    b.   Inflammatory phase, coagulation, scar formation and maturation,
        and granulation phase
    c.   Scar formation and maturation, granulation phase, coagulation
        phase, and inflammatory phase
    d.   Inflammatory phase, granulation phase, coagulation, and scar
        formation and maturation

169.   A patient is taking tetracyclines for an infection. You have to be most
       careful to
    a.   Not expose the patient to excessive light or UV therapy
    b.   Only exercise this patient moderately
    c.   Avoid using the warm therapeutic pool
    d.   Have the patient get up very slowly from a lying position

170.   A patient with lymphedema following breast CA and reconstruction
       requires examination. She is presenting with heaviness, itching, aching
       and redness in her left upper extremity. Your next course of action is to
    a.   Take girth measurements of the arm
    b.   Begin lymph drainage massage
    c.   Take her temperature
    d.   Send her back to physician

171.   Which of the following layers of the epidermis is responsible for the
       constant renewal of epidermal cells?
    a.   Stratum germinativum
    b.   Stratum granulosum
    c.   Stratum lucidum
    d.   Stratum corneum

172.   The right adrenal gland is in contact with the
    a.   Spleen
    b.   Inferior vena cava
    c.   Pancreas
    d.   Stomach

173. Releasing hormones that regulate the anterior lobe of the pituitary gland are synthesized in the
    a. Hypothalamus
    b. Cerebral cortex
    c. Thalamus
    d. Basal ganglia

174. Erythropoietin is a hormone required for the production of red blood cells. It is produced primarily in the
    a. Kidney
    b. Lung
    c. Marrow
    d. Pancreas

175. Which abdominal organs does the thoracic cage protect?
    a. Spleen, liver, adrenal gland, and upper portion of kidneys and stomach
    b. Pancreas, liver, and vermiform appendix
    c. Gallbladder, urinary bladder, liver, and uterus
    d. Spleen, pancreas, adrenal gland, and ovaries

176. Which of the following muscles of the pharynx is supplied by the glossopharyngeal nerve (CN IX)?
    a. Palatopharyngeus
    b. Stylopharyngeus
    c. Superior constrictor
    d. Middle constrictor

177. In abdominal examination, the spleen lies in which of the following quadrants?
    a. Upper left quadrant
    b. Upper right quadrant
    c. Lower left quadrant
    d. Lower right quadrant

178. The majority of disaccharide hydrolysis occurs due to the action of which enzymes?
    a. Enzymes from the pancreatic juice
    b. Enzymes in the brush border of the small intestine
    c. Enzymes found in the saliva
    d. Enzymes in the gastric mucosa

179. The therapist in an outpatient physical therapy clinic receives an order to obtain a shoe orthotic for a patient. After examining the patient, the therapist finds a stage I pressure ulcer on the first metatarsal head. Weight-bearing surfaces need to be transferred posteriorly. Which orthotic is the most appropriate for this patient?
    a. Scaphoid pad
    b. Thomas heel
    c. Metatarsal pad
    d. Cushion heel

180. While obtaining the history, the therapist learns that the patient was recently hospitalized for malfunction of the anterior pituitary gland. Based on this information alone, the therapist knows that there may be problems with the patient's ability to produce which of the following hormones?
    a. Adrenocorticotropic hormone, thyroid-stimulating hormone, growth hormone, follicle-stimulating hormone, luteinizing hormone
    b. Insulin and glucagon
    c. Epinephrine and norepinephrine
    d. Cortisol, androgens, and aldosterone

181. A patient is using a medication for a thyroid condition. Which of the following could be the result of overdosing with the drug and should be mentioned to the physician?
    a. Tachycardia and restlessness when using propylthiouracil
    b. Tachycardia when using a T4 medication
    c. Weight loss when using propylthiouracil
    d. Bradycardia when using a T4 medication

182. A patient using insulin injections before a therapy session must receive special care like
    a. Not massaging the injection site
    b. Recommending the use of glucosamine to increase insulin's effects
    c. Having insulin injected into leg muscles before exercise
    d. All of the above

183. A patient with type 2 diabetes using metformin asks about the use of herbal medications and OTC drugs to be used with his medication. You answer that
    a. Some herbal preparations have been shown to be beneficial
    b. OTC cimetidine can be taken freely without concern
    c. Minerals and chromium might help drug actions
    d. The antacid Tums can be taken but not in excess

184. Which of the following symptoms are most likely to raise suspicion of liver disease?
      a. Fever, melena, urinary frequency
      b. Left shoulder pain, pallor, coffee ground emesis
      c. Jaundice, ascites, asterixis
      d. Left upper quadrant pain, nausea, diaphoresis

185. Which of the following statements about immune disorders is true?
      a. The progression of the disease will not change the clinical presentation of signs and symptoms.
      b. Early diagnosis is not likely to alter the course of the disease.
      c. Direct access will increase the likelihood that a physical therapist might be the first provider to identify potential autoimmune disorders.
      d. The risk factors for immune disorders are clearly understood and will assist in differential diagnosis.

186. An 8-year-old female is admitted to the hospital with hepatosplenomegaly; low grade fever; and swollen and stiff ankle, knee, hip, elbow, and wrist joints. What is the most likely diagnosis?
      a. Systemic onset juvenile rheumatoid arthritis (JRA)
      b. Polyarticular JRA
      c. Pauciarticular JRA
      d. Oligoarticular JRA

187. Lymphedema is
      a. pathologic accumulation of white-blood-cell-filled fluid
      b. accumulation of lymphocytes in the blood and tissues
      c. pathologic accumulation of protein-rich fluid in the tissue
      d. leakage of RBCs into the surrounding tissue

188. The hormones FSH, progesterone, and estrogen do what during the onset of menopause?
      a. Increase
      b. Decrease
      c. Stay the same
      d. Cause CVAs

189. According to the literature, development of bone mass peaks in _____ and begins to decrease in _____.
      a. Early thirties, late forties
      b. Midteens, late thirties
      c. Midtwenties, midforties
      d. Late twenties, late thirties

190. Primary lymphedema occurs in _____ patients who _____ had surgery.
    a. Older, have
    b. Younger, have
    c. Younger, have not
    d. Older, have not

191. A 14-year-old baseball player has type 1 diabetes and uses an insulin pump. His teammates want to know more about this condition. You inform them that all the following statements concerning insulin are true except
    a. It facilitates glucose transport out of the cell and into the blood
    b. It is secreted from b cells in pancreas
    c. It decreases blood glucose levels
    d. It may be present in decreased levels in those with type 2 diabetes mellitus

192. A patient who uses a magnesium-containing antacid at high doses for long periods might experience
    a. Constipation
    b. Diarrhea
    c. Headaches
    d. Muscle cramps

193. A patient on opioid pain medications might experience all of the following except
    a. Seeing poorly in the dark
    b. Some respiratory depression
    c. Motor incoordination
    d. Severe diarrhea

194. Your patient is a 35-year-old female who has been having severe low back pain for the past day. She has no mechanism of injury, but the pain that is located on the left side is greater than that on the right. Her only position of ease is in left fetal position. Her pain has increased in the last day and now is at a constant level that waxes and wanes. She has a mild temperature and has been feeling weak and lethargic since the pain began. She has been experiencing nausea, vomiting, and diarrhea for the past day. What system is mostly likely the source of the patient's symptoms?
    a. Gastrointestinal
    b. Urogenital
    c. Musculoskeletal
    d. Cardiovascular

195. Your patient is a 63 year-old male who presents to you in physical therapy with complaints of right shoulder and abdominal pain. He is having difficulty sleeping and has noticed bilateral tingling in his lateral three fingers. He has been feeling nauseated and has been vomiting lately. He is having muscle tremors and has noticed a dark color in his urine. He has noticed a yellowing of his eyes. What is system is mostly likely the source of the patient's symptoms?
   a. Endocrine
   b. Urogenitial
   c. Hepatic
   d. Gastrointestinal

196. A patient recently informed you that he was diagnosed with a duodenal ulcer and prescribed a proton pump inhibitor. Which of the following is a type of proton pump inhibitor?
   a. Ranitidine
   b. Metoclopramide
   c. Omeprazole
   d. Famotidine

197. Adrenergic receptors
   a. Are subdivided into four major categories
   b. Include the muscarinic and nicotinic receptors
   c. Include the alpha and beta receptors
   d. When blocked, can cause dry mouth, decreased salivation, blurry vision, and constipation

198. Which of the following is an absolute contraindication to initiation of an outpatient cardiac rehabilitation program?
   a. Obesity
   b. Patient currently on dialysis 3 days a week because of renal failure
   c. Asthma
   d. Third-degree heart block

199. Fourteen weeks after surgical repair of the rotator cuff, a patient presents with significant deltoid weakness. Range of motion is within normal limits and equal bilaterally. Internal and external rotation strength is equal bilaterally; flexion and abduction strength is significantly reduced. What is the most likely cause of this dysfunction?
   a. Poor compliance with a home exercise program
   b. Tightness of the inferior shoulder capsule
   c. Surgical damage to the musculocutaneous nerve
   d. Surgical damage to the axillary nerve

200. A patient has recently undergone an acromioplasty. What is the most important goal in early rehabilitation?
   a. Regaining muscle strength
   b. Return to activities of daily living (ADLs)
   c. Endurance and functional progression
   d. Return of normal range of motion (ROM)

201. Inhibition of the internal urethral sphincter allows the body to
   a. Micturate
   b. Defecate
   c. Hold the urine until later
   d. Ejaculate

202. Which of the following hormones stimulates ovulation in the female?
   a. Follicle-stimulating hormone
   b. Growth hormone
   c. Prolactin
   d. Luteinizing hormone

203. Whiplash injury from a rear-end collision would tear the
   a. Posterior longitudinal ligament (PLL)
   b. Anterior longitudinal ligament (ALL)
   c. Ligamentum nuchae
   d. Ligamentum flavum

204. A physical therapist should place the knee in which of the following positions to palpate the lateral collateral ligament (LCL)?
   a. Knee at 60 degrees of flexion and the hip externally rotated
   b. Knee at 20 degrees of flexion and the hip at neutral
   c. Knee at 90 degrees of flexion and the hip externally rotated
   d. Knee at 0 degrees and the hip at neutral

205. A patient on combination contraceptive medication and smoking must be warned that smoking increases the risk of
   a. Thromboembolism
   b. Liver cancer
   c. Internal hemorrhaging
   d. Ovarian cancer

206. A patient on combination contraceptive medication might experience all of the following except
   a. Depressive episodes
   b. Weight gain
   c. Swelling of feet
   d. Joint or muscle pain

207. You notice that a patient looks anemic and when you ask, she tells you that she is self-medicating with iron since she always looses a lot of blood during menstruation. You should respond that she should see a physician since
 a. OTC iron is not effective for anemia
 b. The dose recommended on OTC preparations is much too low
 c. There are different anemias some of which do not respond to iron
 d. Iron alone is not effective but needs additional prescription drugs

208. Your patient is a 33 year-old female who reports to physical therapy with complaints of left low back pain. She has been feeling cramping and has had sweats on and off for the past 3 days. Her symptoms are severe at times, but appear to be coming in waves. She is unable to find a position of comfort. No motion seems to increase the symptoms. She seems to feel an increase in symptoms shortly after drinking water. What system is mostly likely the source of the patient's symptoms?
 a. Urogenital
 b. Gastrointestinal
 c. Hepatic
 d. Musculoskeletal

209. Your patient is a 65-year-old male who reports to you with pain in his right big toe. Symptoms have been off and on for 3 years. He is having difficulty walking, and his great toe is hot and swollen. He has been having right midback pan. He has previously been diagnosed with kidney stones and irritable bowel syndrome. What system is mostly likely the source of the patient's symptoms?
 a. Renal
 b. Musculoskeletal
 c. Gastrointestinal
 d. Cancer

210. A patient requires examination 1 year after a hysterectomy. There is no hormone replacement therapy at this time. She complains of having pain with intercourse and some vaginal burning. What condition does she most likely have?
 a. Atrophic vaginitis
 b. Vulvodynia
 c. Asexually transmitted disease
 d. Complications from the surgery

211. An 80-year-old female complains of daily urinary accidents. She says that when she gets the urge to urinate, she simply cannot get to the bathroom in time. She has had a total hip replacement (6 months ago), has had a long history of getting up in the middle of the night to urinate, and has 3 children and 5 grandchildren with whom she enjoys spending time. What "type" of incontinence would this patient most closely match?
    a. Urge incontinence
    b. Stress incontinence
    c. Functional incontinence
    d. Mixed incontinence

212. A therapist receives an order to examine a patient on the telemetry floor of a hospital. The therapist is informed at the nurses' station that an evaluation will not be necessary because the patient went into shock earlier that morning and died. The patient suffered a myocardial infarction, resulting in damage to the left ventricle. Given information, what is the most likely type of shock?
    a. Vascular shock
    b. Anaphylactic shock
    c. Toxic shock
    d. Cardiogenic shock

213. Children who utilize training programs will not improve
    a. Strength
    b. Anaerobic conditioning
    c. Balance
    d. The ratio of "fast twitch" muscle fibers to "slow twitch" muscle fibers

214. A sports preparticipation examination for prepubescent children is not designed to
    a. Determine the general health of the athlete and detect conditions that place the participant at additional risk and to identify relative or absolute medical contraindications to participation
    b. Identify sports that may be played safely and to educate the athlete
    c. Assess maturity and overall fitness
    d. Assess the eye-hand coordination of the athlete

215. Which of the following is false for the child versus the adult?
    a. Children have less tolerance for exercise in the heat.
    b. Children have similar nutritional requirements.
    c. Children need more hydration in all situations.
    d. Children should follow the same weight-training routines.

216. A patient informs the physical therapist that he self-medicates with over the counter (OTC) drugs and has done so for some time and seems to be doing well. The physical therapist should inform the patient that
    a. This is ok since OTC drugs contain such low drug concentrations they do not cause serious adverse reactions
    b. OTC drugs should not be used for more than 2 weeks without a physician's consent
    c. OTC drug use does not have to be mentioned to a physician, since they are not prescription drugs
    d. This is a waste of money since OTC drugs have been found to be generally ineffective

217. Which of the following are common signs and symptoms seen by a patient using OTC diphenhydramine?
    a. Poor coordination and fatigue
    b. Increased blood pressure and irregular heart beat
    c. Excessive sweating and cold extremities
    d. Weight gain and ankle edema

218. A patient asks if they can use OTC niacin to lower high cholesterol and lipid levels since this has been recommended by friends. How should the physical therapist answer?
    a. Yes, it is ok if the friends feel fine.
    b. No, because niacin is not effective in lowering cholesterol and lipid levels.
    c. Yes, a try can do no harm since it is offered OTC.
    d. No, because the use of niacin requires periodic lab tests to check liver functions.

219. A patient on cancer chemotherapeutic drugs might experience all of the following adverse reactions except
    a. Easy bruising and bleeding
    b. Fatigue and anemia
    c. Constipation with fecal impact
    d. Jaundice and hepatotoxicity

220. A patient on cancer chemotherapy must be careful not to use other drugs including OTC drugs. In particular, you must warn the patient not to use
    a. NSAIDs
    b. Psyllium
    c. Hypnotics
    d. Anxiolytics

221. A patient on long-term corticosteroids during therapy might show all of the following except
    a. Depressed mood
    b. Orthostatic hypotension
    c. Anemia
    d. Muscle loss

222. A patient using diuretics during strenuous exercise might experience all of the following except
    a. Easy bruising
    b. Dehydration
    c. Muscle cramping
    d. Dyspnea

223. An individual consumes one glass of wine (100 ml, 10% alcohol). Most of the alcohol has been metabolized and eliminated after about
    a. 15 min
    b. 1 hr
    c. 2 hr
    d. 4 hr

224. A geriatric patient using OTC cimetidine might experience all of the following except
    a. Confusion
    b. Orthostatic hypotension
    c. Dizziness
    d. Sedation

225. A patient is on long-term NSAIDs therapy. These drugs reduce inflammatory processes by
    a. Inhibiting the enzyme lipoxygenase
    b. Reducing the formation of prostaglandins
    c. Inhibiting formation of inflammatory white blood cells
    d. Stimulating the enzymes COX I and II

226. A patient with severe sleep problems and using sedative/hypnotic drugs should
    a. Preferably be seen in the morning
    b. Preferably be seen in the afternoon
    c. Be advised not to take the medication 2 days before therapy
    d. Be advised that the addition of St. John's wort might help the medications

227. The patient has a dysfunction of the tenth rib; however, he complains of nausea and fullness. This is an example of
    a. Viscero-viscero reflex
    b. Viscero-somatic reflex
    c. Somatic-viscero reflex
    d. Somatic-somatic reflex

228. Knowledge of pharmacology is important to differential diagnosis because
    a. Management of the physical therapy patient cannot be enhanced by medications
    b. Medication side effects can contribute to the signs and symptoms that patients present with
    c. Physical therapists may need to alter the patient's medications to improve disease control
    d. Medications do not provide any additional risk to patient health issues

229. A patient cannot find his dentures when they are on his crowded bedside table. His visual acuity tests at 20/20 with the Snellen eye chart. The physical therapist suspects problems with
    a. Figure-ground discrimination
    b. Body scheme awareness
    c. Agraphia
    d. Vertical orientation

230. You will be performing an examination on a patient diagnosed with Down's syndrome. Which are the correct phenotypic features in Down's syndrome?
    a. Leukemia, hypotonia, joint hypomobility
    b. Developmental delay, simian crease, hypertonia
    c. Large cerebellum and brainstem, atlantoaxial instability, leukemia
    d. Developmental delay, leukemia, atlantoaxial instability

231. A patient who is 3 months pregnant asks advice on activities. Previous prepartum activities included rock climbing, soccer, and hiking. Which of the activities would you recommend?
    a. Rock climbing
    b. Soccer
    c. Nothing, she's pregnant
    d. Hiking

232. Which is NOT a reason for the common postural changes seen during pregnancy?
    a. Ligament laxity
    b. Posterior shift in COG
    d. Enlarging uterus
    c. Increased breast size

233. Which of the following comprise the diagnostic criteria for "female athlete triad" syndrome?
    a. Dieting, dizziness, and weakness
    b. Drop in blood pressure, fatigue, and disordered eating
    c. Stress fracture, fatigue, cold hands and feet
    d. Disordered eating, osteoporosis, amenorrhea

234. In a patient who has a uterine or bladder prolapse, which of the following findings do you expect?
    a. Decreased pelvic floor tone and strength, elongated pelvic floor muscles
    b. Increased pelvic floor tone, good pelvic floor strength
    c. Decreased pelvic floor tone and good pelvic floor strength
    d. Increased pelvic floor tone and poor pelvic floor strength

235. Which of the following will not be compressed with an enlarged uterus (pregnancy)?
    a. Bladder
    b. Vulvar veins
    c. Breasts
    d. Inferior vena cava

236. Which of the following is not a strong predictor of persistent low back pain after pregnancy?
    a. Low BMI
    b. High BMI
    c. Early onset of pain during pregnancy
    d. Hypermobility of the spine

237. Which of the following antibiotics is classified as a beta-lactam?
    a. Penicillin
    b. Levofloxacin
    c. Azithromycin
    d. Tetracycline

238. An athlete is being treated for sinusitis with Augmentin (amoxicillin + clavulanic acid). He mentions that he is allergic to penicillin. He's been taking Augmentin for 2 days now, but his symptoms are not improving, and he's starting to get red, itchy rashes on other parts of his body. What do you tell him?
   a. Even though he's allergic to pencillin, he should not be allergic to Augmentin and he should keep taking it.
   b. Sinusitis is usually a viral infection, so the Augmentin should work and he should keep taking it.
   c. He is probably developing an allergic reaction to the Augmentin and should stop taking it and call his doctor.
   d. He is experiencing a normal side effect of the medication.

239. Nasal decongestants used in the treatments of colds and allergies
   a. Bind to alpha-1 receptors to cause vasoconstriction
   b. Include pseudoephedrine, which is administered as a nasal spray
   c. Cause adverse effects such as drowsiness, lethargy, and dry mouth
   d. Can cause rebound congestion when taken orally

240. Excretion (or elimination) of a drug
   a. Is the removal of the drug from the body
   b. Occurs only via the kidney
   c. Is how the body breaks down medications
   d. Begins only after a toxic amount has accumulated in the body

241. Which drug works by competitively inhibiting the enzyme HMG-CoA reductase to reduce cholesterol levels?
   a. Gemfibrozil (Lopid)
   b. Niacin (Vitamin B12)
   c. Atorvastatin (Lipitor)
   d. Ezetimide (Zetia)

242. Excessive femoral anteversion in children may result in all of the following except
   a. Toeing in during gait
   b. Increased hip internal rotation range of motion
   c. Increased external rotation range of motion
   d. Decreased external rotation range of motion

243. Your patient has a lesion of the left superior gluteal nerve. When your patient is in left unilateral stance you may observe the
   a. Right ASIS is higher than the left ASIS
   b. Right ASIS is anterior to the left ASIS
   c. Trunk side bending to the left
   d. Lumbar spine is side bent to the right

244. Standing on the left leg and flexing your right hip up requires you to use all the following muscles except the
    a. Right lumbar rotators
    b. Left gluteus minimus
    c. Right quadratus lumborum
    d. Left gluteus medius

245. A smaller than normal angle of inclination at the hip is called
    a. Anteversion
    b. Retroversion
    c. Coxa vara
    d. Coxa valga

246. Hip extension may be limited by all of the following tissues except
    a. Iliofemoral ligament
    b. Iliopsoas muscle
    c. Ischiofemoral ligament
    d. Gluteus minimus posterior fibers

247. An angle of 170 degrees to 175 degrees in the frontal plane taken on the lateral side of the knee is considered
    a. Excess genu valgum
    b. Excess genu varum
    c. Normal
    d. Coxa vara

248. The pes anserine insertion is palpable at the _____ and includes the tendons of the _____.
    a. Medial tibia, semimembranosus, semitendinosis, and gracilis
    b. Lateral tibia, biceps femoris, semitendinosus, and iliotibial band
    c. Medial tibia, sartorius, gracilis, and semitendinosus
    d. Medial femur, biceps femoris, semitendinosus, and iliotibial band

249. As the knee extends and the patella moves superiorly in the trochlear groove, the sulcus angle _____ making the patellofemoral joint _____ stable.
    a. Increases, less
    b. Decreases, less
    c. Increases, more
    d. Decreases, more

250. The glenoid faces somewhat
    a. Lateral and inferior and posteriorly
    b. Lateral and superior and anteriorly
    c. Medial and superior and anteriorly
    d. Medial and inferior and posteriorly

251. During normal scapulo humeral rhythm, the
   a. Scapula upwardly rotates 60 degrees and the humeral abducts 120 degrees
   b. Scapula upwardly rotates 2 degrees for every 1 degree of humeral abduction
   c. Scapula abducts 60 degrees and upwardly rotates 120 degrees
   d. Scapula upwardly rotates 120 degrees and the humeral abducts 60 degrees

252. Anterior glenohumeral dislocations are often accompanied by
   a. A stretched subscapularis
   b. A Hill Sachs lesion
   c. A fracture of the greater tubercle
   d. Rotator cuff full-thickness tears

253. Which of the following is false regarding biomechanics of persons with patellofemoral pain?
   a. Weakness of the hip abductors, external rotators, and extensors is frequently present
   b. Excessive hip internal rotation and/or hip adduction is frequently present
   c. Patella alta increases patellar instability
   d. Increased trochlear groove depth increases patellar instability

254. Two drugs, an agonist and a competitive antagonist, are given to a patient. The agonist drug exists at four times the serum concentration of the antagonist. Assuming no other variables are present, what will be the resulting drug effect?
   a. No effect
   b. 20% increased agonist effect
   c. 80% agonist effect
   d. 80% antagonist effect

255. A drug has 60% bioavailability when given orally at the recommended dosage. What does this mean?
   a. 60% of the dose is excreted.
   b. 60% of the drug is available and active in the bloodstream.
   c. 40% will be bound to plasma proteins and active in the serum.
   d. 40% of the drug is available and active in the bloodstream.

256. The half-life of diazepam (Valium) is approximately 12 hours. If a 70-kg patient took 10 mg at 8:00 AM, what amount of drug would be present in his body the next day at 8:00 AM during his scheduled appointment with you?
    a. 5 mg
    b. 2.5 mg
    c. 1.25 mg
    d. 0.625 mg

257. Aspirin, as acetylsalicylic acid, inhibits platelet aggregation like all NSAIDs, but is the drug of choice for thromboprophylaxis because
    a. It has a predictable irreversible mechanism of action
    b. It has a predictable reversible mechanism of action
    c. It has a longer half-life than other NSAID agents
    d. It has no COX II effect

258. In First-order kinetics
    a. A constant percentage of the drug is lost/metabolized per unit time
    b. A variable percentage of the drug is metabolized per unit time
    c. A constant amount *(m)* is metabolized per unit time
    d. A constant first-pass effect is produced

259. Medications within the benzodiazepine (BZD) class of drugs have multiple indications and uses for physical therapy patients. Which of the following is not an indication for use of benzodiazepines?
    a. Alcohol withdrawal
    b. Relief of anxiety
    c. Sleep aid
    d. Analgesia

260. Which of the following benzodiazepine (BZD) medications is properly indicated for relief of anxiety?
    a. Xanax
    b. Valium
    c. Dalmane
    d. Klonopin

261. Angiotensin-converting enzyme (ACE) inhibitors are prone to producing a common, irritating side effect that may necessitate change to another drug agent. What is that side effect?
    a. Dry hacking cough
    b. Peripheral edema
    c. Visual color alteration of blue and green
    d. Atrial fibrillation

262. Which of the following benzodiazepines (BZD) is contraindicated in the elderly because of an extremely long half-life?
    a. Alprazolam
    b. Lorazepam
    c. Temazepam
    d. Flurazepam

263. Which of the following benzodiazepine medications is most properly indicated for outpatient-based treatment of convulsive disorders?
    a. Xanax
    b. Valium
    c. Dalmane
    d. Klonopin

264. Skeletal muscle relaxant agents fall into two main categories. Which of the following choices are those categories?
    a. Beta-1 and beta-2
    b. COX-1 and COX-2
    c. Prostaglandin and prostacyclin agonists
    d. Centrally and peripherally acting

265. A key side effect of Flexeril, Soma, Robaxin, and Norflex and other centrally acting skeletal muscle relaxants of note to therapists is
    a. Sedation
    b. Drug-induced spasticity in spinal cord patients
    c. Paralysis
    d. Rhabdomyolyis

266. In what way is Flexeril (cyclobenzaprine) somewhat unique among muscle relaxants that affect the central nervous system?
    a. Flexeril has more peripheral effect.
    b. Flexeril shares pharmacologic characteristics with the tricyclic antidepressant agents.
    c. Flexeril is a GABA-agonist similar to barbiturates.
    d. Flexeril acts at the acetylcholine (Ach) receptors, producing neuromuscular blockade.

267. Side effects of note among patients taking Baclofen include
    a. Drowsiness and memory impairment
    b. Weight gain
    c. Weight loss
    d. Beta-1 suppression of maximum heart rate

268. Opium, derived from the poppy flower, contains two main natural opiates. What are they?
      a. Codeine and demerol
      b. Heroin and codeine
      c. Hydrocodone and hydroxycodone
      d. Codeine and morphine

269. The primary side effect, common among almost all oral hypoglycemic agents, of particular note during active physical therapy is
      a. Hypoglycemia
      b. CNS depression
      c. Nephrolithiasis
      d. Increased deep tendon reflexes

270. A Tylenol with codeine #3 tablet (TC3) contains how much codeine?
      a. 60 mg
      b. 30 mg
      c. 15 mg
      d. 7.5 mg

271. Talwin and Stadol are examples of which opiate analgesic class?
      a. Antagonist
      b. Agonist-antagonist
      c. Competitive agonist
      d. Agonist

272. Which of the paired drug interactions between an opiate and second drug agent is INCORRECT?
      a. Alcohol/increased respiratory depression
      b. Tricyclic antidepressants/increased constipation
      c. Cigarette smoking/decreased opiate analgesic effect
      d. Diuretic agents/hypertensive crisis

273. Demerol (Meperidine) is combined with Vistaril (Hydroxyzine HCl) (an antihistamine), producing an enhanced analgesic effect of demerol. This allows decreased dosage and potential deleterious effects. This is an example of what drug interaction?
      a. Additive
      b. Reversible antagonism
      c. Potentiation
      d. Antagonism

274. Which of the following is the only skeletal muscle relaxant that acts on the peripheral nervous system?
    a. Diazepam (Valium)
    b. Baclofen (Lioresol)
    c. Orphenadrine (Norgesic)
    d. Dantrolene (Dantrium)

275. Cyclo-oxygenase II (COX-2) specific agents are now indicated only for patients with
    a. History of GI or renal disorders
    b. Patients with hypersensitivity to aspirin
    c. Patients in need of postoperative thromboprophylaxis
    d. Patients hypersensitive to acetaminophen

276. The chief difference between acetaminophen and the nonsteroidal anti-inflammory drugs (NSAIDs) is that acetaminophen has no _____ or _____ effect.
    a. Analgesic/antithrombotic
    b. Antipyretic/antithrombotic
    c. Anti-inflammatory/antithrombotic
    d. Antipyretic/anti-inflammatory

277. Your patient is unlikely to be compliant with a short half-life NSAID, so you select a long-acting agent. Which of these NSAID agents has the longest half-life?
    a. Aspirin
    b. Feldene
    c. Naproxyn
    d. Daypro

278. An example of the most common FIRST-LINE diuretic used in the treatment of hypertension would be
    a. Hydrochlorothiazide (HCT)
    b. Lasix
    c. Spironolactone
    d. ACTH

279. Your 31-year-old male patient presents with his third episode of extreme pain at the first metatarsal phalangeal joint of the right foot. Clinical examination and laboratory results indicate gouty arthritis as the diagnosis. Which drug is LEAST appropriate for acute care?
    a. Colchicines
    b. Indomethacin
    c. Probenecid
    d. Ibuprofen

280. Side effects of physical therapy concern with use of angiotensin-converting enzyme (ACE) inhibitor agents include all of the following EXCEPT
   a. Headache
   b. Dizziness
   c. Postural hypotension
   d. Potassium depletion

281. Furosimide, 40 mg twice a day, is prescribed for your congestive heart failure (CHF) patient who is also taking Lanoxin. What is your chief monitoring concern?
   a. Hypervolemia
   b. Hypokalemia
   c. Hypercalcemia
   d. Hyperkalemia

282. Of what significance is the Edinger-Westphal response to you in monitoring your patient prescribed an opiate analgesic?
   a. The Edinger-Westphal response suggests opiate overdose.
   b. The Edinger-Westphal response suggests opiate antagonist effect.
   c. The Edinger-Westphal response correlates with concurrent Dantrium.
   d. The Edinger-Westphal response indicates the patient is receiving insufficient dosage for analgesic effect of the opiates.

283. The angiotensin-receptor blockers (ARB agents) act by what mechanism of action?
   a. Antagonize Na+ ion receptors
   b. Angiotensin-receptor antagonism
   c. Angiotensin-converting enzyme antagonism
   d. Dilation of vascular smooth muscle

284. The main advantage of aldactone over thiazide is that aldactone is/causes
   a. Potassium sparing
   b. Less hypotension
   c. Less hypertension
   d. Receptor site specificity of alpha$_1$ receptors

285. The biguanide group of oral hypoglycemic agents includes metformin. Metformin has what characteristic of note to physical therapists?
   a. No hypoglycemic effect
   b. Interferes with carbohydrate absorption
   c. Delays carbohydrate absorption
   d. Will not cause nausea

286. What is true of the thiazolidinediones?
    a. Thiazolidinediones will not cause hypoglycemia.
    b. Thiazolidinediones' effect is independent of insulin production.
    c. Thiazolidinediones decrease insulin receptor site activity.
    d. Thiazolidinediones decrease lipids.

287. Side effects of progestin include all of the following EXCEPT
    a. Weight gain
    b. Edema
    c. Manic episodes
    d. Possible mild androgenic effects

288. What side effect is shared by all benzodiazepine agents?
    a. Muscle weakness
    b. Hypertension
    c. Sedation
    d. Cross-sensitivity with penicillin-derived antibiotics

289. The nonsteroidal anti-inflammatory drugs impede COX-2 activity. COX-2 produces inflammatory prostaglandins via biosynthesis of what substance?
    a. Serotonin
    b. Substance P
    c. Arachidonic acid
    d. Gamma butyric acid

Answers

1. b. The sinoatrial node is located in the right atrium of the heart. It serves as the pacemaker for the heart. Impulses generated there are passed on from right to left and inferiorly to the atrioventricular node in the lower end of the interatrial septum.

2. b. The vessels of various sizes provide transmission conduits for body fluids, but the exchange described takes place between cell surfaces and the interstitial fluid.

3. d. During the isovolumetric ventricular relaxation phase, all of the ventricular volume has been ejected. The semilunar and AV valves are closed, and no volume is changing in the ventricles. This phase has the lowest volume.

4. b. The SA node has a frequency of 70 to 80 depolarizations per minute; the AV node frequency is 40 to 60; and the Purkinje cell frequency is 15 to 40; the myocardium is even slower. This question refers to how often these fibers will have action potentials, not how fast they travel.

5. b. Cranial nerve X stimulation causes bradycardia by inhibiting automaticity of the SA node. Tachycardic effects are caused by inhibiting, not stimulating, the vagus. Cardiac rigor is a consequence of hypercalcemia and causes the heart to stop in systole.

6. b. Inspiratory capacity is the volume of air moved going from normal expiration to full forced inspiration. Total lung capacity is the volume of air in the lung on full forced inspiration and cannot be measured on spirometry. Inspiratory reserve volume is the volume of air moved going from normal inspiration to full forced inspiration.

7. a. Cardiac output and stroke volume both increase during exertion. Increased cardiac cycle time is just another way of saying the heart is beating slower, which is the opposite of what occurs with exertion.

8. c. Orthopnea, which is dyspnea in the recumbent position, is a typical symptom of chronic left heart failure. All of the other symptoms and signs are due to right heart failure.

9. b. Verapamil reduces contractility of the heart and increases coronary artery dilation, resulting in decreased cardiac workload and increased blood flow to the heart muscle.

10.   a.   Cycling 11 mph is approximately 6 to 7 METs. Walking 4 mph is approximately 4.6 METs. Driving a car is approximately 2 METs. Weeding a garden is approximately 3 to 5 METs.

11.   a.   In the case of a reciprocal click, the initial click is created by the condyle slipping back into the correct position under the disk with opening of the mouth. In this disorder, the condyle is resting posterior to the disk before jaw opening. With closing, the click is caused by the condyle slipping away from the disk.

12.   d.   The supraspinatus tendon is best palpated by placing the patient's involved upper extremity behind the back in full internal rotation.

13.   c.   The superior pole is in most contact at approximately 90 degrees of knee flexion.

14.   d.   Choice D describes an expiratory reserve volume. Choice A is residual volume, choice B is tidal volume, and choice C is vital capacity.

15.   c.   Epinephrine, digitalis, and norepinephrine increase heart rate. Quinidine is an antiarrhythmic drug.

16.   c.   Choice C provides correct instructions. The patient is often instructed to begin this technique in the supine position and progress to the sitting position. This technique should be practiced for approximately 5 minutes several times per day.

17.   b.   The sedentary patient's cardiovascular response increases faster than the trained patient's if the workloads are equal.

18.   b.   The pattern described in the question—a gradual increase in the rate and depth of respirations followed by periods of absent breathing—is known as *Cheyne-Stokes breathing.* Small breaths followed by inconsistent periods of absent breathing are known as a Biot's breathing pattern. Deep gasping breaths are known as a *Kussmaul's breathing pattern.* Awakening during the night because of periods of absent breathing is known as *paroxysmal nocturnal dyspnea.*

19.   c.   Residual volume, the amount of air left in the lungs after a forceful expiration, increases with age.

20.   c.   The heart receives nerve impulses that travel through the sinoatrial node to the ventricles by way of the atrioventricular node, bundle branches, and Purkinje fibers.

21. c. Deconditioned people benefit initially from low-intensity exercise with multiple sessions per day and per week.

22. d. The posterior cruciate ligament becomes tight in full knee extension. This assists the tibia in external rotation, which is needed for the screw home mechanism with open-chain activities.

23. b. Antihypertensive medication may cause a sharp drop in blood pressure when getting up quickly or leaving a warm pool, which causes vasodilation. This is most evident at the beginning of therapy. Patients must be supervised and warned to get up slowly, to hold on to something firm, and to sit down when leaving the pool.

24. c. Beta blockers block the beta receptors on the heart; they also block sympathetic nerve impulses and reduce heart rate and contractility. The other drugs have no effects, or they might increase heart rate.

25. a. A beta agonist stimulates cardiac beta receptors, leading to an increase in heart rate and blood pressure.

26. a. In a small percentage of patients, statin drugs can cause liver damage (liver function tests are required) and muscle pain, which can lead to rhabdomyolisis (dark urine due to muscle breakdown), a potentially life-threatening condition. The other signs/symptoms are usually not drug related.

27. c. Statin drugs inhibit HMG-CoA reductase and lower cholesterol levels most effectively (about 30 % or more), while the other drugs interfere with absorption and lipase activity.

28. d. All of the listed reactions can be observed, with joint and muscle pain being the exception.

29. b. While the use of an inhaler is user specific, it is generally recommended to have the patient inhale about 20 minutes before exercise, particularly in a cool environment, which seems to aggravate existing asthma.

30. b. The reactions described in choices A and C can be expected because of blockade of beta receptors in the lungs and heart, and drowsiness is perhaps caused by a central action. No muscle cramps and pain should be expected.

31. d. Beta receptor blockade, both peripherally and perhaps centrally, causes the blood pressure reducing effects, but peripheral resistance is not reduced but rather might be slightly increased (patient might complain about cold extremities).

32. c. Calcium channel blockers will cause all of the listed reactions, except tremors, by interfering with calcium fluxes in blood vessels and cardiac muscle.

33. b. A local anesthetic that might leak into the general blood circulation can affect the cardiac (bradycardia, hypotension) and central nervous systems (restlessness, tremors, seizures) and can interfere with the functions of sensory nerves and motor neurons.

34. c. Nitroglycerin dilates coronary blood vessels and provides more blood and oxygen to the heart and also reduces peripheral resistance, making it easier for the heart to pump. Both actions eliminate the pain. If no relief is obtained, then this could be a true heart attack.

35. a. All of the symptoms could potentially be related to musculoskeletal problems within the shoulder, but several factors make the cardiovascular system the best answer. The symptoms began insidiously, and many musculoskeletal shoulder issues can be traced back to a single incident or repetitive motions that aggravate and result in damage to musculoskeletal tissue. The patient cannot remember any incident that triggered the symptoms. Most of the symptoms that the patient is reporting can be attributed to the cardiovascular system. Lifting heavy objects, shoveling dirt, walking fast, high blood pressure, and shortness of breath are all symptoms indicative of cardiovascular system involvement.

36. b. Although some of the symptoms could be the result of musculoskeletal system involvement (i.e., rib fracture) or the cardiovascular system (left-sided pain), the best answer is the pulmonary system. The blood in the sputum is an indicator that the ribs may have punctured the lungs. This evidence, coupled with the breathing problems, should move the pulmonary system up as your top hypothesis.

37. b. Aspirin and clopidogrel act as anticlotting/anticoagulant medications by preventing platelets from clumping together, thereby making it harder to form a clot.

38. d. Sublingual nitroglycerin acts very quickly to relieve anginal pain by relaxing blood vessels to allow more blood to flow to the heart. Nitroglycerin patches are used to prevent an angina attack but sublingual nitroglycerin is most effective once an attack occurs.

39. a. The bronchioles are the smallest branches of the airways and are surrounded by smooth muscle. During an asthma attack, inflammation and muscle contraction occur, narrowing these airways and causing asthma symptoms.

40. a.   Angina is caused by decreased blood flow to the heart resulting in pain. Nitrates relax blood vessels, allowing more blood to flow to the heart and thereby decreasing pain.

41. a.   Beta-blockers block beta$_1$-and beta$_2$-receptors, resulting in decreased heart rate and dilation of blood vessels, which helps decrease hypertension. Unfortunately, they could also trigger an asthma attack in susceptible persons by blocking the beta$_2$-receptors in the lungs.

42. d.   Short-acting beta-agonists, also known as "rescue" meds, act very quickly by binding to the beta$_2$-receptors in the bronchioles, causing relaxation of the airways. They are indicated for asthma attacks and are not useful for long-term control of asthma symptoms.

43. a.   Healing time is unchanged with this patient population.

44. b.   Femoral anteversion is the only one that would account for the internal rotation seen in toe in.

45. c.   The medial femoral condyle is the most common area for osteochondritis dissecans, although it can occur in the femoral capital epiphysis.

46. c.   The knee is most common with this diagnosis followed by the ankles and elbows.

47. d.   Pauciarticular juvenile rheumatoid arthritis (RA) occurs in 50% to 60% of the cases, followed by polyarticular RA and then systemic RA.

48. a.   The healing phase of ligaments is divided into the following categories: inflammatory phase (first few days after injury, proliferative phase (1 to 6 weeks after injury), and remodeling phase (begins at 7 weeks postinjury).

49. b.   Since eccentric exercise makes the muscle work the hardest, this type of exercise will exacerbate DOMS. DOMS symptoms are alleviated in 2 to 3 days with stretching and ice application.

50. b.   Healing phases of bone after fracture are divided into the following categories: Inflammatory phase (immediately after injury), soft callous phase (1 to 6 weeks postinjury), hard callous phase (4 to 6 weeks after injury), and remodeling phase (6 weeks to several months postinjury).

51. c. Dense regular connective tissue includes ligaments and tendons, and dense irregular connective tissue includes joint capsules, periosteum, and aponeurosis. Choice D does not exist.

52. d. The aged are more likely to have osteophyte formation. All other populations can have rotator cuff damage, but it will most likely come from another source.

53. b. A steroid injection can weaken tendons and ligaments; thus, the joint must be moved carefully.

54. d. Thyroid hormone is not used but the parathyroid hormone is used in cases of certain calcium imbalances. All of the listed agents are used with bisphosphonates to be taken on an empty stomach and sitting or standing for at least 30 min.

55. d. Acetaminophen has analgesic and antipyretic but no antiinflammatory properties. It is not indicated in rheumatoid arthritis, which is an inflammatory condition; however, it can be used in osteoarthritis, which is not an inflammatory problem.

56. a. Some patients use certain aspects of spasticity to maintain balance; weakening of this spasticity could interfere with their balance. Skeletal muscle relaxants (except botulinus toxin) weaken but do not paralyze muscles, and some may cause physical dependence, which prohibits abrupt cessation of their long-term use. Numerous studies have confirmed the effectiveness of skeletal muscle relaxants.

57. b The line of vision dictates head and neck posture. If the screen is too low or too far away from the face, the user must flex the neck and trunk. If the head is held forward, cervical muscles become fatigued.

58. d. The tuberosity of the fifth metatarsal is at the base of the metatarsal. The base of the metatarsal is proximal and the head is distal. The medial cuneiform is on the high medial side of the transverse arch of the foot. The cuboid bone is on the lower lateral side of the foot.

59. c. Metacarpophalangeal joints are condyloid joints. These are biaxial joints that allow flexion/extension around one axis and abduction/adduction around another axis.

60. b. These actions can be easily demonstrated and palpated. Resisting anterior movement of the arm abducted to 60 degrees tests the sternocostal head of the pectoralis major; the clavicular head is tested after the arm is abducted to 90 degrees.

61. c. The structures that pass through the foramen magnum include the spinal cord, the meninges, the spinal components of cranial nerve XI, and the vertebral arteries. Cranial nerve XII exits the skull through the hypoglossal canals.

62. a. The longus capitis, longus colli, and sternocleidomastoid muscles are all associated with the anterior aspect of the cervical vertebrae and thus produce flexion of the head.

63. a. The nucleus pulposus is thickest in the lumbar spine, followed by the cervical region; it is thinnest in the thoracic spine.

64. a. The speed of contraction is directly related to the resting length of the muscle fiber, whereas the force of contraction depends upon the cross-sectional diameter. Creatine phosphate content ensures availability of ATP for the contraction-relaxation cycles, and glycolytic capacity is important for endurance.

65. c. This is the normal anatomy, lateral to medial of the proximal row of the carpus. The distal row, lateral to medial, is the trapezium, trapezoid, capitate, and hamate.

66. d. The long toe extensors represent the spinal cord segment L5. The iliopsoas represents L2. The quadriceps are innervated by L3 and the tibialis anterior is innervated by L4.

67. b. Bifid spinous processes (spinous processes that are split) are found only in the cervical spine.

68. c. In static standing, the line of gravity is posterior to the hip joint. The body relies on the anterior pelvic ligaments and the hip joint capsule. The iliopsoas may be recruited at times, but anterior ligaments are used first to keep the trunk from extending in static stance.

69. b. The area of contact between the humerus and the glenoid fossa is maximal in this position.

70. d. The subscapularis, teres minor, and infraspinatus muscles oppose the superior pull of the deltoid muscle. The supraspinatus does not oppose the pull of the deltoid but is important because (along with the other cuff muscles) it provides a compression force to the glenohumeral joint.

71. a. Only the edges of the adult meniscus are vascularized by the capillaries from the synovial membrane and joint capsule.

72. a. The intervertebral disc has the greatest amount of fluid at the time of birth. The fluid content decreases as a person ages.

73. d. The metacarpophalangeal joint is enclosed in a joint capsule and therefore is considered a diarthrodial joint.

74. b. Choice B best describes the position that causes injury only to the ACL. In most cases an audible pop indicates a tear of the ACL. Varus or valgus blows to the knee injure the collateral ligaments and possibly the ACL.

75. a. Torticollis involving the right sternocleidomastoid would cause right lateral cervical flexion and left cervical rotation.

76. b. Genu valgum is a term used to describe a deformity of the knee causing an inward bowing of the legs. Genu varus is an outward bowing of the legs. Coxa valgum is a deformity at the hip in which the angle between the axis of the neck of the femur and the shaft of the femur is greater than 135 degrees. In coxa varus this angle is less than 135 degrees. Pes cavus is an increase in the arch of the foot. Pes planus is flat foot.

77. c. This is the loose-packed position of the hip.

78. a. The second cuneiform of the foot articulates with the first cuneiform, second metatarsal, third cuneiform, and navicular.

79. b. Viscosity is the friction of fluids. Buoyancy is the property that pushes up on the part immersed with a pressure that is equal to the weight of the amount of water displaced by that part. Relative density states that if the specific gravity of an object is less than one, it will float, and if it is greater than one, it will sink. Hydrostatic pressure is the property of water that places pressure equally on the immersed part.

80. a. Flexion and extension of the thumb are performed in a plane parallel to the palm of the hand. Abduction and adduction are performed in a plane perpendicular to the palm of the hand.

81. d. Acetic acid is sometimes used in attempts to dissolve a calcium deposit and is driven by the negative pole. Dexamethasone is an anti-inflammatory driven by the negative pole. Magnesium sulfate is used to decrease muscle spasms and is driven by the positive pole. Hydrocortisone is also used to treat inflammation and is driven by the positive pole.

82. a. The popliteus, biceps femoris, and iliotibial band offer active restraint for the lateral side of the knee joint. The gastrocnemius assists in active restraint of the posterior side of the knee joint.

83. b. The anterior cruciate ligament is located within the articular cavity but outside the synovial lining. The anterior and posterior cruciate ligaments have their own synovial lining.

84. b. Plantar flexors have to contract in quiet standing. Other muscles are recruited with movement of the center of gravity.

85. a. The talus is palpated just anterior and lateral to the medial malleolus. Supination is excessive lateral deviation of the talus, and pronation is excessive medial deviation.

86. c. The triangular fibrocartilage complex is made up of the dorsal radioulnar ligament, ulnar collateral ligament, ulnar articular cartilage, volar radioulnar ligament, ulnocarpal meniscus, and sheath of the extensor carpi ulnaris.

87. d. The muscle spindles are responsible for the stretch reflex. When a muscle is stretched too quickly, the muscle spindles cause the muscle to contract and shorten (which is called the stretch reflex). The Golgi tendon organs are responsible for the inverse stretch reflex. They are located in the junction between the muscle and tendon and detect changes in tension. When a tendon is stretched too quickly, the Golgi tendon organs cause the muscle to relax.

88. c. Forty millimeters is the normal end range of opening.

89. c. Dental trismus may be due to spasm or to abnormally short jaw muscles. There is an inability to open the jaw fully.

90. d. The condyle glides anterior translatory down the eminence (26 mm to 50 mm of opening) with the disc in the upper joint compartment. Occasionally the disc is displaced anteriorly, and adhesions may occur that produce an anterior displaced disc without reduction (locked joint).

91. b Reduction indicates that the condyle is able to slide under the disc (reduce), causing a clicking noise.

92. d. Ipsilateral rotation and contralateral translation describe lateral jaw movement.

93. a. Bilateral anterior translation describes jaw protrusion.

94. b. A combination of rotation occurs during the first 26 mm, then anterior translation describes wide jaw opening.

95. c. Pressure in right side-lying would create pressure on the right greater trochanter and right lateral mallelous. No pressure is put on the occiput or ischial tuberosity in side-lying

96. c. Shortened hip flexors and lengthened anterior abdominals will contribute to an anterior tilt. Choices A and D would create a posterior pelvic tilt, and choice B will likely present with a more neutral position of the pelvis.

97. c. Patella cartilage cannot be the source of the pain. Every structure in the knee has pain nerve fibers except the articular cartilage.

98. b. Synovial fluid has been shown to inhibit healing of ligament tissues.

99. d. Jumping (plyometrics) can generate up to 7 times body weight at the patella. Running is next most stressful at 3.5 times body weight.

100. a. Rotator cuff tear is rare under the age of 40. It can occur from either side and is very common. Cadaver studies confirm that cuff tear is not usually symptomatic.

101. d. Traction from operative positioning, retractor placement, or lengthening of the leg leads to most cases of sciatic traction neurapraxia and foot drop.

102. a. Sever's apophysitis is a physeal stress injury. Tight Achilles tendons are uniformly seen and frequently there is tendinitis.

103. b. Pes planus is common and usually painless. Hyperlaxity is a powerful risk factor for development of pes planus. In most cases, no treatment is necessary.

104. c. Passive insufficiency of the pronator teres. The question asks specifically about passive limitations to elbow extension. The pronator teres is a polyarticular muscle crossing anterior to the elbow joint.

105. b. Choice B, flexion, biceps femoris, is the correct answer. A hip flexion contracture increases flexor torque across the anterior hip. This increases muscle demand on the hip extensors. The biceps femoris is an extensor of the hip.

106. b. Weak left gluteus medius with left trunk lean to move center of mass towards weaker side is the correct hypothesis. A pelvic drop in single limb midstance is a classic positive Trendelenberg sign of gluteus medius weakness. The compensatory trunk lateral lean is to bring the center of mass closer to the weaker side to decrease the external moment arm on the weak muscle.

107. b. Left lateral trunk flexion is limited primarily by the rib cage because of multiple attachments. The thoracic spine has frontal plane facet alignment. The lumbar spine facets are oriented in the sagittal plane. The left quadratus lumborum is on slack during left lateral flexion.

108. d. According to Cyriax's classical description, flexion in the hip is limited the greatest in its capsular pattern.

109. a. Of the choices listed, cranial nerve II or the optic nerve functions to constrict the pupil and vision. Ischemia, resulting from stroke or head injury, or pressure from tumors can adversely affect the function of the nerve. Visual field loss depends on the location of the lesion. A lesion occurring before the optic chiasm results in loss of vision in the fields on the same side. After the optic chiasm, a lesion will cause loss of vision in both fields. The visual field affected will be opposite the side of the lesion and is also known as homonymous hemianopsia.

110. d. Risk factors for osteoporosis include advanced age, being thin, positive family history, exposure to certain medications, and ancestry (Caucasian or Asian).

111. d. Physical therapy intervention for individuals with osteoporosis has several goals: optimization of bone formation, fall prevention, fracture prevention, postfracture rehabilitation, and treatment of musculoskeletal conditions that place the individual at risk for falls in the future. Ultrasound is contraindicated over a fracture site.

112. c. Opioids belong to a class of drugs that provide pain relief by binding to opioid receptors. Ibuprofen and aspirin are nonsteroidal anti-inflammatory (NSAID) medications, while acetaminophen is in a class of its own; however, none of these three medications bind to opioid receptors.

113. c. Drowsiness, blurred vision, and dry mouth are side effects of the anticholinergic properties that muscle relaxants possess. These side effects are also the ones patients complain about most often.

114. b. All NSAIDs inhibit the enzyme cyclooxygenase (COX), thereby decreasing the inflammatory reaction.

115. d. Celecoxib is unique from the other NSAIDs in that it specifically inhibits COX-2. One of the most worrisome side effects of NSAIDs is the potential for ulcers since nonselective COX inhibitor NSAIDs block the production of prostaglandins that provide a protective effect against acids in the stomach. COX-2 specific NSAIDs do not inhibit the production of these protective prostaglandins.

116. d. The saphenous nerve lies just anterior to the medial malleolus alongside the great saphenous vein. This nerve is most likely to be injured by the sutures.

117. b. The phrenic nerve arises from ventral rami of C3, C4, and C5 spinal nerves. The sensory neurons of the dorsal root ganglia of C3, C4, and C5 supply axons for somatic pain from the named area of parietal serous membranes. C3, C4, and C5 also supply the shoulder with the cutaneous innervation by the supraclavicular nerves. This is why pericardial or diaphragmatic pain will refer to the shoulder.

118. b. The neural canal (vertebral canal) is largest and most triangular in the cervical region and smallest and most circular in the thoracic region.

119. a. The white matter of the spinal cord carries ascending (sensory) tracts and descending (motor) tracts.

120. c. The four cranial nerves that contain parasympathetic fibers are oculomotor, facial, glossopharyngeal, and vagus nerves.

121. c. Norepinephrine can be a motor neurotransmitter at myoneural junctions of postganglionic sympathetic neurons, but the term "motor endplate" is reserved for only skeletal muscles. Dopamine is a neurotransmitter in the basal ganglia, which is part of the motor system but nowhere near the myoneural junction. Myasthenia gravis is a condition of impaired neurotransmitter reception at the motor endplate, which is not what the question asked about.

122. a. Generally, GABA (gamma-aminobutyric acid) is an inhibitory neurotransmitter in the CNS, whereas epinephrine, glutamate, and norepinephrine are excitatory.

123. c. Parkinson's disease and dementia are disorders involving the brain. Myasthenia gravis is a problem with acetylcholine receptors at the neuromuscular junction.

124. a. I—No response. II—Generalized response. III—Localized responses. IV—Confused agitated. V—Confused inappropriate. VI—Confused appropriate. VII—Automatic appropriate. VIII—Purposeful and appropriate.

125. c. Choice A is incorrect because the patient should be able to learn how to be independent with activities of daily living. Choice B is incorrect because the patient can learn to drive an automobile independently with the assistance of hand controls. Choice C is correct because total balance of a wheelchair using a wheelie is an unrealistic goal. After proper rehabilitation, these patient's should be independent with a manual cough.

126. b. A beta fibers are the largest in diameter and conduct faster than C fibers and A delta fibers.

127. b. The fifth lumbar nerve root is impinged because it arises from the spinal column superior to the L4-L5 lumbar disc.

128. b. The responses of the patient represent the lowest possible score on the Glasgow Coma Scale. One point is given for each of the listed responses (or lack thereof).

129. c. Choice C describes the symmetric tonic neck reflex. With passive cervical extension, an infant displays upper extremity extension and lower extremity flexion.

130. a. Infants accomplish this task between approximately 5 and 10 months of age. The response in Choice A would prevent the parent from excessive unnecessary worry. Sources vary widely about the exact month when developmental milestones are reached, but A is the correct choice in this scenario.

131. c. The common peroneal nerve travels over the lateral knee. It is the least likely to be injured. The other structures are either within the knee or directly posterior.

132. d. The radial side is the lateral side of the forearm, which is innervated by the musculocutaneous nerve. The lateral antebrachial cutaneous nerve is a continuation of the musculocutaneous nerve.

133. d. This patient has a lesion at the level of C7.

134. c. Increasing motor ability is not independent of motor learning. A therapist must facilitate motor learning with proper sensory cues and by promoting appropriate motor activity. Choice D is true because infants begin spontaneous movement, which later develops into more deliberate movement. Choice A is true because reflex movement can be used to develop more deliberate movement.

135. a. Isometric control develops before isotonic control.

136. c. Postural reactions and motor milestone development occur in the same sequence as with normal infants, but the progression of an infant with Down's syndrome is slower.

137. c. Involvement of the basal ganglia results in dyskinesia or athetosis. Cerebellar lesions produce ataxia, or unstable movement. The corpus callosum is not involved.

138. a. Axonotmesis involves disruption of axons while the neural sheath remains intact. Nueropraxia is a temporary nerve conduction block with intact axons. The term *axonopraxia* does not exist.

139. b. Myelodysplasia can involve the entire spinal cord, not just the anterior cord. Teratogens are any agents that cause a structural abnormality during pregnancy. Excessive alcohol and drug intake have been shown to cause myelodysplasia. Although the lower spinal region is more likely to be effected in myelodysplasia, it can refer to defects in any part of the spinal column.

140. c. Exteriorization of neuralgic function can occur throughout life, and gait abnormalities are often the first complaint. Scoliosis can be slow in developing and should be monitored by the physical therapist.

141. a. This result is typical in normal development.

142. a. Ballistic movements are high velocity movements requiring antagonist muscle groups to contract. Coactivation would not produce movement, and visual guidance is not needed for random, ballistic movements. Propriocetion is not an issue.

143. d. Since the head is large (compared to the body) at this stage of development, weight must be shifted to the thighs and lower abdomen to raise the head in a prone position.

144. a. Contractions of antagonistic muscle groups produce reciprocal patterns. This is not seen in children with cerebral palsy.

145. d. These movements remain until 5 months when they become associated with a lack of movement of the extremities to midline.

146. d. Newborns do not move to stationary objects as in Choice A, nor can they grasp as in choice B. Light avoidance also occurs later in the development process.

147. c. In normal development, gaining the ability of postural control allows for more rapid change of positions. This change will allow more normal movement patterns. An infant may not be able to understand feedback, and a single way of performing the skill is not advisable.

148. d. Often children learn by trial and error. Age and weight are not strong predictors of walking skill.

149. b. Four year olds typically can manage buttons, and 3 year olds still show dysmetria with block stacking. Infants that are just beginning the skill of walking are unafraid of falling.

150. d. Levodopa/carbidopa can cause all of the listed effects except bradycardia. Due to the off-effect, the patient might have to be scheduled at times when he or she is in the on-phase.

151. a. It is known that flickering lights or repetitive noises can trigger epileptic episodes. Although anticonvulsants are quite effective, it is recommended to avoid such aversive stimuli in these patients.

152. a. Lithium has a very small margin of safety and can be quickly under- or overdosed requiring frequent drug blood level determinations. Ataxia, tremors, increased deep tendon reflexes, confusion and later seizures are indications of lithium overdose.

153. a. All of these movement disorders can occur but tardive dyskinesia is irreversible and might possibly require an immediate change in the drug prescribed.

154. c. Neuralgia and myopathies are encountered during antiviral treatments while all of the other reactions are rare. For some drugs, it is important to ask the patient to drink a lot of water during strenuous exercise to prevent dehydration and drug precipitations in the kidney.

155. a. The most common adverse reactions are sedation, confusion, and psychomotor impairment while erratic heartbeat might be of other origins.

156. a. Cholinergic agonists stimulate muscarinic receptors and cause diarrhea, sweating, salivation, bradycardia, some decreased blood pressure, and miosis.

157. b. GABA is one of the main inhibitory neurotransmitters in the CNS. Some sedatives, anxiolytics, skeletal muscle relaxants, and anticonvulsants cause their therapeutic effects by increasing its actions.

158. b. Choice B, perception of spatial relationships, is the correct answer. The parietal lobes function to integrate sensory information for perception of spatial relations.

159. d. Choice D, spasticity, hyperreflexia, positive Babinski sign, is the correct answer. Fasciculations are also a sign of lower motor neuron disorders as they represent denervation hypersensitivity of the lower motor neuron. UMN syndrome does not produce rigidity. Rigidity is a sign of basal ganglia disease. Hyporeflexia is a sign of lower motor neuron lesions.

160. c. The Landau reflex is not fully integrated until the child's second year.

161. b. A nerve regenerates at an approximate rate of 1 inch per month.

162. c. The most common injury of the brachial plexus is to the upper roots, C5-C6, resulting in an Erb's palsy.

163. a. An injury to the C5-C6 nerve roots results in an Erb's palsy. The flexor carpi ulnaris is innervated by C8-T1.

164. a. Atrial fibrillation is a relative contraindication for therapy. Exercise should start at a lower intensity and be progressed slowly if the ventricular ate remains controlled. There is no contraindication against upper extremity exercise.

165. b. In a complete supine position, patients with this diagnosis will have excess fluid move from the lower body to the chest cavity. This causes a decrease in heart and lung function and efficiency.

166. b. This patient is likely to experience a decrease in the number of red blood cells. All of the other statements are correct. Fibrinogen drops initially but then rises throughout recovery.

167. c. Choice C is more common than the other choices.

168. a. This is the correct order of incision or wound healing after surgery.

169. a. Tetracyclines cause mostly a toxic photosensitization and sun light or UV light should be avoided. They should also not be given to children because of bone and teeth problems, and they should not be taken with antacids, which prevent their absorption.

170. d. Signs and symptoms of lymphangitis (infection) may include some or all of the following: rash; red, blotchy skin; itching of the affected area; discoloration; increase of swelling and/or temperature of the skin; heavy sensation in the limb (more so than usual); pain; and, in many cases, a sudden onset of high fever and chills. Treatment for infections is to immediately discontinue ALL current lymphedema treatment modalities (including manual lymphatic drainage, bandaging, pumps, and wearing of compression garments), and contact your physician as soon as possible.

171. a. The stratum germinativum (basale) contains stem cells characterized by intense mitotic activity indicative of cellular division since the main function of this layer is the continual renewal of epidermal cells.

172. b. The right adrenal gland is in contact with the inferior vena cava anteromedially. It is separated from the pancreas by the duodenum. The left adrenal is in contact with the posterior wall and the stomach and the body-tail of the pancreas.

173. a. The anterior lobe of the pituitary gland is regulated by releasing hormones produced by the hypothalamus. These hormones are sent to the anterior lobe via the hypophyseal-portal vascular system. The other three components of the central nervous system do not affect or connect to the anterior lobe.

174. a. Eighty percent to ninety percent of erythropoietin is formed in the kidney, with the remainder coming from the liver. Marrow responds to this hormone.

175. a. The abdominal cavity extends superiorly into the thoracic cage. Subsequently, the ribs protect several abdominal organs. These are the spleen, liver, adrenal gland, and upper portions of the kidneys and stomach.

176. b. All the pharyngeal muscles are supplied by the vagus nerve (CN X) except the stylopharyngeus muscle, which is supplied by the glossopharyngeal nerve (CN IX).

177. a. The spleen lies in the upper left quadrant or left hypochondrium of the abdomen under the diaphragm, adjacent to the ninth, tenth, and eleventh ribs.

178. b. Enzymes responsible for the breakdown of disaccharides are located in the brush border.

179. c. Metatarsal pads successfully transfer weight onto the metatarsal shafts of this patient. A Thomas heel and a scaphoid pad are for patients with excessive pronation. A cushion heel absorbs shock at contact.

180. a. Adrenocorticotropic hormone, thyroid-stimulating hormone, growth hormone, follicle-stimulating hormone, and luteinizing hormone are all produced by the anterior pituitary gland. Insulin and glucagon are produced in the pancreas. Epinephrine and norepinephrine are produced in the adrenal medulla. Cortisol, androgens, and aldosterone are produced by the adrenal cortex.

181. b. Tachycardia could be the result of taking too much thyroid hormone, and a dose adjustment may be needed. Overdosing with propylthiouracil might cause lethargy and weight gain.

182. a. Massaging the injection site can increase insulin absorption and cause hypoglycemia. Glucosamine can interfere with insulin effects, and injections into the abdomen are recommended when exercising.

183. d. OTC cimetidine and chromium have been shown to interfere with the action of metformin, while herbal medications have not been found to be of significant benefit.

184. c. The liver is located in the right upper quadrant making pain referral more common to the right shoulder. Coffee ground emesis or melena are generally associated with GI disorders, as liver disease tends to create gray-colored stools and dark urine.

185. c. Direct access will increase the likelihood of therapists being the first provider for many conditions. Risk factor assessment is helpful in identifying immune problems, but the cause and risk for many conditions is still unknown. Disease progression is common with different signs and symptoms, and early recognition of immune dysfunction can improve the course of the disease.

186. b. A patient with polyarticular JRA presents with acute or insidious symmetrical arthritis of the large and small joints of the upper and lower extremities, with more than four joints involved. The joints are swollen and warm, but rarely red. The systemic symptoms are usually mild and include low grade fever, mild to moderate hepatosplenomegaly, and lymphadenopathy.

187. c. Lymphedema is swelling that occurs when protein-rich lymph fluid accumulates in the interstitial tissue. This lymph fluid may contain plasma proteins, extravascular blood cells, excess water, and parenchymal products.

188. b. The most dramatic bone loss in women occurs in the years immediately after menopause and its associated abrupt decline in estrogen production. Menopause begins naturally when your ovaries start making less estrogen and progesterone, the hormones that regulate menstruation.

189. d. Peak bone mass is usually attained by age 30, and then begins a slow decline that will continue throughout life. Women lose 1% to 2% of bone mass per year (compared to 0.3% to 1% in men), ultimately losing 30% to 50% of their initial bone mass (compared to 20% to 30% in men).

190. c. Primary lymphedema is an inherited disorder resulting from abnormal formation of lymphatic vessels before birth. These malformations most commonly cause swelling that affects the feet and legs.

191. a. Insulin works to decrease blood glucose levels by transporting glucose out of the bloodstream and into cells.

192. b. Although a patient should not self-medicate with large dose of antacids over long periods of time, such a use of magnesium-containing antacids can lead to diarrhea and use of aluminum-containing antacids can lead to constipation. Patients have experienced muscle weakness with magnesium-containing antacids perhaps because of interference with the neurotransmitter-releasing action of calcium at the neuromuscular junction.

193. d. Opioid analgesics stimulate opioid receptors leading to analgesia, sedation, miosis (vision problems in the dark since pupils cannot dilate), respiratory depression, sometimes nausea (less in supine position), and constipation.

194. a. The best answer is the gastrointestinal system. Musculoskeletal and urogenital both can cause similar symptoms, but the musculoskeletal system usual is painful in response to mechanical changes in the body. This pain is relatively constant. The urogenital system is potentially the source, but symptoms are often central, and urogenital pathology does not usually result in nausea and diarrhea. The gastrointestinal system is the best answer because all of the patient's symptoms can be attributed to gastrointestinal dysfunction.

195. c.   All of these symptoms could produce pain in the right low back. The symptoms that increase the likelihood that the hepatic system is the source of the symptoms are the patient's complaints of muscle tremors, dark urine, nausea, vomiting, and yellowing of the eyes. All of these symptoms are indicative of liver or gallbladder pathology. Both of these are a part of the hepatic system.

196. c.   Omeprazole is a proton pump inhibitor that inhibits the enzyme in the gastric parietal cells. When this enzyme (proton pump) is stopped, acid secretion decreases.

197. c.   All of the other characteristics are those of cholinergic receptors, with the exception of A, which is not a characteristic of any receptor group.

198. d.   A third-degree heart block can appear as dizziness and fatigue and may require a pacemaker. Patients with asthma and obesity should be monitored closely but should be permitted to exercise. Dialysis should be scheduled on nondialysis days.

199. d.   The axillary nerve is in close proximity to the surgical field in this patient. ROM is normal so choice B is incorrect; poor compliance would lead to a multitude of problems rather than just deltoid weakness. The musculocutaneous nerve is not involved with this procedure, and it innervates muscles involved in elbow flexion.

200. d.   The other choices will be important later in the rehabilitation of this diagnosis. ROM is important early to reduce abnormal scar tissue formation.

201. a.   Parasympathetic fibers inhibit the smooth muscles of the internal urethral sphincter, which allows urine to flow into the urethra.

202. d.   During the preovulatory phase of the menstrual cycle, follicle-stimulating hormone is the dominant hormone. The feedback mechanism of high levels of estradiol cause a midcycle surge in luteinizing hormone (LH). About 24 hours after the surge in LH, the follicle ruptures and ovulation occurs. LH also maintains the function of the corpus luteum in the postovulatory phase.

203. b.   Whiplash injury includes hyperextension of cervical vertebrae that may tear the anterior longitudinal ligament that limits extension of the cervical spine. All of the other ligaments limit flexion of the cervical spine; accordingly, they may be torn in hyperflexion injuries.

204. c. The lateral collateral ligament of the knee is best palpated with the patient in the sitting position. The patient then places the foot of the involved lower extremity on the knee of the uninvolved lower extremity. This maneuver places the involved knee in 90 degrees of flexion and the hip in external rotation.

205. a. Contraceptive combination medications increase the risk of thromboembolism, which is markedly enhanced by smoking. All the others should not occur or should not be affected.

206. d. All of the listed reactions can occur except joint or muscle pain.

207. c. Iron deficiency anemia responds to iron supplementation, but there are other anemias, including folic acid or B12 deficiency anemias, which only respond to folic acid or B12 administration.

208. a. The patient's symptoms do not appear to be provoked by movement or activities; therefore, the musculoskeletal system is probably not the top hypothesis. Hepatic symptoms usually appear on the right side and this patient has left-sided low back pain. Gastrointestinal and urogenital systems can both produce pain in the left low back. The fact that the symptoms appear to increase with the intake of fluid makes the urogenital system the best answer.

209. a. Gastrointestinal pathology rarely results in great toe pain. The musculoskeletal system and cancer can both impact the great toe, but with the patient's 3-year history of waxing and waning symptoms, as well as his history of kidney disease places gout at the top of the hypothesis list. Gout occurs when excess uric acid (a normal waste product) accumulates in the body, and crystals deposit in the joints. This may happen because either uric acid production increases or, more often, the kidneys are unable to remove uric acid from the body adequately.

210. a. Also referred to as "urogenital atrophy," atrophic vaginitis has an incidence level somewhere between 10% to 40% of postmenopausal women. Both vaginal and urethral tissue is estrogen dependent. A history of smoking, nonvaginal deliveries, certain immune disorders, and noncoital status are some of the risk factors for developing atrophic vaginitis.

211.   c.   Though this patient may have some symptoms that also match *urge incontinence*, the definition of functional incontinence is the following: *Functional incontinence* occurs when a person recognizes the need to urinate, but cannot physically make it to the bathroom in time because of limited mobility. Causes of functional incontinence include confusion; dementia; poor eyesight; poor mobility; poor dexterity; and unwillingness to toilet because of depression, anxiety, or anger, or being in a situation in which it is impossible to reach a toilet.

212.   d.   A myocardial infarction that involves the left ventricle is likely to cause cardiogenic shock. Cardiogenic shock is a rapid decline in cardiac output. Vascular shock is widespread vasodilation. Toxic and anaphylactic shock occur when the body is exposed to a toxin or allergin, respectively.

213.   d.   Improvement in strength, anaerobic conditioning, balance, and many other areas can be gained with the proper training program in all ages. A child is "born with" a fixed ratio of fast/slow twitch fibers. Athletes can improve reaction time with proper training.

214.   d.   Preparticipation screenings accomplish all the objectives mentioned in the question. Many times children with serious medical conditions are barred from athletic participation. Eye-hand coordination is beyond the scope of the preparticipation examination in this population.

215.   b.   Children require more caloric intake (and hydration as well) than an adult in athletics. Children have a greater surface area per body weight and a decreased ability to sweat versus an adult. This makes exercise in the heat more of a concern for the adolescent athlete. An adult weight training program should be much more aggressive than a child's program. Aggressive weight training in children can cause many musculoskeletal dysfunctions.

216.   b.   It is recommended that OTC drugs should not be used for more than 2 weeks without the advice of a physician since they are effective but can mask a serious problem, interact with prescription drugs, and have adverse reactions.

217.   a.   Diphenhydramine is an antihistamine that blocks histamine or H1 receptors and is being used for allergic conditions (type I only). It can cause sedation, dry mouth, blurred vision, dry mouth and skin, contact lens intolerance, constipation and urinary hesitancy (mostly via its anticholinergic actions, which are more pronounced in the elderly).

218. d. OTC niacin is effective, but its use requires periodic lab tests that only a physician can order.

219. c. All the listed adverse reactions can occur due to suppression of platelet and red blood cell formation and liver damage (some drugs only), but GI problems include diarrhea, which can often be severe.

220. a. Chemotherapy affects the GI tract and problems are made worse by NSAIDs, which also affect and irritate the stomach. The others should not present problems.

221. b. All of the listed effects can be expected plus fat shifts (moon face, buffalo hump), hypertension, muscle wasting, cataracts, increased intraocular pressure and osteoporosis but not orthostatic hypotension.

222. a. Easy bruising would not be expected, but dehydration with electrolyte changes, muscle cramping, and dyspnea are expected.

223. b. A glass of wine (100 ml) contains about 10 ml of alcohol or ethanol (about 10%). The average person metabolizes about 10 ml within an hour.

224. b. Cimetidine is an H2 blocker that blocks acid-releasing H2 receptors in the stomach and is associated with all of the listed reactions except orthostatic hypotension.

225. b. NSAIDs inhibit the enzymes COX I and II (except celecoxib, which only acts on II) and reduce formation of pain, fever, and inflammation-causing prostaglandins, but they also reduce their protective effects in the stomach.

226. b. Sleep drugs can cause some residual effects or some drowsiness in the morning. If so, schedule the patient in the afternoon. Do not recommend St. John's wort.

227. c. It is possible to get these reflexes because the somatic and visceral afferents enter the spinal cord at the same level. Somatic sources that create visceral symptoms are known as somatic-visceral reflexes.

228. b. Medications are an integral part of current medical practice, and therapists need to be aware of the use, benefits, and risks associated with these medications. Part of our responsibility is to monitor patients for potential side effects, but it is generally not in the physical therapist's scope of practice to change the medications.

229. a. Figure-ground discrimination. The patient has difficulty finding an item within a crowded visual field. This is figure-ground discrimination. Agraphia is the inability to write. Vertical orientation and body scheme awareness relate to the patient's self-awareness.

230. d. The phenotypic features in Down Syndrome are flat facial profile, low nasal bridge, shortened palate, joint hypermobility, hypoplastic pelvis, atlantoaxial instability, simian creases, ventricular septal defect, patent ductus arteriosus, tetralogy of Fallot, hypotonia, mental retardation, developmental delay, small cerebellum and brainstem, and leukemia.

231. d. A review of current "safe exercise guidelines" would indicate avoiding exercises that risk direct trauma to the abdominal region. However, continuing an exercise program, in moderation, is highly recommended for both the health of the baby and mom during the pregnancy.

232. b. A posterior shift in the center of mass would create the opposite presentation in terms of posture. Secondary to anterior weight gain, a posterior shift does not make sense in this case.

233. d. Frequently missed by coaches and health professionals, choice D is the definition of female athlete triad. Consequences of this disorder include early osteoporotic fractures, delayed healing, and an inability to regain appropriate bone mineral density.

234. a. Uterine prolapse occurs when pelvic floor muscles and ligaments stretch and weaken, providing inadequate support for the uterus. The uterus then descends into the vaginal canal.

235. c. Owing to the location of the baby, all but the breasts may be compressed at some point during a pregnancy.

236. a. Predictors include significantly earlier onset of pain during pregnancy, higher maternal age, higher body mass index (BMI), and a higher proportion of women with joint hypermobility are affected.

237. a. Beta-lactam antibiotics are so named because of a unique chemical ring structure that all drugs in this class possess. Oftentimes, beta-lactams are referred to as the penicillins, penicillin being the first drug in this class to be described. Levofloxacin is a flouroquinolone; azithromycin is a macrolide, and tetracycline is the prototype tetracycline.

238. c. Hypersensitivity reactions to penicillin are the most common side effect of this antibiotic. Amoxicillin falls into the class of penicillins (or beta-lactam antibiotics), and therefore, the rash is most likely the result of an allergic reaction to the amoxicillin. Sinusitis is a type of bacterial infection; therefore, treatment with an antibiotic is justified.

239. a. Abnormal swelling of the vessels in the nasal cavity usually causes nasal congestion. Treatment with a medication that binds to alpha-receptors will cause these vessels to contract or shrink and will help improve symptoms. Pseudoephedrine is only taken orally. Rebound congestion is only seen with nasal sprays. All drugs in this category are more likely to cause CNS stimulation, excitability, nervousness rather than drowsiness, or dry mouth (these are typical anti-cholinergic side effects).

240. a. Excretion is the pharmacokinetic term used to describe how the body removes drugs from the body. Drugs can be eliminated in a variety of ways including via urine, sweat, feces, bile, and other means. Excretion is not a static process and occurs as soon as the drug is able to be eliminated.

241. c. The "statins" are a group of drugs that inhibit the rate-limiting step in cholesterol synthesis. The enzyme HMG-CoA reductase catalyzes this rate-limiting step.

242. c. Increased external rotation range of motion. Excessive femoral anteversion has been shown to be related to increased internal rotation and decreased external rotation ROM. Also, it has been shown that it results in a reduced hip abductor moment arm.

243. c. Trunk side bending to the left. The superior gluteal nerve innervates the gluteus medius muscle. A lesion would result in a Tredelenberg stance, leading to left side bending of the spine (to maintain an upright posture).

244. a. Choice A, right lumbar rotators, is the correct answer. The single leg stance would result in activation of all of the left-sided hip abductors and the right quadratus lumborum.

245. c. Choice C, coxa vara, is the correct answer. Coxa valga would be a larger than normal angle of inclination at the hip. Anteversion is the angle made by the femoral neck and the femoral condyles (as measured from the coronal plane). Excessive medial rotation is anteversion, and excessive lateral rotation is retroversion.

246. d. Choice D, gluteus minimus posterior fibers, is the correct answer. Hip abductors and hip extensors do not limit hip extension. All the other choices may limit hip extension.

247. c. Choice C, normal, is the correct answer. Genu valgum is an abnormal inward "bowing" of the knees (knock knee). Genu varus is an outward anatomic presence of the knee (bow-legged).

248. c. Choice C, medial tibia, sartorius, gracilis, and semitendinosus, is the correct answer. An interesting pneumonic to remember the pes anserine insertion is "Say Grace before SupperTime" Say = sartoriuos, Grace = gracilis, SupperTime = semitendinosus.

249. a. Choice A, increases, less, is the correct answer. As the patella rides superiorly out of the trochlear groove, the joint becomes less stable because less of the patella is in contact with the trochlear groove.

250. b. Choice B, lateral and superior and anteriorly, is the correct answer. This is the normal anatomic presentation of the glenoid.

251. a. The scapula upwardly rotates 60 degrees and the humeral abducts 120 degrees. The scapula upwardly rotates 1 degree for every 2 degrees of humeral abduction. Abnormalities of this relationship could signal deficiencies in the rotator cuff musculature.

252. b. a Choice A, Hill-Sachs lesion, is the correct answer. While many of these injuries are seen with sholder dislocation, a Hill-Sachs lesion is by far the most common. A Hill-Sachs lesion to the humerus is caused when the smooth surface of the humerus hits the outer rim of the glenoid fossa.

253. d. Increased trochlear groove depth increases patellar instability. An internally rotated femur causes the patella to track laterally. A lateral patella is unstable. Weakness of the hip external rotators will lead to a more internally rotated femur. A superior patella (as in patella alta), will move the patella out of the trochlear groove. However, increased trochlear groove depth makes the patella MORE stable.

254. c. The competitive antagonist will occupy 20% of available receptor sites because four parts agonist/one part antagonist = 80% agonist effect.

255. b. Bioavailability refers to the drug fraction available to produce the desired effect.

256. b. A 24-hour period has elapsed, which is 2 half-lives. The serum drug concentration will be reduced by half during the first half-life period and half again during the second half-life time period. $\frac{1}{2} \times 10$ mg $= 5$ mg, $\frac{1}{2} \times 5$mg $= 2.5$mg.

257. a. Aspirin is unique among the NSAID agents in that its impact on thromboxane biosynthesis and platelet aggregation is an irreversible effect. The thromboprophylactic effect following aspirin administration therefore lasts about 8 to 10 days, the lifespan of a platelet.

258. a. First-order kinetics refers to drugs metabolized in half-life patterns. Fifty percent of active drug is metabolized each half-life.

259. d. BZD agents do not produce analgesia.

260. a. Xanax is specifically indicated for treatment of anxiety. Klonopin is indicated for convulsive disorders and Valium for skeletal muscle spasm and convulsive disorders. It is not a first-line agent for anxiety because of sedation and its long half-life.

261. a. The dry hacking cough is a major irritant and problem with the ACE agents that often results in a change to an ARB class agent.

262. d. Flurazepam (Dalmane) has an extended half-life (12 to 24 hours), which is even longer in the elderly. Some sources note Dalmane may never be eliminated from the body of an elderly patient.

263. d. Klonopin is indicated as a first-line agent for treatment of convulsive disorders. Valium may be used in emergency room settings to treat status epilepticus, but it is not a first-line agent for outpatient care.

264. d. Skeletal muscle relaxants are primarily classified by the site of action. This is either the central nervous system (CNS) or peripheral nervous system (myoneural junction).

265. a. All centrally acting muscle relaxants, by definition, produce CNS sedation.

266. b. Flexeril is related to the tricyclic antidepressant agents and may share some side effects including anticholinergic activity.

267. a. Baclofen does not alter weight or have beta-1 adrenergic activity.

268. d. The two naturally occurring opiates within the poppy flower are codeine and morphine.

269. a. With few exceptions, the oral hypoglycemic agents may produce hypoglycemia. Patients should be monitored to ensure dietary glucose intake is appropriate to their hypoglycemic agent dosage.

270. b. The old apothecary system used the grain as a unit of weight. One grain is approximately 63 mg. A Tylenol with codeine #4 contains 1 grain, nominally 60 mg. A #3 is half that amount, 30 mg; a #2 contains 15 mg; and a #1 contains 7.5 mg.

271. b. Both of these agents are classified as agonist-antagonist opiate agents and are among the more common seen in practice.

272. d. Combining an opiate with a diuretic agent will not increase blood pressure but rather reduce blood pressure by virtue of ethanol's ability to relax vascular smooth muscle.

273. c. Two dissimilar drugs one with the ability to multiply a specific effect of the other is potentiation.

274. d. The only skeletal muscle relaxant that acts directly on muscle is dantrolene.

275. a. Current prescribing protocol notes the only indication for a COX-2 agent is a patient with a GI or renal disorder. Even then, COX-2 agents are not the first-line drug because of their mild effect on both GI and renal function.

276. c. Acetaminophen has no peripheral anti-inflammatory effect and does not impede biosynthesis of thromboxane and therefore has no impact on platelet aggregation.

277. d. Daypro exhibits one of the longest NSAID half-lives, over 50 hours.

278. a. HCT is a common first-line agent for initial treatment of hypertension. It is relatively safe and effective and may be combined with second-line agents if needed.

279. c. Probenicid acts by a different mechanism of action and is used to reduce uric acid synthesis as a means of preventing recurrent attacks rather than treatment of acute attacks of gouty arthritis. The other listed agents are used to treat acute episodes.

280. d. The ACE inhibitors inhibit biosynthesis of angiotensin II and have no impact on potassium levels as do the thiazide and loop diuretics.

281. b. Fursosemide is a loop diuretic and will cause significant potassium loss in the urine. Potassium supplements are sometime required. Patients should be monitored for hypokalemia.

282. a. The Edinger-Westphal response is a direct drug action, rather than a side effect. Bilateral myosis suggests opiate overdosage.

283. b. ARB agents are similar in effect to the ACE group but their mechanism of action is at the angiotensin II receptor site rather than enzymatic production of angiotensin.

284. a. Patients prone to hypokalemia or potassium-sensitive agents such as digoxin may require use of a "potassium-sparing agent" such as aldactone.

285. a. Metformin is unique among oral hypoglycemic agents in that it does not produce hypoglycemia.

286. c. This newer class of oral hypoglycemic agents exerts its effect at the peripheral insulin receptor, resulting in increased active diffusion of insulin across the cell membrane.

287. d. Progestin is progesterone and will not produce male secondary sex characteristics.

288. c. Sedation is the shared side effect of all BZD agents of note to PTs.

289. c. All NSAID agents exert their myriad effects by blocking COX-1 and/or COX-2 biosynthesis from their precursor, arachidonic acid, which is naturally found on most cell surfaces in the body.

CHAPTER 2

Examination

1. A patient who suffered a myocardial infarction is participating in an exercise test. The therapist notes ST-segment depression of 1.7 mm on the patient's current rhythm strip. What is the most appropriate course of action?
    a. Stop the exercise session immediately and send the patient to the emergency room.
    b. Continue with the exercise session.
    c. Contact the patient's cardiologist about continuing exercise.
    d. Stop the exercise session to take the patient's heart rate and blood pressure.

2. The therapist is treating a patient who received an above-elbow amputation 2 years ago. The prosthesis has a split cable that controls the elbow and the terminal device. With this type of prosthesis, the patient must first lock the elbow to allow the cable to activate the terminal device. This is accomplished with what movements?
    a. Extending the humerus and elevating the scapula
    b. Extending the humerus and retracting the scapula
    c. Extending the humerus and protracting the scapula
    d. Extending the humerus and depressing the scapula

3. A physical therapist is treating a patient who is participating in cardiac rehabilitation. Because the patient complains of chest pain, the therapist attempts to assess heart sounds with a stethoscope. Which of the following is true about the first sound during auscultation of the heart?
    a. The first sound is of the closure of the aortic and pulmonic valves.
    b. The first sound is of the closure of the mitral and tricuspid valves.
    c. The first sound is of the beginning of ventricular diastole.
    d. The first sound is usually the loudest.

4. A 53-year-old man with chronic obstructive pulmonary disease reports to an outpatient cardiopulmonary rehabilitation facility. Pulmonary testing reveals that forced expiratory volume in 1 second (FEV1) and vital capacity (VC) are within 60% of predicted values. What is the appropriate exercise prescription?
   a. Exercise at 75% to 80% of the target heart rate 3 times/week.
   b. Begin exercise with levels of 1.5 METs and increase slowly 3 times/week.
   c. Exercise at 75% to 80% of the target heart rate 7 times/week.
   d. Begin exercise with levels of 1.5 METs and increase slowly 7 times/week.

5. A patient reports throbbing pain in the lower extremities accompanied by trophic changes and diminished pulses. The pain is aggravated by activity and was not influenced by spinal movements. What source of pain is most likely responsible for these complaints?
   a. Peripheral neuropathy
   b. Restless leg syndrome
   c. Vascular pain
   d. Neurogenic pain

6. A physical therapist is working with a patient who has chronic obstructive pulmonary disease. If the patient's level of oxygen being carried by arterial blood is measured, a Pao_2 finding of _____ _____ is considered normal.
   a. 35 to 45 mm Hg
   b. 60 to 80 mm Hg
   c. 80 to 100 mm Hg
   d. 100 to 120 mm Hg

7. Whiplash injury from a rear-end collision would tear which of the following ligaments?
   a. Posterior longitudinal ligament (PLL)
   b. Anterior longitudinal ligament (ALL)
   c. Ligamentum nuchae
   d. Ligamentum flavum

8. Where is the most common site of fracture in osteoporosis?
   a. Metacarpals
   b. Skull
   c. Proximal radius
   d. Vertebral bodies

9. Which one of the following conditions is characterized by reduced osteoclastic bone resorption?
   a. Paget's disease of the bone
   b. Osteoporosis
   c. Osteopetrosis
   d. Osteomalacia

10. Which of the following conditions is descriptive of osteoarthritis?
    a. It provokes giant cell pigmented villonodular synovitis.
    b. It is associated with decreased type II collagen, cytokines, and chondrolysis.
    c. Ankylosis and follicular inflammation are predominant.
    d. It is associated with increased cartilage matrix synthesis and deposition.

11. An overweight 12-year-old presents with hip pain and weight-bearing difficulties. These symptoms presented rapidly following physical activity. On examination, limping is observed and passive ranges of motion are limited and painful. Which of the following is the MOST probable diagnosis?
    a. Legg-Calvé-Perthes disease
    b. Transient hip synovitis
    c. Congenital hip dysplasia
    d. Slipped femoral capital epiphysis

12. A defining symptom of fibromyalgia is
    a. Fatigue
    b. Diffuse pain
    c. Regional pain
    d. Unexplained weight loss

13. Morton's neuroma is usually located between which metatarsal heads?
    a. First and second
    b. Second and third
    c. Third and fourth
    d. Fourth and fifth

14. A 50-year-old, slightly obese man presents with a 1-month history of right hip pain without radiation, a protective limp, and activity-induced symptoms. He improves with rest and has some mild morning stiffness. Examination reveals restricted and painful internal rotation of the hip. What is the MOST likely diagnosis?
    a. Inflammatory arthritis
    b. Osteoarthritis
    c. Osteoporotic hip fractures
    d. Iliopsoas tendinosis

15. What is the MOST common myofascial pain syndrome of the low back?
    a. Piriformis
    b. Quadratus lumborum
    c. Iliopsoas
    d. Tensor fascia latae

16. What shoulder view BEST demonstrates the greater tubercle?
    a. External rotation
    b. Internal rotation
    c. Baby arm
    d. Transthoracic

17. The Waddell tests are used to identify
    a. Pain of a nonorganic origin
    b. Space-occupying lesions
    c. Balance and coordination functions
    d. History of alcohol or substance abuse

18. While assessing the standing posture of a patient, the therapist notes that a spinous process in the thoracic region is shifted laterally. The therapist estimates that T2 is the involved vertebra because he or she notes that it is at the approximate level of the
    a. Inferior angle of the scapula
    b. Superior angle of the scapula
    c. Spine of the scapula
    d. Xiphoid process of the sternum

19. While ambulating a stroke patient (the right side is the involved side), the therapist notes increased circumduction of the right lower extremity. Which of the following is an unlikely cause of this deviation?
    a. Increased spasticity of the right gastrocnemius
    b. Increased spasticity of the right quadriceps
    c. Weak hip flexors
    d. Weak knee extensors

20. The therapist is treating a 52-year-old woman after right total hip replacement. The patient complains of being self-conscious about a limp. She carries a heavy briefcase to and from work every day. The therapist notes a Trendelenburg gait during ambulation on level surfaces. What advice can the therapist give the patient to minimize gait deviation?
    a. Carry the briefcase in the right hand.
    b. Carry the briefcase in the left hand.
    c. The patient should not carry a briefcase at all.
    d. It does not matter in which hand the briefcase is carried.

21. Which of the following actions places the greatest stress on the patellofemoral joint?
   a. When the foot first contacts the ground during the gait cycle
   b. Exercising on a stair-stepper machine
   c. Running down a smooth decline of 30 degrees
   d. Squats to 120 degrees of knee flexion

22. While observing the ambulation of a 57-year-old man with an arthritic right hip, the therapist observes a right lateral trunk lean. Why does the patient present with this gait deviation?
   a. To move weight toward the involved hip and increase joint compression force
   b. To move weight toward the uninvolved hip and decrease joint compression force
   c. To bring the line of gravity closer to the involved hip joint
   d. To take the line of gravity away from the involved hip joint

23. A therapist has been treating a patient who received a rotator cuff surgical repair with sessions consisting only of passive range of motion (for an extended period). The patient has just returned from a follow-up doctor's visit with an additional order to continue with passive range of motion only. Which of the following is the best course of action for the therapist?
   a. Continue with passive range of motion as instructed, and call the physician to consult with him or her about the initiation of active range of motion.
   b. Begin active range of motion within the pain-free range, and continue passive range of motion.
   c. Continue passive range of motion, and do not question the physician's decision.
   d. Perform passive range of motion and any other exercise that is within the normal protocol for this diagnosis.

24. A patient's lawyer calls the therapist requesting his or her client's clinical records. The lawyer states that he or she needs the records to pay the patient's bill. What is the best course of action?
   a. Tell the lawyer either to have the patient request a copy of the records or to have the patient sign a medical release.
   b. Fax the needed chart to the lawyer.
   c. Mail a copy of the chart to the patient.
   d. Call the patient and tell him or her of the recent development.

25. A 35-year-old woman with a diagnosis of lumbar strain has a physician's prescription with a frequency and duration of 3 sessions/week for 6 weeks. The physical therapy examination reveals radiculopathy into the L5 dermatome of the right lower extremity, increased radiculopathy with lumbar flexion, decreased radiculopathy with lumbar extension, poor posture, and hamstring tightness bilaterally at 60 degrees. What is the best course of treatment?
    a. Lumbar traction, hot packs, and ultrasound
    b. McKenzie style lumbar extensions, a posture program, hamstring stretching, and a home exercise program
    c. McKenzie style lumbar extensions, a posture program, hamstring stretching, home program, hot packs, and ultrasound
    d. Lumbar traction, hot packs, ultrasound, and hamstring stretching

26. Which of the following does the therapist observe if a patient is correctly performing an anterior pelvic tilt in standing position?
    a. Hip extension and lumbar flexion
    b. Hip flexion and lumbar extension
    c. Hip flexion and lumbar flexion
    d. Hip extension and lumbar extension

27. At what point in the gait cycle is the center of gravity the lowest?
    a. Double support
    b. Terminal swing
    c. Deceleration
    d. Midstance

28. A 14-year-old girl with right thoracic scoliosis is referred to physical therapy. The therapist should expect which of the following findings?
    a. Left shoulder high, left scapula prominent, and right hip high
    b. Left shoulder low, right scapula prominent, and left hip high
    c. Right shoulder high, right scapula prominent, and right hip high
    d. Right shoulder low, right scapula prominent, and left hip high

29. What is the most likely cause of anterior pelvic tilt during initial contact (heel strike)?
    a. Weak abdominals
    b. Tight hamstrings
    c. Weak abductors
    d. Back pain

30. A posterior lateral herniation of the lumbar disc between vertebrae L4 and L5 most likely results in damage to which nerve root?
    a. L4
    b. L5
    c. L4 and L5
    d. L5 and S1

31. During examination of a patient, the therapist observes significant posterior trunk lean at initial contact (heel strike). Which of the following is the most likely muscle that the therapist needs to focus on during the exercise session in order to minimize this gait deviation?
    a. Gluteus medius
    b. Gluteus maximus
    c. Quadriceps
    d. Hamstrings

32. A patient presents to an outpatient physical therapy clinic with a 140 degrees kyphoscoliotic curve. What is the therapist's greatest concern?
    a. The patient's complaint of low back pain
    b. Gait deviations
    c. Pulmonary status
    d. Poor upright standing posture

33. After performing an examination, a therapist notes the following information: severe spasticity of plantar flexors in the involved lower extremity; complete loss of active dorsiflexion in the involved lower extremity; minimal spasticity between 0 degrees and 5 degrees of dorsiflexion, with increased spasticity when the ankle is taken into more than 5 degrees of dorsiflexion. Which ankle-foot orthosis (AFO) is most likely contraindicated for the patient, an 87-year-old man who had a stroke 4 weeks ago?
    a. Dorsiflexion spring assist AFO
    b. Posterior leaf spring AFO
    c. Hinged AFO
    d. Spiral AFO

34. The therapist is performing an orthopedic test on a 25-year-old man with the chief complaint of low back pain. The patient has a positive Thomas test. With this information, what might the therapist need to include in the treatment plan?
    a. Stretching of the hip abductors
    b. Stretching of the hip adductors
    c. Stretching of the hip extensors
    d. Stretching of the hip flexors

35. A patient is positioned by the therapist with the cervical spine rotated to the right. The patient then extends the neck as the therapist externally rotates and extends the right upper extremity. The patient is then instructed to hold a deep breath. The radial pulse is palpated in the right upper extremity by the therapist. What type of special test is this, and for what condition is it testing?
    a. Adson's maneuver, cervical disc herniation
    b. Lhermitte's sign, cervical disc herniation
    c. Adson's maneuver, thoracic outlet syndrome
    d. Lhermitte's sign, thoracic outlet syndrome

36. The therapist observes a patient with the latter stages of Parkinson's disease during ambulation. Which of the following characteristics is the therapist most likely observing?
    a. Shuffling gait
    b. Increased step width
    c. Wide base of support
    d. Increased cadence especially at the onset of gait

37. A therapist is examining the gait pattern of a patient and notes that the pelvis drops inferiorly on the right during the midswing phase of the right lower extremity. The patient also leans laterally to the left with the upper trunk during this phase. Which of the following is the most likely cause of this deviation?
    a. Weak right gluteus medius
    b. Weak right adductor longus
    c. Weak left gluteus medius
    d. Weak left adductor longus

38. The therapist is performing an orthopedic test that involves (1) placing the patient in a side-lying position, (2) placing the superior lower extremity in hip extension and hip abduction, (3) placing the knee of the superior lower extremity in 90 degrees of flexion, and (4) allowing the superior lower extremity to drop into adduction. Failure of the superior lower extremity to drop indicates a tight
    a. Iliopsoas
    b. Rectus femoris
    c. Iliotibial band
    d. Hamstring

39. A therapist is assessing radial deviation range of motion at the wrist. The correct position of the goniometer should be as follows: the proximal arm is aligned with the forearm and the distal arm is aligned with the third metacarpal. What should be used as the axis point?
    a. Lunate
    b. Scaphoid
    c. Capitate
    d. Triquetrum

40. The therapist is assessing a patient's strength in the right shoulder. The patient has 0 degrees of active shoulder abduction in the standing position. In the supine position, the patient has 42 degrees of active shoulder abduction and 175 degrees of pain-free passive shoulder abduction. What is the correct manual muscle testing grade for the patient's shoulder abduction?
    a. 3−/5 (fair −)
    b. 2+/5 (poor +)
    c. 2−/5 (poor −)
    d. 1/5 (trace)

41. A therapist is examining a patient with poor motor coordination. The therapist observes that when the patient is standing erect and still, she does not respond appropriately when correcting a backward sway of the body. With the body in a fully erect position a slight backward sway should be corrected by the body firing specific muscles in a specific order. Which list is the correct firing order?
    a. Bilateral abdominals, bilateral quadriceps, bilateral tibialis anterior
    b. Bilateral abdominals, bilateral tibialis anterior, bilateral quadriceps
    c. Bilateral tibialis anterior, bilateral abdominals, bilateral quadriceps
    d. Bilateral tibialis anterior, bilateral quadriceps, bilateral abdominals

42. A physical therapist is performing a functional capacity evaluation on a patient with a L4-L5 herniated disc. Part of the evaluation consists of performing floor to waist lifts using 30 pounds as resistance. During the first trial, the physical therapist notices that the patient exhibits decreased anterior pelvic tilt. What should the physical therapist do during the second trial?
    a. The therapist should correct the deviation verbally before the lift.
    b. The therapist should correct the deviation with manual contact during the lift.
    c. The therapist should correct the deviation both verbally and manually during the lift.
    d. The therapist should not attempt to correct the lift.

43. A physical therapist is examining a patient with muscular dystrophy. The patient seems to "waddle" when she walks. She rolls the right hip forward when advancing the right lower extremity and the left hip forward when advancing the left lower extremity. Which of the following gait patterns is the patient demonstrating?
    a. Gluteus maximus gait
    b. Dystrophic gait
    c. Arthrogenic gait
    d. Antalgic

44. A 48-year-old woman is being examined by a physical therapist. Her diagnosis is right rotator cuff tendinitis. She reports right shoulder weakness and pain for the past 2 months. The patient describes "pins and needles" over the lateral right shoulder and upper extremity, extending into the thumb. She also reports no causative trauma. Manual muscle testing in the right upper extremity reveals the following data: flexion = 4/5, extension = 3+/5, abduction = 3+/5, adduction = 4/5, internal rotation = 3+/5, and external rotation = 3+/5. Manual muscle testing in the left upper extremity reveals the following data: flexion = 4+/5, extension = 5/5, abduction = 5/5, adduction = 4+/5, internal rotation = 4+/5, and external rotation = 4+/5. Active and passive shoulder range of motion is within normal limits and equal bilaterally. All thoracic outlet tests are negative. All shoulder special tests are negative. Which of the following steps would most likely assess the source of the patient's problems?
     a. Elbow strength and range of motion testing
     b. Grip strength testing
     c. Cervical spine testing
     d. Scapular muscle strength testing

45. A therapist is screening a patient complaining of pain at the anterior left shoulder region. The pain is increased when the examiner instructs the patient to position the left arm by his side with the elbow flexed at 90 degrees and to actively supinate the forearm against resistance (provided by the examiner). What test is being performed?
     a. Froment's sign
     b. Yergason's test
     c. Waldron test
     d. Wilson test

46. A therapist is examining a patient with traumatic injury to the left hand. The therapist asks the patient to place the left hand on the examination table with the palm facing upward. The therapist then holds the second, third, and fifth digits in full extension. The patient is then asked to flex the fourth digit. What movement would be expected by a patient with an uninjured hand, and what muscle or muscles is the therapist restricting?
     a. The fourth finger would flex at the distal interphalangeal (DIP) joint only, and the muscle being restricted would be the flexor digitorum superficialis.
     b. The fourth finger would flex at the proximal interphalangeal (PIP) joint only, and the muscle being restricted would be the flexor digitorum profundus.
     c. The fourth finger would flex at the DIP joint only, and the muscles being restricted would be the lumbricals.
     d. The fourth finger would flex at the PIP joint only, and the muscles being restricted would be the palmar interosseous.

47. A patient is in prone position with his head rotated to the left side. The left upper extremity is placed at his side and fully internally rotated. The left shoulder is then shrugged toward the chin. The therapist then grasps the midshaft of the patient's left forearm. The patient is then instructed to "try to reach your feet using just your left arm." This movement is resisted by the therapist. This test is assessing the strength of what muscle?
    a. Upper trapezius
    b. Posterior deltoid
    c. Latissimus dorsi
    d. Triceps brachii

48. Which of the following is the normal end-feel perceived by an examiner assessing wrist flexion?
    a. Bone to bone
    b. Soft tissue approximation
    c. Tissue stretch
    d. Empty

49. A physical therapist is beginning an examination of a patient with a diagnosis of "knee strain." Range of motion limitation does not follow the normal capsular pattern of the knee. Which of the following are possible causes of the restriction in range of motion?
    a. Ligamentous adhesions
    b. Internal derangement
    c. Extra-articular lesions
    d. All of the above

50. Which of the following statements best describes lower extremity positioning in standing during the first 2 years of life of a child with no dysfunction?
    a. Femoral anteversion, femoral external rotation, foot pronation
    b. Femoral anteversion, femoral internal rotation, foot supination
    c. Femoral retroversion, femoral external rotation, foot pronation
    d. Femoral retroversion, femoral internal rotation, foot supination

51. A patient with decreased function of the gluteus minimus is referred to physical therapy for gait training. During the examination, the therapist places the patient in prone position and instructs the patient to extend the hip. Knowing that the gluteus minimus is extremely weak, which of the following is most likely to happen?
   a. The patient will abduct the hip more than usual when attempting to perform hip extension.
   b. The patient will externally rotate the hip excessively when attempting to perform hip extension.
   c. The patient will excessively flex the knee when attempting to perform hip extension.
   d. The patient will not have difficulty performing straight hip extension.

52. A patient is placed in supine position with the knee in 90 degrees of flexion. The foot is stabilized by the therapist's body on the examination table. The therapist then wraps his fingers around the proximal tibia so that the thumbs are resting along the anteromedial and the anterolateral margins. The therapist then applies a force to pull the tibia forward. What special test is being performed?
   a. Pivot shift
   b. Lachman's test
   c. Anterior drawer
   d. Posterior drawer

53. A therapist is examining a patient who complains of frequent foot, ankle, and knee pain. The therapist asks the patient to assume a standing position with the knees slightly flexed. The therapist then demonstrates active bilateral foot pronation to the patient. When asked to perform this task, the patient has difficulty. Which of the following limitations is a possible cause of the patient's difficulty in performing this task?
   a. Restriction limiting plantar flexion and lateral rotation of the talus
   b. Restriction limiting dorsiflexion and medial rotation of the talus
   c. Restriction limiting eversion of the calcaneus and medial rotation of the talus
   d. Restriction limiting inversion of the calcaneus and lateral rotation of the talus

54. Of the following, which is the earliest period after surgery that an 18-year-old boy who received an uncomplicated partial meniscectomy of the right knee can perform functional testing, such as a one-leg hop test, for distance?
   a. 1 week after surgery
   b. 2 weeks after surgery
   c. 6 weeks after surgery
   d. 12 weeks after surgery

55. A patient presents to therapy with an ankle injury. The therapist has determined that the injury is at the junction of the distal tibia and fibula. Which of the following functions the most in preventing excessive external rotation and posterior displacement of the fibula?
   a.   Anterior inferior tibiofibular ligament
   b.   Posterior inferior tibiofibular ligament
   c.   Interosseous membrane
   d.   Long plantar ligament

56. A physical therapist is examining a patient who complains of posterior ankle pain. The patient is positioned prone with the feet extended over the edge of the mat. The therapist squeezes the involved gastrocnemius over the middle third of the muscle belly. What test is the therapist performing? What indicates a positive test?
   a.   Thompson's test, plantar flexion of the ankle
   b.   Homan's test, plantar flexion of the ankle
   c.   Thompson's test, no ankle movement
   d.   Homan's test, no ankle movement

57. Which of the following is the correct method to test for interossei muscular tightness of the hand?
   a.   Passively flex the proximal interphalangeal (PIP) joints with the metaphalangeal (MP) joints in extension, then passively flex the PIP joints with the MP joints in flexion. Record the difference in PIP joint passive flexion.
   b.   Passively extend the PIP joints with the MP joints in extension, then passively extend the PIP joints with the MP joints in flexion. Record the difference in PIP joint passive flexion.
   c.   Passively flex the PIP joints with the MP joints in extension, then passively extend the PIP joints with the MP joints in flexion. Record the difference in PIP joint passive flexion.
   d.   Passively extend the PIP joints with the MP joints in extension, then passively flex the PIP joints with the MP joints in flexion. Record the difference in PIP joint passive flexion.

58. A therapist is beginning an examination of a 34-year-old woman with a diagnosis of carpal tunnel syndrome. Part of the evaluation consists of grip strength testing. To accurately test strength of the flexor digitorum profundus, where should the grip dynamometer's adjustable handle be placed?
   a.   1 inch from the dynamometer's nonadjustable handle
   b.   3 inches from the dynamometer's nonadjustable handle
   c.   1.5 inches from the dynamometer's nonadjustable handle
   d.   4 inches from the dynamometer's nonadjustable handle

59. A physical therapist is examining a 17-year-old distance runner with complaints of lateral knee pain. During the evaluation, the therapist performs the following test: The patient is placed in supine position with the hip flexed to 45 degrees and the knee to 90 degrees. The therapist then places firm pressure over the lateral femoral epicondyle and extends the patient's knee. Pain is felt by the patient at the point of palpation when her knee is 30 degrees from full knee extension. The positive result of this test suggests which of the following structures as the source of pain?
    a. Iliotibial band
    b. Biceps femoris
    c. Quadriceps
    d. Lateral collateral ligament

60. When ambulating on uneven terrain, how should the subtalar joint be positioned to allow forefoot rotational compensation?
    a. The subtalar joint should be placed in pronation.
    b. The subtalar joint should be placed in supination.
    c. The subtalar joint should be placed in a neutral position.
    d. The position of the subtalar joint does not influence forefoot compensation.

61. A physical therapist begins gait training for a patient with bilateral knee flexion contractures at 30 degrees at a long-term care facility. The therapist knows that the patient will have a forward trunk lean during gait because the patient's line of gravity
    a. Is anterior to the hip
    b. Is anterior to the knee
    c. Is posterior to the ankle
    d. Is posterior to the hip

62. What motion takes place at the lumbar spine with right lower extremity single limb support during the gait cycle?
    a. Left lateral flexion
    b. Right lateral flexion
    c. Extension
    d. Flexion

63. An outpatient physical therapist is gait-training a patient recently discharged from the hospital. The inpatient therapist's notes describe a decrease in left stride length due to pain with weight bearing on the right lower extremity. The outpatient therapist knows that the patient's gait deviation is an abnormally short
    a. Distance from the left heel strike and the successive right heel strike
    b. Amount of time between the left heel strike and the successive right heel strike
    c. Amount of time in stance phase on the left lower extremity
    d. Distance between the left heel strike and the successive left heel strike

64. In the terminal swing phase of gait, what muscles of the foot and ankle are active?
    a. Extensor digitorum longus
    b. Gastrocnemius
    c. Tibialis posterior
    d. Flexor hallucis longus

65. A physical therapist is beginning a gait examination. During heel strike to foot flat on the right lower extremity, which of the following does not normally occur?
    a. The left side of the pelvis initiates movement in the direction of travel.
    b. The right femur medially rotates.
    c. The left side of the thorax initiates movement in the direction of travel.
    d. The right tibia medially rotates.

66. When the knee is at its maximal amount of flexion during the gait cycle, which of the following muscles are active concentrically?
    a. Hamstrings
    b. Gluteus maximus
    c. Gastrocnemius
    d. Flexor hallucis longus

67. When comparing the gait cycle of young adults to the gait cycle of older adults, what would a therapist expect to find?
    a. The younger population has a shorter step length.
    b. The younger population has a shorter stride length.
    c. The younger population has a shorter period of double support.
    d. The younger population has a decrease in speed of ambulation.

68. A therapist is treating a patient with a venous insufficiency ulcer over the medial mallelous. The wound is moist and not infected. The involved lower extremity is swollen, and the patient reports no pain around the wound. The physician has ordered wound care 3 times/week. Which of the following should be used in intervention of this wound?
    a. Warm whirlpool
    b. Sharp debridement
    c. Intermittent compression pump
    d. Hot packs to the wound

69. A physical therapy examination of an infant with osteogenesis imperfecta should include all of the following except
    a. Pain
    b. Passive ROM
    c. Caregiver's handling
    d. Active functional movement

70. During therapy, a patient with Parkinson's disease on levodopa/carbidopa therapy might experience all of the following except
    a. The "off" phase
    b. Dizziness
    c. Involuntary movements
    d. Marked bradycardia

71. The alar ligament stress test is considered positive if
    a. Laxity is felt in neutral
    b. Laxity is felt in extension
    c. Laxity is felt in flexion
    d. Laxity is felt in both flexion and extension

72. A springy block end-feel in a joint is indicative of
    a. Normal end feel
    b. An inflamed capsule
    c. A meniscal tear
    d. An unstable joint

73. A physical therapist is examining a patient reporting knee pain. The patient is positioned in a prone position, and the physical therapist passively flexes the knee to end range. Based on the examination technique, which of the following structures would not be expected to limit movement?
    a. Joint capsule
    b. Vastus intermedius
    c. Sciatic nerve
    d. Rectus femoris

74. A physical therapist is assessing the posture of a 12-year-old female with cystic fibrosis. All of the following are common postural abnormalities except
    a. Thoracic kyphosis
    b. Forward head posture
    c. Scapular retraction
    d. Cervical lordosis

75. A child loses balance and falls down whenever she tries to catch a ball thrown in her direction; otherwise the child can sit, stand, and walk well. The physical therapist would determine that the child has a problem with
    a. Development of higher-level balance skills
    b. Protective reactions
    c. Anticipatory postural control
    d. Labyrinthine head righting

76. A grasp that is often used to control tools or other objects is the
    a. Hook grasp
    b. Power grasp
    c. Lateral pinch
    d. Tip pinch

77. Nerve conduction velocity/EMG studies of motor nerves are NOT able to differentiate
    a. Peripheral nerve disease from anterior horn cell disease
    b. The specific location cord, nerve, root, plexus, or peripheral nerve
    c. Neuromuscular junction disease from peripheral nerve disease
    d. The specific cause or nature of the neural lesion

78. What is the difference in testing motor function when examining for a nerve root deficit versus a peripheral nerve deficit?
    a. In peripheral nerve deficit, the motor weakness is evident more rapidly when applying resistance compared with nerve root deficit.
    b. In nerve root deficit, the motor weakness is evident more rapidly when applying resistance compared with peripheral nerve deficit.
    c. In peripheral nerve deficit, the motor weakness is only evident when applying resistance without gravity.
    d. In nerve root deficit, the motor weakness is only evident when applying resistance without gravity.

79. Which impairment occurs in carpal tunnel syndrome?
    a. Atrophy of the hypothenar eminence
    b. Paresthesias over the dorsal aspect of the hand
    c. Decreased resisted thumb abduction
    d. Decreased resisted forearm pronation

80. The L4 deep tendon reflex is elicited at the
    a. Achilles tendon
    b. Femoral tendon
    c. Medial hamstring tendon
    d. Patella tendon

81. A 25-year-old football player fell on his shoulder vertically and violently stretched his neck in the opposite direction. He was later diagnosed with a brachial plexus injury (Erb-Duchenne paralysis). His arm is hanging at his side in medial rotation in the "waiter's tip" position. What results are expected from the neurologic examination?
    a. Paralysis of the deltoid, triceps, wrist extensors (long and short carpi radialis), and finger extensors
    b. Paralysis of all intrinsic muscles of the hand, flexors muscles (claw hand), loss of sensation over C8-T1 dermatomes, and Horner's syndrome
    c. Hypesthesia over C5-C6 and weakness of the deltoid, supraspinatus and infraspinatus, biceps, and brachioradialis muscles
    d. Klumpke paralysis caused by forced hyperabduction of the arm

82. A patient presents to an outpatient physical therapy clinic with a severed ulnar nerve of the right upper extremity. What muscle is still active and largely responsible for the obvious hyperextension at the metacarpophalangeal (MCP) joints of the involved hand?
    a. Dorsal interossei
    b. Volar interossei
    c. Extensor carpi radialis brevis
    d. Extensor digitorum

83. A patient presents to an outpatient facility with complaints of pain in the groin area (along the medial left thigh). With manual muscle testing of the involved lower extremity, a therapist determines the following: hip flexion = 4+/5, hip extension = 4+/5, hip abduction = 4+/5, hip adduction = 2+/5, hip internal rotation = 2+/5, and hip external rotation = 2+/5. Which nerve on the involved side is most likely injured?
    a. Lateral cutaneous nerve of the upper thigh
    b. Obturator nerve
    c. Femoral nerve
    d. Ilioinguinal nerve

84. A mother comes to a therapist concerned that her 4-month-old infant cannot sit up alone yet. Which of the following responses is the most appropriate for the therapist?
    a. "Your infant probably needs further examination by a specialist because, although it varies, infants can usually sit unsupported at 2 months of age."
    b. "Your infant probably needs further examination by a specialist because, although it varies, infants can usually sit unsupported at 3 months of age."
    c. "This is probably nothing to be concerned about because, although it varies, most infants can sit unsupported at 8 months of age."
    d. "This is probably nothing to be concerned about because, although it varies, most infants can sit unsupported at 5 months at age."

85. In the geriatric population, _____ usually occurs after _____ is present.
    a. Spondylolisthesis, spondylolysis
    b. Spondylolysis, spondylolisthesis
    c. Spondyloschisis, spondylolysis
    d. Spondylolisthesis, spondyloschisis

86. A patient is referred to the therapist with a diagnosis of arthritis. What type of arthritis would the therapist expect if the patient presented with the following signs and symptoms? (1) Bilateral wrists and knees are involved, (2) pain at rest and with motion, (3) prolonged morning stiffness, and (4) crepitus.
    a. The patient has osteoarthritis.
    b. The patient has rheumatoid arthritis.
    c. The patient has degenerative joint disease.
    d. It is not possible to determine with the given information.

87. A patient presents to an outpatient clinic with complaints of shoulder pain. The therapist observes a painful arc between 70 degrees and 120 degrees of active abduction in the involved shoulder. This finding is most indicative of what shoulder pathology?
    a. Rotator cuff tear
    b. Acromioclacivular joint separation
    c. Impingement
    d. Labrum tear

88. A tennis player receives a surgical repair of the annular ligament. Where should the therapist expect to note the most edema?
    a. Radial ulnar joint
    b. Olecranon bursa
    c. Ulnohumeral joint
    d. Lateral triangle

89. A physical therapist is assessing a 40-year-old man's balance and coordination. The following instructions are given to the patient: "Stand normally, with your eyes open. After fifteen seconds, close your eyes and maintain a normal standing posture." Several seconds after closing his eyes, the patient nearly falls. What type of test did the patient fail?
    a. Postural sway test
    b. Nonequilibrium test
    c. Romberg test
    d. One-legged stance test

90. A physical therapist is performing electromyographic testing. During a maximal output test of the patient's quadricep muscle, 25% of the motor unit action potential is polyphasic. What is the significance of this finding?
    a. It is normal in the quadricep.
    b. It is normal in the triceps brachii, not in the quadricep.
    c. It is normal in the biceps brachii, not in the quadricep.
    d. It is abnormal in any muscle.

91. A physical therapist is ordered to examine a patient in the late stages of amyotrophic lateral sclerosis. In the patient's chart is an electromyography report and nerve conduction velocity test. What should the physical therapist not expect to find in these test results?
    a. Decreased amplitude of motor unit action potential
    b. Decreased duration of motor unit action potential
    c. Decreased sensory evoked potentials
    d. Decreased polyphasic action potentials

92. A physical therapist is asked by a coworker to finish examining a patient because an emergency requires the therapist to leave. The coworker agrees and resumes the examination. The first therapist left notes titled, "sensory assessment." Two wooden blocks identical in appearance but 1 pound different in weight are on the table in front of the patient. What test was the prior therapist most likely performing?
    a. Barognosis test
    b. Stereognosis test
    c. Graphesthesia test
    d. Texture recognition

93. A patient is referred to physical therapy with a history of temporomandibular joint pain. The therapist notices that the patient is having difficulty closing his mouth against minimal resistance. With this information, which of the following muscles would not be a target for strengthening exercise to correct this deficit?
    a. Medial pterygoid muscle
    b. Temporalis
    c. Masseter
    d. Lateral pterygoid muscle

94. A physical therapist is reviewing the chart of a 24-year-old woman with a diagnosis of L2 incomplete paraplegia. The physician noted that the left quadricep tendon reflex is 21. What does this information relay to the therapist?
    a. No active quadricep tendon reflex
    b. Slight quadricep contraction with reflex testing
    c. Normal quadricep tendon reflex
    d. Exaggerated quadricep tendon reflex

95. A physical therapist performs the following test during an examination: With the patient lying in supine position, the therapist traces a diamond shape around the patient's umbilicus with a sharp object. What reflex is being assessed, and what is the significance if the patient's umbilicus does not move in response to the stimulus provided by the therapist?
    a. Cremaster reflex, suggests upper motor neuron involvement
    b. Superficial abdominal reflex, suggests upper motor neuron involvement
    c. Cremaster reflex, suggests lower motor neuron involvement
    d. Superficial abdominal reflex, suggests lower motor neuron involvement

96. A physical therapist is asked to examine a 37-year-old man with right-side sciatica. The therapist performs a passive straight leg raise test of the right lower extremity with the knee and ankle in neutral position. In performing this test on a patient with an L5 disc protrusion, what is the lowest degree at which the therapist would expect to reproduce the patient's symptoms?
    a. At 0 degrees of hip flexion
    b. At 35 degrees of hip flexion
    c. At 70 degrees of hip flexion
    d. At 90 degrees of hip flexion

97. Using tests of neurologic status and motor function, an experienced physical therapist or pediatrician should be able to accurately diagnose cerebral palsy in all but the mildest cases by
    a. 3 months of age
    b. 6 months of age
    c. 1 year of age
    d. 2 years of age

98. Which of the following muscles would you not expect to be affected by a C6-C7 lesion?
    a. Biceps brachii
    b. Anterior deltoid
    c. Infraspinatus
    d. Triceps brachii

99. Indicators of complex regional pain syndrome include all of the following except
    a. Pain from superficial touch
    b. Profuse sweating
    c. Skin color changes
    d. Increased uptake on bone scan

100.   What is the BEST order of these tests during neurologic patient examination?
   a.   Cognition, sensation, range of motion (ROM), reflexes, spasticity testing, manual muscle testing (MMT)
   b.   Reflexes, MMT, cognition, sensation, ROM, spasticity testing
   c.   Cognition, sensation, spasticity testing, ROM, MMT, reflexes
   d.   ROM, reflexes, sensation, MMT, ROM, spasticity testing, cognition

101.   The patient has dysdiadochokinesia. What is the best measure of patient function?
   a.   Drawing figure eight
   b.   Alternating pronation/supination
   c.   Rebound test
   d.   Static balance

102.   Upon observation, the patient has unilateral LEFT facial weakness. He is unable to smile or show his teeth on the left side. However, he is able to raise his left eyebrow. The physical therapist suspects
   a.   Peripheral cranial nerve 5 lesion
   b.   Central cranial nerve 5 lesion
   c.   Peripheral cranial nerve 7 lesion
   d.   Central cranial nerve 7 lesion

103.   During physical therapy examination, the patient has full ROM bilaterally. Muscle tone at rest appears normal bilaterally. Reflexes on the right side are 21. On the left they are 11. What is the next thing you should test for?
   a.   Repeat reflex testing with Jendrassik maneuver to enhance deep tendon reflex on the left
   b.   Spasticity testing on the left due to increased reflexes
   c.   Assess for associated reactions as patient has upper motor neuron syndrome findings on the left.
   d.   Cognition, as the patient may have been confused with reflex testing so results could be unreliable

104.   When performing an examination on a patient after traumatic spinal cord injury to determine the American Spinal Injury Association (ASIA) sensory level of injury a clinician tests
   a.   Proprioception
   b.   Kinesthesia
   c.   Pain
   d.   Reflexes

105. During your cranial nerve examination of extraocular muscle function, you note that your patient has vertical nystagmus during smooth pursuits. You suspect
    a. Lesion of optic nerve (cranial nerve II)
    b. Posterior canal BPPV
    c. Acoustic neuroma
    d. Central nervous system lesion

106. Your patient presents with a nerve injury that causes the thenar eminence to be flattened because of muscle atrophy. The thumb is adducted and extended. You would want to test the muscles supplied by the
    a. Ulnar nerve
    b. Antebrachial nerve
    c. Median nerve
    d. Radial nerve

107. Your patient is a framer on a construction project. He has been wearing a heavy carpenter's belt for the last month. He now complains of painful hyperthesias on the proximal anterior lateral thigh. He gets relief with sitting, and walking seems to aggravate his symptoms. The structure most likely producing these symptoms is the
    a. Lateral femoral cutaneous nerve
    b. Motor branch of the femoral nerve
    c. Medial femoral cutaneous nerve
    d. Inguinal nerve

108. Your patient complains of neck pain and peripheral symptoms. Radiographs revealed narrowing of the C4-C5 intervertebral foramen. The nerve root most likely involved would be the
    a. C5 nerve root
    b. C4 nerve root
    c. C6 nerve root
    d. Sensory branch of C4

109. A physical therapist is conducting a screening examination on a patient with a suspected upper motor neuron lesion. In the presence of an upper motor neuron lesion, deep tendon reflexes will be
    a. Hypoactive
    b. Absent
    c. Diminished
    d. Hyperactive

110. You are performing an examination on a 2-month-old infant diagnosed with Klumpke's palsy. The classic physical findings of a Klumpke's palsy are
    a. Lack of forearm supination, elbow extension, and wrist flexion
    b. Lack of forearm supination, elbow flexion, and wrist extension
    c. Lack of shoulder external rotation, elbow flexion, and wrist extension
    d. Lack of elbow extension, forearm pronation, and wrist flexion

111. A 16-year-old male is diagnosed with a spinal tumor and has undergone surgery to resect the mass. After the procedure, the patient presents with variable motor paralysis and loss of pain and temperature sensation below the level of the injury. The patient would be diagnosed with what spinal cord syndrome?
    a. Brown-Sequard
    b. Anterior Cord
    c. Posterior Cord
    d. Cauda Equina

112. A 5-year-old male had an undiagnosed arteriovenous malformation and is recently hospitalized because of an acute brain bleed. The patient is not acknowledging individuals who stand on the left side of his bed, he does not respond to sensory stimuli that is applied to the left side of his body, and he displays visual spatial deficits. What lobe of the brain has been affected by the stroke?
    a. Right parietal
    b. Left temporal
    c. Frontal
    d. Occipital

113. An infant is able to transition from quadruped to sitting, demonstrate protective extension reactions in all directions except backwards, and pivots on belly in a prone position. This infant is demonstrating gross motor skills at what chronologic age?
    a. 3 to 4 months
    b. 5 to 6 months
    c. 7 to 8 months
    d. 11 to 12 months

114. A two-month-old infant is diagnosed with left congenital muscular torticollis, which has resulted in plagiocephaly. This would result in
    a. Flattening of the left frontal and left occipital regions
    b. Flattening of the right frontal and left occipital regions
    c. Flattening of the right frontal and right occipital regions
    d. Flattening of the left frontal and right occipital regions

115. A therapist is asked to estimate the percentage of a patient's body that has been burned. The patient is a 32-year-old man of normal size. Burns are located along the entire anterior surface of the face. The patient also burned the entire anterior portion of the right upper extremity in an attempt to guard himself from flames. Using the rule of nines, what percentage of the patient's body is burned?
    a. 9%
    b. 18%
    c. 4.5%
    d. 27%

116. The patient with the least chance of survival of the following injuries is an
    a. 18-month-old male, s/p 40% total body surface area (TBSA), third-degree scald
    b. 13-year-old male, s/p 60% TBSA, indeterminate flame burns with inhalation injury
    c. 8-year-old female, s/p motor vehicle accident MVA with 20% deep burns to face, neck, chest, hands, and pelvic fractures
    d. 4-year-old male, s/p 80% TBSA, severe sunburn with blisters

117. A 10-year-old female has been diagnosed with a stage IV pressure sore on the sacrum. She was transferred to the hospital from a subacute facility and is being followed by the wound care team. After 2 weeks of wound care treatment, the physical therapist is reassessing the wound and determines that the bone is no longer visible. How would the physical therapist document the stage of the wound at this time?
    a. Stage IV
    b. Stage III
    c. Stage II
    d. Stage I

118. Signs and symptoms of hypertrophic burn scar include all of the following except
    a. Increasing itching and redness in a healed burn
    b. Increasing difficulty in achieving a full stretch of the burned area
    c. Fever and malaise
    d. Raised edges around a newly healed graft

119. To decrease the risk of hypoglycemia in a patient with type 1 insulin-dependent diabetes, which of the following is inappropriate?
    a. Eat or drink a snack high in carbohydrates 30 minutes before exercise.
    b. Exercise muscles that have not had an insulin injection recently.
    c. A carbohydrate snack for each 30 to 45 minutes of exercise.
    d. Exercise at the peak time of insulin effect.

120. Which of the following is false regarding T2-weighted MRI images?
    a. Synovial fluid displays high signal intensity.
    b. Cortical bone displays high signal intensity unless fat-suppression techniques are used.
    c. Bone marrow edema-like lesions (when present) are commonly seen in these images.
    d. Cerebral spinal fluid displays high signal intensity.

121. Your patient presents with radiating pain down the right posterior leg, which is aggravated by running and seated hip internal rotation. What is the most likely cause?
    a. Right semimembranosus tendonitis causing posterior leg pain
    b. Right piriformis syndrome resulting in sciatica
    c. Lumbar central stenosis with L4 radiculopathy
    d. Right lumbar intervertebral foramen stenosis with radiculopathy

122. When discussing magnetic resonance imaging (MRI) images, all observations of tissue appearance should be described in terms of
    a. Lucency
    b. Window
    c. Density
    d. Signal intensity

123. Edema on a T2 weighted MRI image will appear as_____ signal intensity (SI).
    a. Low signal intensity (SI)
    b. High signal intensity
    c. Radiopacity
    d. Radiolucent

124. While evaluating a shoulder split tau inversion recovery (STIR) sequence MRI study, you note increased SI on the images within the region. This suggests
    a. Fibrosis
    b. Organized hematoma
    c. Edema or effusion
    d. Calcification of the tendon

125. Musculoskeletal MRI "fluid sensitive" sequences include all of the following except
    a. STIR
    b. T1 weighted
    c. T2 weighted
    d. Proton density

126. What is correct regarding the atlanto-dens interval?
    a. The atlanto-dens interval is measured on AP projections.
    b. The atlanto-dens interval is measured on lateral views.
    c. An abnormality of the atlanto-dens interval may correlate with compromise of the ligamentum nuchae.
    d. Normal measurement is the same for adults and children.

127. An MRI study of the shoulder typically includes three anatomic planes of study. Image slices taken perpendicular to the long axis of the scapular spine are identified as what plane of study?
    a. Coronal oblique
    b. Axial
    c. Sagittal oblique
    d. Lateral

128. A commonly encountered MRI sequence in PT practice is FS PD FSE. This sequence is most often used to display
    a. Abnormal fat tissues
    b. Brain trauma or hemorrhage
    c. Orthopedic pathology
    d. Details of cortical bone

129. The "FS" in and FS PD FSE sequence refers to
    a. Fat presaturation technique
    b. Fast spin echo
    c. Use of contrast media
    d. Functional MRI sequence

130. Normal high SI tissues on T1 weighted images include
    a. Acute edema
    b. CSF
    c. Fat
    d. Synovial fluid

131. CT studies of the knee typically include three planes of study. Which choice is not one of the conventional planes?
    a. Condylar oblique
    b. Sagittal
    c. Coronal
    d. Axial

132. A high repetition time (TR) combined with low echo time (TE) setting noted on the scout film would indicate what common orthopedic sequence?
a. T1
b. T2
c. Proton density
d. STIR

133. MRI studies of the knee typically include three planes of study. Which choice is not one of the conventional planes?
a. Medial oblique
b. Sagittal
c. Coronal
d. Axial

134. A "window" in computerized tomography (CT) terminology refers to
a. Lucent regions of the lung
b. Lytic lesions of bone
c. Hounsfeld units
d. CT machine setting for enhancement of contrast

135. The left posterior oblique (LPO) cervical spine projection specifically allows study of what anatomic structures?
a. Intervertebral disk
b. Left side intervertebral joints
c. Right side intervertebral foramina
d. Left side intervertebral foramina

136. Which radiologic terms are incorrectly paired?
a. Density/opacity
b. Density/sclerosis
c. Lucency/high density
d. Lucency/low density

137. Increased bone density viewed on plain film x-rays would appear as ____ bone on T1 weighted MRI images.
a. Low SI
b. High SI
c. Radiopacity
d. None of these

138. A scaphoid fracture is suspected on plain film x-ray but not clearly demonstrated. The imaging technology most commonly employed for further evaluation and diagnosis is
    a. Positron emission tomography
    b. MRI
    c. Plain film x-ray with contrast media
    d. Computerized tomography

139. Standard nomenclature used to describe radiodensity employed when reading plain film x-rays include all of the following except
    a. Ligamentous density
    b. Air
    c. Bone density
    d. Fat density

140. On plain film x-ray a black or dark gray lesion within a normally white region such as cortical bone would be termed a region of
    a. Density
    b. Opacity
    c. Sclerosis
    d. Lucency

141. Radiology reports using the terms, *sequestra* and *involucrum* are referring specifically to what diagnosis of concern to a treating physical therapist?
    a. Bone cancer
    b. Osteomyelitis
    c. Fracture
    d. Spondylolisthesis

142. Superimposition of soft tissue structures on plain film images creates the illusion of
    a. Increased density
    b. Decreased density
    c. Abnormal lucency
    d. Gas bubbles

143. A lateral x-ray projection of a dorsal phalangeal avulsion fracture reveals sagittal plane dislocation. What standard view should be ordered to assess possible coronal plane dislocation?
    a. AP
    b. PA
    c. Oblique
    d. Opposite side lateral

144. Cortical bone as viewed on CT scans within a "bone window" will appear as
    a. Low density
    b. High density
    c. Low SI
    d. Hyperintense signal

145. Which structure is most poorly studied or assessed on an AP lumbar spine projection?
    a. Intervertebral disk height of superior lumbar vertebra
    b. Superior end plates
    c. Pars interarticularis
    d. Inferior end plates

146. The celebrated "Scotty Dog" appears on what x-ray projections?
    a. Lumbar AP
    b. Lumbar oblique
    c. Coned lateral
    d. Lumbar lateral

147. The front leg of the celebrated "Scotty Dog" is what anatomic structure?
    a. Inferior articular process
    b. Superior articular process
    c. Pars interarticularis
    d. Transverse process

148. The spinolaminar line employed in evaluation of a lateral view of the cervical spine is drawn immediately anterior to the
    a. Posterior aspect of central canal
    b. Anterior aspect of vertebral bodies
    c. Posterior aspect of vertebral bodies
    d. Superior to C3 uncus if present

149. Normal articular cartilage appears as _____ on plain film x-ray?
    a. Radiodense
    b. Water or mid-density
    c. Lucent or lung density
    d. Opaque or bone density

150. Degenerative arthritic changes viewed on x-ray images may typically include all of the following except
    a. Subchondral sclerosis
    b. Osteophyte formation
    c. Periarticular osteopenia
    d. Loss of joint space

151. Your patient has low back pain that you diagnose clinically as degenerative disease of the left side L4-L5 facet. Which lumbar spine projection would best support your clinical impression?
   a. Right posterior oblique
   b. Left posterior oblique
   c. Right lateral
   d. Left lateral

152. Osteoarthritis may be differentiated from rheumatoid arthritis (RA) on x-ray by the observation of
   a. Loss of joint space
   b. Periarticular osteopaenia
   c. Asymmetric joint involvement
   d. Osteophyte formation

153. Cortical bone appears as _____ on virtually all MRI sequences because of low water content.
   a. Radiopaque
   b. Radiolucent
   c. Low signal intensity
   d. High signal intensity

154. You are examining a child with a fractured distal femur. The fracture begins at the medial aspect of the distal diaphyseal region, progresses distal-laterally through the metaphysis, epiphyseal plate, and epiphyseal region, exiting into the knee joint surface. This would be classified as a Salter Harris type ____ fracture.
   a. 1
   b. 2
   c. 3
   d. 4

155. Following a suspected stress fracture of the third metatarsal bone, bone callus would normally first become radiographically visible at about
   a. 3 to 4 days
   b. 10 to 14 days
   c. 2 to 4 months
   d. 6 to 18 months

156. Lumbar spondylolisthesis is best evaluated on what x-ray projection?
   a. Lateral
   b. AP
   c. PA
   d. Anterior oblique

157. When an adult lumbar spine degenerating disk breaks through either the superior or inferior end plate it is referred to as a(n)
    a. Napoleon's hat sign
    b. Schmorl's nodule
    c. Salter-Harris 5 fracture
    d. Osteoblastoma

158. Anteriorly located anatomic structures appear larger than posterior structures on anteroposterior (AP) x-ray projections because of what form of X-ray distortion?
    a. Superimposition
    b. Enlargement
    c. Foreshortening
    d. Compression

159. As a cardiopulmonary specialist observing a patient's chest x-ray you note radiolucency within the lung fields. This is most likely to be
    a. Heterotopic ossification
    b. Tuberculosis
    c. Collapse of lung
    d. Normal air density lung

Answers

1. b. Exercise testing should be terminated at 2 mm of ST depression.

2. d. To lock the elbow with this type of prosthesis, the patient must extend the humerus and depress the scapula.

3. b. The first sound heard corresponds with the closing of the mitral and tricuspid valves. The second sound corresponds to closing of the aortic and pulmonic valves. Therefore, the first sound is indicative of the onset of ventricular systole, and the second sound is indicative of the onset of ventricular diastole. The first sound is usually lower in pitch and longer than the second.

4. d. This patient has moderate lung disease. Because the intensity of exercise is low, frequency should be increased to 5 to 7 times/week.

5. c. This scenario describes vascular claudication. The lack of pain or symptoms with spinal movements rules out peripheral neuropathy. Neurogenic pain is usually represented by a stocking distribution around the ankle, and restless leg syndrome occurs during periods of rest only.

6. c. Normal Pao_2 ranges from 80 to 100 mm Hg and is an important determinant of when it is safe to exercise a patient either with or without supplemental oxygen. Pao_2 is determined by examining the concentration of oxygen present in arterial blood. Understanding the parameters under which a patient may safely perform exercise is important.

7. b. Whiplash injury includes hyperextension of cervical vertebrae that may tear the anterior longitudinal ligament that limits extension of the cervical spine. All of the other ligaments limit flexion of the cervical spine; accordingly, they may be torn in hyperflexion injuries.

8. d. Osteoporosis affects all bones of the body, but most commonly it produces symptoms in the major weight-bearing bones.

9. c. Osteopetrosis is a genetic disorder characterized by osteoclast dysfunction that leads to excessive osteoid tissue formation. Paget's disease is an acquired disease in which the osteoclast dysfunction initially causes excessive removal of bone (osteolysis). Osteomalacia is the softening of bone due to poor and delayed calcification. Osteoporosis is due to more than one etiological factor, acquired and genetic, accompanied by reduced amount of osteoid tissue.

10.   b.   Osteoarthritis is induced by aging, trauma, and genetic factors. Hence, fibrillation, osteophytes, and decreased collagen II synthesis are the main features. In contrast, synovitis and inflammation occur in other forms, such as rheumatoid and giant villonodular arthritis.

11.   d.   Slipped femoral capital epiphysis is the most common hip condition in adolescent boys (10 to 16 years old). Fifty percent of cases present with a traumatic history. Traumatic slipped femoral capital epiphysis is considered a Salter-Harris type I epiphyseal fracture.

12.   b.   Diffuse pain is a defining criterion of fibromyalgia. According to the American College of Rheumatologists' 1990 criteria for the classification of fibromyalgia, widespread pain must be present for at least 3 months. Pain is considered widespread when all of the following are present: pain in the left side of the body, pain in the right side of the body, pain above the waist, pain below the waist, and axial skeletal pain. Pain in 11 of 18 tender point sites on digital palpation must also be present in order to establish the diagnosis of fibromyalgia.

13.   c.   A painful neuroma in the space between the third and the fourth metatarsal heads is a Morton's neuroma.

14.   b.   Patients older than 40 years of age with a new episode of hip pain presents evidence of osteoarthritis in 44% of cases. Restricted and painful internal rotation is highly suggestive of osteoarthritis, and three-plane range of motion limitation is less sensitive but more specific.

15.   b.   Travell and Simons report that myofascial pain syndrome of the quadratus lumborum muscle is the most common myofascial pain syndrome of the lower back.

16.   a.   Due to the anatomic location of the greater tubercle, external rotation positions it in profile for best visualization.

17.   a.   Waddell testing is used to identify patients suffering from pain of a nonorganic origin.

18.   b.   The superior angle of the scapula commonly rests at the same level as vertebra T2. The spine of the scapula is approximately at T3. The inferior angle of the scapula and xiphoid process represent T7.

19.   d.   Choices A, B, and C would increase the functional length of the right lower extremity and possibly cause a circumduction during gait. Choice D would not change the functional leg length.

20. a. The briefcase should be carried in the right hand. Carrying the briefcase in the left hand would increase the amount of force that the right gluteus medius would have to exert to maintain a stable pelvis during gait.

21. d. Patellofemoral joint reaction forces increase as the angle of knee flexion and quadriceps muscle activity increase. Choice D involves the greatest knee flexion angle and quadriceps activity.

22. c. Leaning the trunk over the involved hip decreases joint reaction force and strain on the hip abductors. These factors together decrease pain in the involved hip.

23. a. It is best to consult with the physician because of an extended amount of passive range of motion. A therapist should not deviate from a physician's order, but a telephone call to clarify the order is necessary when the therapist feels that another treatment plan is more appropriate.

24. a. A patient can obtain his or her medical records simply by signing a release form. Charts and records should never be given or faxed to an attorney unless the patient has signed a release.

25. b. Hot packs are not indicated because there is no mention of abnormal muscle tone. The entire lumbar area is too much surface area for ultrasound. An argument could be made for lumbar traction, but it is paired with heating modalities in all of the answers.

26. b. Choice B is the correct answer. Choice A is a posterior pelvic tilt.

27. a. The lowest point in the gait cycle occurs when both lower extremities are in contact with the ground (double support).

28. b. The patient probably has a low left shoulder, prominent right scapula, and high left hip.

29. a. Abdominal muscles attach to the lower border of the ribs and the superior surface of the pelvis. Strong abdominals prevent excessive anterior rotation of the pelvis during gait.

30. b. The fifth lumbar nerve root is impinged because it arises from the spinal column superior to the L4-L5 lumbar disc.

31. b. This gait deviation is caused by the patient leaning back to decrease the flexion moment created at the hip at initial contact. The gluteus maximus is most responsible for counteracting this flexion moment.

32.   c.   A curve greater than 120 degrees is often associated with restrictive lung dysfunction. The other factors listed are not life threatening.

33.   a.   Choice A probably would activate increased tone because of the resistance to plantar flexion offered by the spring.

34.   d.   The Thomas test is a screen to determine whether the hip flexors are too tight.

35.   c.   Adson's maneuver tests for thoracic outlet syndrome. Lhermitte's sign tests for dural irritation in the cervical spine.

36.   a.   A shuffling gait and difficulty with initiating gait are typical signs of Parkinson's disease. This population would also present with a small base of support.

37.   c.   The pelvis is dropping on the right side because the left gluteus medius is weak. The patient also may lean toward the left hip joint to move the center of gravity, making it easier to hold up the right side of the pelvis.

38.   c.   This is called Ober's test, which screens for a tight iliotibial band.

39.   c.   The capitate is the axis.

40.   c.   Because the patient does not have 50% of normal range of motion in the gravity eliminated position, $2-/5$ is the appropriate grade. Some therapists argue that this is an example of a $1+/5$ grade. Sources used in preparation of this exam indicate that there is no grade of $1+/5$ with manual muscle testing.

41.   d.   This sequence assists in propelling the center of gravity forward to maintain balance after a backward sway.

42.   d.   During a functional capacity evaluation, the physical therapist should not correct postural abnormalities. The therapist should only observe and record.

43.   b.   This is a description of a dystrophic gait pattern, also called penguin gait. Patients with muscular dystrophy commonly demonstrate this gait pattern. A gluteus maximus gait presents with the patient leaning the trunk back while striking the heel on the involved side (or lurching). An arthrogenic gait pattern presents with the patient circumducting and elevating the hip on the involved side. This pattern is present with severe stiffness or a fused joint in the involved lower extremity. An antalgic gait pattern is exhibited when a person has pain with weight bearing on the involved lower extremity.

44. c. The subjective complaints of "pins and needles" suggest that the source of the problem is either vascular or neurologic. Because thoracic outlet syndrome has been cleared, focus should be placed on the cervical spine.

45. b. Yergason's test detects tendinitis of the long head of the biceps. Froment's sign is a test to determine adductor pollicis weakness due to ulnar nerve dysfunction. In the Waldron test, the patient performs squats while the therapist assesses the patella region for crepitus or pain. A positive test indicates possible chondromalacia. A positive Wilson test indicates possible osteochondritis dissecans. The test is performed by asking the patient to extend the knee in the seated position with internal rotation and again with external rotation of the tibia. The test is positive if there is pain with internal rotation and no pain with external rotation of the tibia.

46. b. The flexor digitorum profundus has four tendons, each attaching to the distal phalanx. If the three mentioned in the question are restricted, flexion at the distal interphalangeal joint in the normal hand would not be possible.

47. c. This test assesses the strength of the latissimus dorsi. One of the functions of the latissimus is to push up from a sitting position. This test simulates that movement.

48. c. A tissue stretch end-feel is also felt with ankle dorsiflexion. An example of a bone-to-bone end-feel is with knee or elbow extension. Knee flexion is an example of soft tissue approximation. In an empty end-feel, a patient stops the movement due to pain.

49. d. All of the choices are capable of causing a noncapsular pattern.

50. a. After the first 2 years of life, the femurs rotate to a more neutral position, and the amount of anteversion decreases.

51. b. The patient is prone to excessive external rotation when attempting to extend the involved hip because the gluteus minimus counteracts the lateral rotational force created by the gluteus maximus.

52. c. The tests in Choices A, B, and C assess the integrity of the anterior cruciate ligament. The pivot shift test is performed with the patient in supine position. The therapist applies a valgus stress with the lower leg internally rotated while passively flexing and extending the knee. A positive test is associated with instability with this motion. Lachman's test is similar to the anterior drawer test, but the knee is in slight flexion. In performing a posterior drawer test, the positioning is the same as for performing an anterior drawer test, but a posterior force is applied to the tibia to assess posterior cruciate ligament integrity. When performing these tests, the therapist is assessing the end-feel and amount of joint play to determine the integrity of the ligament.

53. c. During pronation of the feet, the calcaneus everts, and the talus medially rotates and plantar flexes.

54. c. At 1 to 2 weeks after surgery, the patient has an inflamed knee, and no functional testing can take place. Six weeks is an appropriate amount of time to allow inflammation to decrease enough for functional testing. Patients who have received a partial meniscectomy do not require as much healing time as patients who have received a meniscus repair.

55. a. This is the primary function of the anterior inferior tibiofibular ligament.

56. c. Thompson's test checks the integrity of the Achilles' tendon. When this test is performed on an ankle with no dysfunction, squeezing the gastrocnemius causes passive plantar flexion of the ankle.

57. a. Because the interossei cross the MP joints and the PIP joints, the PIP joints should be flexed with the MP joints in flexion and extension.

58. b. The last position (3 inches) of the grip strength dynamometer tests the extrinsic muscles of the hand (muscles located in the forearm). The closer positions test the intrinsic muscles.

59. a. The patient has an irritation of the iliotibial band as it passes over the lateral femoral epicondyle. This occurs at approximately 30 degrees from full knee extension.

60. a. When the hindfoot is pronated, the forefoot (transverse tarsal joints) can compensate for uneven terrain. If the hindfoot is supinated, the forefoot also is likely to supinate and possibly cause damage to the lateral ankle ligaments.

61. d. A patient with severe knee flexion contractures has a line of gravity that is anterior to the hip, posterior to the knee, and anterior to the ankle. This causes a flexion moment at the hip, knee, and ankle.

62. b. To maintain balance, the lumbar spine must laterally flex toward the supporting lower extremity during single-limb support.

63. d. Choice D is the length of stride during one gait cycle. Choice A describes a decreased step length, choice B describes a decrease in step duration, and choice C describes a decrease in single-limb support time.

64. a. The tibialis anterior, extensor digitorum longus, and extensor hallucis longus contract concentrically to achieve a neutral ankle position before initial contact.

65. c. The right shoulder and thorax begin to move forward at heel strike (initial contact).

66. a. The hamstrings bring the knee to approximately 60 degrees of flexion during acceleration. The hip flexors, ankle dorsiflexors, and toe extensors are also active.

67. c. The geriatric population would have a longer period of double support in an attempt to maintain balance. They also would have a shorter step and stride length.

68. c. A warm whirlpool with the lower extremity in a dependent position is likely to increase the edema. The addition of moist heat is contraindicated for the same reason. There is no need for sharp debridement on a clean wound. A compression pump is often used for increased edema in the extremities.

69. b. Since pain responses may be unreliable in this population, PROM is contraindicated. AROM may be measured. Functional ROM is the most important measure at this point.

70 d. LevoDOPA/carbidopa can cause all of the listed effects except bradycardia. Due to the off-effect the patient might have to be scheduled at times when he or she is in the on-phase of the drug

71. d. The test is only considered positive if it is lax in two or more planes. This is due to the variation of direction of the fibers as they connect to the alar ligament.

72. c. Cyriax's classical description describes the obvious cause of a springy end-feel as being that of a torn part of a meniscus in the knee engaging between the bone ends, blocking extension.

73. c. Passive flexion of the knee would be expected to place stress on the muscles acting to extend the knee and the joint capsule. The only tissue structure that would be placed on "slack" would be the sciatic nerve, which runs along the posterior aspect of the femur.

74. c. Children with cystic fibrosis commonly have cervical lordosis resulting from thoracic kyphosis. This leads to the scapulae and shoulders to be pushed forward and anteriorly.

75. c. Children with limited anticipatory postural control have difficulty catching, reaching, or throwing in any posture, as a result of a poor feed-forward control. Protective reactions are mainly to protect the infant from a fall. A problem with development of higher-level balance skills is evidenced by inability to stand on one limb, walk on a balance beam, or hop.

76. b. The power grasp often is used to control tools or other objects. The hook grasp is used when strength of grasp must be maintained to carry objects. Lateral pinch is used to exert power on or with a small object. Opposition of the thumb tip and the tip of the index finger, forming a circle, describes the tip pinch which is used to get small objects.

77. d. Nerve conduction/EMG studies are useful for identifying the possible injury site along the lower motor nerve reflex but cannot provide a definitive clinical diagnosis.

78. a. A lesion of a peripheral nerve produces a complete paralysis of the muscles innervated by this nerve. Weakness is immediately apparent when testing the motor function. A lesion of a unique nerve root produces paresis of the myotome (group of muscles innervated by a single nerve root) innervated by this nerve root. Some time is necessary for the weakness to become apparent when testing for motor function. The isometric contraction must be held for a minimum of 5 seconds.

79. c. Atrophy of the hypothenar eminence is a sign of ulnar nerve lesion, while paresthesias over the dorsal aspect of the hand are symptoms of radial nerve lesion. Decreased resisted thumb abduction and forearm pronation are signs of median nerve lesion, but the motor branches of pronator teres and pronator quadratus arise before the median nerve enters the carpal tunnel.

80. d. According to Hoppenfeld, the patella deep tendon reflex muscles (the quadriceps muscle group) are innervated by the L4 nerve root via the femoral nerve.

81. c. The mechanism of injury indicates implication of the superior plexus of C5-C6, causing diffuse arm weakness not fitting typical radicular presentation (involvement of one myotome). Nerve regeneration is still possible when only the endonurium and capillary complex are disrupted ("a burner"). However, when the perineurium (funiculus) or epinurium is disrupted (brachial neuropraxia), useful regeneration is not expected. This requires urgent neurosurgical intervention to prevent permanent neurologic deficit.

82. d. An ulnar nerve–compromised hand presents as a "claw" hand after a prolonged amount of time because of atrophy of the interossei. The extensor digitorum takes over and pulls the MCPs in hyperextension.

83. b. The oburator nerve innervates the adductor brevis, adductor longus, adductor magnus, oburator externus, and gracilis muscles. Choice A has no motor function. Choice C innervates the sartorius, pectineus, iliacus, and quadriceps femoris. The ilioinguinal nerve innervates the obliquus internus abdominis and transversus abdominis.

84. c. Although sources vary widely, a child can sit unsupported usually between 4 and 8 months of age. Choices A and B are incorrect. Choice D would possibly cause the parent to worry prematurely.

85. a. A defect in the lamina of a vertebrae usually occurs first. This defect is called spondylolysis. The vertebrae may then slip because of shear forces; this slippage is called spondylolisthesis.

86. b. Rheumatoid arthritis is a systemic condition commonly involving joints bilaterally. Crepitus can be associated with osteoarthritis or rheumatoid arthritis, but rheumatoid arthritis is the most likely in this case.

87. c. The "painful arc" is most indicative of shoulder impingement. The soft tissues of the shoulder are pinched under the acromion process at approximately 60 degrees to120 degrees of abduction. Pain throughout abduction active range of motion suggests acromioclavicular joint dysfunction.

88. d. The lateral triangle (composed of the radial head, olecranon process, and lateral epicondyle) is the most likely of the choices to exhibit joint edema. Joint edema is common after a surgical procedure.

89. c. The Romberg test is a type of equilibrium test. Equilibrium tests are usually conducted with the patient in a standing position, whereas nonequilibrium tests are performed with the patient in the supine position. Postural sway tests involve the patient standing on a computerized platform and electronically measuring the amount of sway the patient exhibits. One-legged stance tests obviously involve the patient attempting to stand on one leg during the test.

90. d. More than 10% of polyphasic potentials in the total output of muscle is considered abnormal.

91. c. In performing these tests on patients who have this disorder, sensory potentials are generally unchanged. Motor unit potentials are increased in amplitude and duration because of variable impulse conduction time in sprouting axon terminals. Increased polyphasic potentials are usually found with increased duration.

92. a. Barognosis is the ability to differentiate between different weights. Stereognosis is the ability to differentiate between different sizes and shapes. Graphesthesia is the ability to identify letters, numbers, or designs traced on the skin. Texture recognition is the ability to differentiate between textures such as cotton, wool, and silk.

93. d. All of the listed muscles participate in mandibular elevation with the exception of the lateral pterygoid muscle. The lateral pterygoid muscle and the suprahyoid muscles participate in mandibular depression.

94. c. No activity = 0. Slight contraction = 1+. Normal response = 2+. Exaggerated response = 3+. Severely exaggerated = 4+.

95. b. When the test is performed on a patient with no motor neuron lesion, the umbilicus should move toward the stimulus. Unilateral movement suggests lower motor neuron involvement. A cremaster reflex is performed by stroking the medial thigh of a male with a sharp object. A normal response consists of superior movement of the scrotum on the ipsilateral side. An abnormal response is absence of scrotal movement on one side, which indicates possible lower motor neuron involvement. Bilateral absence of movement indicates upper motor neuron involvement.

96. b. During a unilateral straight leg raise of the involved lower extremity, tension is placed on the sciatic nerve at approximately 35 degrees of hip flexion. At 0 degrees of hip flexion, tension is minimal to none, and tension is maximal above 70 degrees of hip flexion.

97. b. A variety of tests can be used to determine the proper diagnosis by 6 months of age.

98. d. Choices A, B, and C all receive innervation from that branch of the brachial plexus. The triceps brachii is innervated by C7-C8.

99. b. CRPS symptoms do not include sweating, but rather dryness compared to the normal side.

100. a. Cognition, sensation, ROM, reflexes, spasticity testing, MMT is the best order. Sensory testing results can only be considered accurate if a patient's cognitive status is known. Spasticity and manual muscle testing results are based on range of motion, so ROM must come first.

101. b. Alternating pronation/supination is the correct answer. Dysdiadochokinesia is difficulty with rapid alternating motions such as pronation and supination. A drawing does not capture the rapid motion. The rebound test measures graded muscle response to stimulus. Static balance does not involve rapid alternating motion patterns.

102. d. The therapist suspects central cranial nerve 7 lesion because the facial nerve 7 innervates the motions described. A peripheral lesion results in complete loss to one side of the face. Sparing of the frontalis is a sign of a central lesion due to bilateral corticobulbar innervation of that muscle.

103. a. Repeat reflex testing with Jendrassik maneuver to enhance DTR on the left. This answer is correct because you have no reason to suspect abnormal reflexes (normal muscle tone), so tester error is the most likely first hypothesis. Reflexes of 2+ are normal, and 1+ is hyporeflexia, not increased or a sign of upper motor neuron syndrome. Cognition will not change findings with reflex testing, as it is a test of an unconscious spinal reflex arc.

104. c. Pain as measured by pinprick and light touch are used to determine sensory level for ASIA guidelines.

105. d. Central nervous system lesion. Central nervous system nystagmus has a more vertical component. Peripherally generated nystagmus is typically horizontal and rotary in nature. A lesion of optic (cranial nerve II) would cause only sensory changes. It has no motor component. BPPV would not be triggered with testing because no head motions are occurring. An acoustic neuroma would also not cause nystagmus during smooth pursuit, as no head motion is occurring.

106. c. The ape or simian hand described is indicative of a median nerve palsy.

107. a. This case represents a classic presentation of meralgia parasthetica, which involves the lateral femoral cutaneous nerve. The other choices are not in the area.

108. a. It is well known that the C5 nerve root exits the C4-C5 intervertebral space. The other choices exit above and below this level.

109. d. Upper motor neuron lesions involve damage to neural pathways above the level of the motor neuron. Such lesions typically result in a constellation of symptoms that include increased or hyperactive deep tendon reflexes, the appearance of pathologic reflexes, tonal increases, and weakness. Muscle wasting is not common. Increased deep tendon reflexes can be one finding in determining the need for referral or differential diagnosis.

110. d. A Klumpke's palsy involves injury to the lower roots, C8-T1 (occasionally C7 is also involved) and results in weakness of the triceps, forearm pronators, and wrist flexors.

111. b. Damage to the anterior cord results in loss of motor function and pain/temperature sensation. There will be preservation of light touch, proprioception, and vibratory sense.

112. a. A lesion to the parietal lobe results in loss of contralateral stimulus location and intensity, impairment of two-point discrimination, tactile and visual agnosia, visual disorientation, and neglect of contralateral self and surroundings.

113. c. The 7 to 8 month old will be able to transfer from quadruped to sitting; pivot on belly in a prone position; and demonstrate protective extension reactions downward, sideways, and forward. Backward reactions will begin around 9 months.

114. d. Left torticollis and resultant plagiocephaly would cause flattening of the left frontal and right occipital regions with bulging of the opposite areas.

115. a. The anterior surface of the face and the upper extremity are each considered 4.5% of the body, according to the rule of nines. The anterior trunk is 18%. Each anterior surface of the lower extremities is 9%. The posterior side is the same, respectively. The total groin area is 1%.

116. b. The injuries of the patient in choice B, involve the lungs. This patient would not have a good chance of being weaned from the ventilator. The other choices are medical emergencies, but choice B has the least chance of survival.

117. a. The wound would be documented as a healing stage IV pressure sore. You cannot reverse staging of pressure sores. Healing of pressure ulcers should be documented by objective parameters such as size, depth, amount of necrotic tissue, amount of exudate, presence of granulation tissue, and so on.

118. c. Fever and malaise might be signs of infection or other medical complications. They are not signs of hypertrophic scarring.

119. d. Exercising at the peak time of insulin effect causes hypoglycemia. Insulin causes the liver to decrease sugar production. The body needs increased levels of blood glucose during exercise.

120. b. Cortical bone displays high signal intensity unless fat-suppression techniques are used. T2 weighted images show fluid as bright. In addition, fat will show up fairly bright in the bone marrow unless suppressed. Bone has extremely short T2 times and never displays high signal intensity in the absence of pathology (fracture, etc).

121. b. Right piriformis syndrome resulting in sciatica is the most likely cause. The aggravating activities implicate the piriformis, which becomes an INTERNAL rotator at hip angles above 60 degrees (i.e., in sitting). The pattern of symptoms is consistent with sciatic nerve involvement.

122. d. MRI images are produced by radiofrequency signals. All visual findings are referred to in terms of signal intensity.

123. b. T2 weighted images are "fluid sensitive," meaning that fluid such as edema produces high signal intensity. A common mnemonic used in radiology is "WW II," water is white on T2.

124. c. STIR, a common MRI sequence seen in orthopedic PT practice (split tau inversion recovery), is extremely fluid sensitive so edema will be observed as a region of high signal intensity.

125. b. T1 weighted images favor recording of fast recovery protons such as in fat tissues, which therefore appear as high signal intensity. Fluids on T2 images display mid- to low-signal intensity.

126. b. The atlanto-dens interval is the distance between the anterior aspect of the dens and the posterior aspect of the anterior neural arch of C1. It is measured only on a lateral projection.

127. c. Shoulder studies are based on the scapular plane, a sagittal study that is also called a sagittal oblique study; it will display images oriented perpendicular to the long axis of the scapular spine.

128. c. FS (fat saturation) PD (proton density) FSE (fast spin echo) sequences are excellent for evaluation of articular cartilage, joint structures, and edema and are therefore quite common in orthopedic evaluation.

129. a. Fat saturation or presaturation is abbreviated "FS" and referred to verbally as "fatsat."

130. c. High signal intensity of a T1 weighted image corresponds to fat tissues.

131. a. CT employs views on the three anatomic planes; there is no condylar oblique view.

132. c. TR and TE settings will vary with PD sequences, but the universal finding is high TR and low TE.

133. a. *Medial oblique* is a term used for specific plain film x-ray views. It is not appropriate nomenclature for any MRI study.

134. d. The window of CT images refers to the tissue density range being computer enhanced. Bone, brain, soft tissue, or lung are common CT windows.

135. c. Posterior oblique views of the cervical spine demonstrate contralateral intervertebral foramina.

136. c. Lucent areas on x-ray are regions of low density.

137. a. Increased mineral content in bone will show decreased SI on MRI because of decreased or absent fluid and fat hydrogen nuclei.

138. d. CT is excellent for study of occult fractures and is the imaging modality of choice if plain film x-ray findings are inconclusive.

139. a. Ligaments fall into the generic description of "soft tissue" or "mid-density" on plain film x-ray.

140. d. Lucency refers to an area of low density (i.e., molecular weight), thus producing a black or dark gray lesion within normal dense bone. A lytic lesion would be identified as lucent.

141. b. Both terms refer specifically to bacterial infections of bone. Sequestra refers to pieces of necrotic bone and involucrum refers to reactive bone formation in response to bacterial bone destruction.

142. a. Multiple layers of any soft tissue structure increases apparent, not true, radiodensity.

143. b. A PA view demonstrates coronal plane relationships.

144. b. A bone window enhances radiographic contrast of bone; therefore, cortical bone appears very radiodense or white.

145. c. The pars interarticularis is superimposed on the vertebral body in the AP projection and therefore nearly impossible to visualize.

146. b. Lumbar oblique, both anterior and posterior, visualize the "Scotty Dog."

147. a. The ipsilateral inferior articular process is seen as the front leg.

148. a. The spinolaminar line represents the posterior aspect of the central canal.

149. b. Articular cartilage is histologically mostly water and appears as mid-density or water density.

150. c. Periarticular osteopenia is a classic sign of rheumatoid arthritis due to hyperperfusion due to inflammation of the synovium.

151. b. Posterior oblique views of the lumbar spine demonstrate ipsilateral posterior elements of the vertebra.

152. d. Osteophyte formation is typical of osteoarthritis, whereas loss of bone density is observed in RA.

153. c. Cortical bone has little water or fat so few hydrogen nuclei are available to record radiofrequency signal in MRI images.

154. d. A Salter-Harris IV fracture passes through both the metaphyseal and epiphyseal portions of the bone along with, of course, the epiphyseal plate.

155. b. Calcification of the organized hematoma begins at about 10 to 14 days after injury. The hematoma, organized hematoma, and fibrous hematoma are soft tissue and not radiographically visible. Calcium deposition marks the onset of x-ray visibility of callus formation.

156. a. Spondylolisthesis, is best viewed and measured on lateral views only.

157. b. Schmorl's nodules are regions of lucency usually seen at the vertebral end plate where the degenerating disk is penetrating into bone material. Napoleon's hat sign is indicative of severe spondylolysthesis, and a Salter-Harris fracture type 5 is present in the pediatric population only. Osteoblastoma is a benign bone-forming tumor.

158. b. Enlargement exaggerates the size of structures located closest to the x-ray beam source.

159. d. Radiolucency refers to low density areas such as the lung. The lung is normally radiolucent.

CHAPTER 3

Foundations for Evaluation, Differential Diagnosis, and Prognosis

1. The most serious complication of lower extremity thrombophlebitis is
   a. Cerebral infarction
   b. Pulmonary infarction
   c. Myocardial infarction
   d. Kidney infection

2. A 50-year-old man has a persistent cough, purulent sputum, abnormal dilation of bronchi, more frequent involvement of the left lower lobe than the right, hemoptysis, and reduced forced vital capacity. What is the most likely pulmonary dysfunction?
   a. Chronic bronchitis
   b. Emphysema
   c. Asthma
   d. Bronchiectasis

3. Which of the following are tests for peripheral arterial involvement in a patient with complaints of calf musculature pain?
   a. Claudication time
   b. Homan's sign
   c. Percussion test
   d. Hoffa's test

4. A patient presents to a clinic with decreased tidal volume (TV). What is the most likely cause of this change in normal pulmonary function?
   a. Chronic obstructive pulmonary disease
   b. Restrictive lung dysfunction
   c. Emphysema
   d. Asthma

5. A patient presents with tachypnea, corpulmonale, hypoxemia, rales on inspiration, and decreased diffusing capacity. What is the probable cause?
    a. Restrictive lung dysfunction
    b. Chronic obstructive pulmonary disease
    c. Asthma
    d. Emphysema

6. A physician instructs the therapist to educate a patient about the risk factors of atherosclerosis. Which of the following is the most inappropriate list?
    a. Diabetes, male gender, and excessive alcohol
    b. Genetic predisposition, smoking, and sedentary lifestyle
    c. Stress and inadequate exercise
    d. Obesity, smoking, and hypotension

7. A therapist is ordered by a physician to treat a patient with congestive heart failure in an outpatient cardiac rehabilitation facility. Which of the following signs and symptoms should the therapist not expect?
    a. Stenosis of the mitral valve
    b. Orthopnea
    c. Decreased preload of the right heart
    d. Pulmonary edema

8. At a team meeting, the respiratory therapist informs the rest of the team that the patient, just admitted to the subacute floor, experienced breathing difficulty in the acute care department. The respiratory therapist describes the breathing problem as a pause before exhaling after a full inspiration. Which of the following is the therapist describing?
    a. Apnea
    b. Orthopnea
    c. Eupnea
    d. Apneusis

9. A therapist is performing chest physiotherapy on a patient who is coughing up a significant amount of sputum. The therapist later describes the quality of the sputum in his notes as mucoid. This description tells other personnel which of the following?
    a. The sputum is thick.
    b. The sputum has a foul odor.
    c. The sputum is clear or white in color.
    d. The patient has a possible bronchopulmonary infection.

10. A therapist is sent to provide passive range of motion to a patient in the intensive care unit. The chart reveals that the patient is suffering from pulmonary edema. The charge nurse informs the therapist that the patient is coughing up a thin, white sputum with a pink tint. Which of the following terms best describes this sputum?
    a. Purulent
    b. Frothy
    c. Mucopurulent
    d. Rusty

11. Strengthening exercises for persons with hemophilia should
    a. Begin as soon as a joint bleed is recognized
    b. Never include isokinetic exercises
    c. Be increased using high repetition, low load PREs
    d. Only occur in joints that demonstrate muscle weakness

12. A patient with cryoglobulinemia presents to outpatient physical therapy with complaints of lumbar pain. Which of the following should the physical therapist avoid during intervention for this diagnosis?
    a. Moist heat packs
    b. Weight-bearing exercises
    c. Muscle energy techniques
    d. Cold pack application

13. A physical therapist is assessing the endurance of a 12-year-old female with cystic fibrosis. Which objective screening tool would be most appropriate to quantify the patient's endurance level?
    a. Six-minute walk test
    b. Tinetti Performance-Oriented Mobility Assessment
    c. Vo_2 Max Test
    d. Romberg test

14. A physical therapist is performing an examination for an infant that has recently been diagnosed with a congenital heart defect. Which of the following clinical signs would not likely be present?
    a. Bradycardia
    b. Poor weight gain
    c. Decreased respiratory rate
    d. Lower extremity swelling

15. Besides the anterolateral abdominal muscles, which muscle assists in forced expiration, coughing, sneezing, vomiting, urinating, defecating, and fixation of the trunk during strong movements of the upper limb?
    a. Piriformis
    b. Pelvic diaphragm
    c. Trapezius
    d. Gluteus maximus

16. Which muscle does NOT flex the knee and extend the hip?
    a. Semitendinosus
    b. Hamstring portion of the adductor magnus
    c. Long head of the biceps femoris
    d. Semimembranosus

17. History taking revealed that a patient experiences pain after horseback riding or skating. The pain is located over the anteromedial thigh and is aggravated by resisted abduction. What is the MOST likely preliminary diagnosis?
    a. Piriformis syndrome
    b. Trochanteric bursitis
    c. Adductor longus strain/tendonitis/tendinosis
    d. Avascular necrosis

18. A patient has dull posterior hip pain radiating down the leg. He says that he has a limp and that his pain is aggravated by turning his leg outside or with deep pressure near the middle of the right buttock. What is the MOST likely preliminary diagnosis?
    a. Piriformis syndrome
    b. Trochanteric bursitis
    c. Adductor longus strain/tendonitis/tendinosis
    d. Avascular necrosis

19. What is the BEST imaging modality for detecting the changes in the articular cartilage seen with chondromalacia patella?
    a. Plain film radiography
    b. Bone scan
    c. Magnetic resonance imaging (MRI)
    d. Computed tomography (CT)

20. Which of the following imaging modalities does NOT give a radiation dose to the patient?
    a. MRI
    b. CT
    c. Mammography
    d. Bone scan

21. A therapist is examining a 3-year-old child, who is positioned as follows: supine, hips flexed to 90 degrees, hips fully adducted, and knees flexed. The therapist passively abducts and raises the thigh, applying an anterior shear force to the hip joint. A click at 30 degrees of abduction is noted by the therapist. What orthopedic test is the therapist performing, and what is its significance?
   a. Ortolani's test, hip dislocation
   b. Appley's compression/distraction test, cartilage damage
   c. McMurray test, cartilage damage
   d. Piston test, hip dislocation

22. A teenager comes to an outpatient facility with complaints of pain at the tibial tubercle when playing basketball. The therapist notices that the tubercles are abnormally pronounced on bilateral knees. What condition does the patient most likely have?
   a. Jumper's knees
   b. Anterior cruciate ligament sprain
   c. Osgood-Schlatter disease
   d. Sever's disease

23. A patient presents to physical therapy with complaints of pain in the right hip due to osteoarthritis. Which of the following is not true about this type of arthritis?
   a. Osteoarthritis causes pain that is usually symmetric because it is a systemic condition.
   b. Osteoarthritis is not usually more painful in the morning.
   c. Osteoarthritis commonly involves the distal interphalangeal joint.
   d. Osteoarthritis mainly involves weight-bearing joints.

24. Which of the following is used to treat a patient referred to physical therapy with a diagnosis of Dupuytren's contracture?
   a. Knee continuous passive motion (CPM)
   b. Work simulator set for squatting activities
   c. Hand splint
   d. A 2-pound dumbbell

25. A 17-year-old football player is referred to the outpatient physical therapy clinic with a diagnosis of a recent third-degree medial collateral ligament sprain of the knee. The patient wishes to return to playing football as soon as possible. Which protocol below is the best?
    a. Fit the patient with a brace that prevents him from actively moving the knee into the last available 20 degrees of extension. Prescribe general lower extremity strengthening with the exception of side-lying hip adduction.
    b. Do not fit the patient with a brace. All lower extremity strengthening exercises are indicated.
    c. Fit the patient with a brace that prevents him from actively moving the knee into the last available 20 degrees of extension. Avoid all open-chain strengthening for the lower extremity.
    d. Do not fit the patient with a brace. Prescribe general lower extremity strengthening with the exception of side-lying hip adduction.

26. During an examination, the therapist taps on the flexor retinaculum of the patient's wrist, which causes tingling in the thumb. What test is this? For what condition does it screen?
    a. Phalen's test, carpal tunnel
    b. Finkelstein test, de Quervain's disease
    c. Tinel's sign, de Quervain's disease
    d. Tinel's sign, carpal tunnel

27. A physical therapist is treating a patient with balance deficits. During treatment, the physical therapist notes that large-amplitude changes in the center of mass cause the patient to lose balance. The patient, however, can accurately compensate for small changes nearly every time a change is introduced. What muscles most likely need to be strengthened to help alleviate this dysfunction?
    a. Tibialis anterior, gastrocnemius
    b. Peroneus longus/brevis, tibialis posterior
    c. Rectus abdominis, erector spinea
    d. Iliopsoas, gluteus maximus

28. The physical therapist is reading the physician's interpretation of an x-ray that was taken of the left humerus of a 7-year-old patient. The physician notes in the report the presence of an incomplete fracture on the convex side of the humerus. Which type of fracture is the physician describing?
    a. Comminuted
    b. Avulsion
    c. Greenstick
    d. Segmental

29. A physical therapist is beginning an examination of a 5-year-old boy. The mother indicates that she pulled the child from a seated position by grasping the wrists. The child then experienced immediate pain at the right elbow. The physician's orders are for right elbow range of motion and strengthening. Which of the following is the most likely diagnosis?
    a. Radial head fracture
    b. Nursemaid's elbow
    c. Erb's palsy
    d. Ulnar coronoid process fracture

30. A child presents to physical therapy with a diagnosis of right Sever's disease. What joint should be the focus of the therapist's examination?
    a. Right knee joint
    b. Right hip joint
    c. Right wrist joint
    d. Right ankle joint

31. A 10-year-old boy presents to outpatient physical therapy with complaints of diffuse pain in the right hip, thigh, and knee joint. The patient was involved in a motor vehicle accident 3 weeks ago. He is also obese and has significant atrophy in the right quadricep. The right lower extremity is held by the patient in the position of flexion, abduction, and lateral rotation. Which of the following is most likely the source of the patient's signs and symptoms?
    a. Greater trochanteric bursitis
    b. Avascular necrosis
    c. Slipped femoral capital epiphysis
    d. Septic arthritis

32. A high-school athlete is considering whether to have an anterior cruciate ligament reconstruction. The therapist explains the importance of this ligament, especially in a person that is young and athletic. Which of the statements below is correct in describing part of the function of the anterior cruciate ligament?
    a. The anterior cruciate ligament prevents excessive posterior roll of the femoral condyles during flexion of the femur at the knee joint.
    b. The anterior cruciate ligament prevents excessive anterior roll of the femoral condyles during flexion of the femur at the knee joint.
    c. The anterior cruciate ligament prevents excessive posterior roll of the femoral condyles during extension of the femur at the knee joint.
    d. The anterior cruciate ligament prevents excessive anterior roll of the femoral condyles during extension of the femur at the knee joint.

33. Which tendon is most commonly involved with lateral epicondylitis?
    a. Extensor carpi radialis longus
    b. Extensor carpi radialis brevis
    c. Brachioradialis
    d. Extensor digitorum

34. A patient who has suffered a zone 2 rupture of the extensor tendon of the third digit presents to physical therapy. This patient had a surgical fixation of the avulsed tendon. During the period of immobilization, which of the following deformities is most likely to develop?
    a. Boutonniére deformity
    b. Claw hand
    c. Swan neck deformity
    d. Dupuytren's contracture

35. Which of the following muscle tendons most commonly sublux in patients who suffer from rheumatoid arthritis?
    a. Flexor digitorum profundus
    b. Extensor carpi ulnaris
    c. Extensor carpi radialis longus
    d. Flexor pollicis longus

36. A therapist is scheduled to examine a patient with a chronic condition of "hammer toes." Where should the therapist not expect to find callus formation?
    a. The distal tips of the toes
    b. The superior surface of the interphalangeal joints
    c. The metatarsal heads
    d. The inferior surface of the interphalangeal joints

37. Each of these factors influences the probability of scoliosis curve progression in the skeletally immature patient except
    a. Magnitude
    b. Gender
    c. Race
    d. Age

38. The child with clubfoot will have
    a. A larger than normal calcaneus
    b. Forefoot valgus
    c. Significant tibial shortening
    d. Fixed equinas

39. Differential diagnosis in the infant born with severe calcaneovalgus includes
    a. Congenital vertical talus
    b. Metatarsus adductus
    c. Accessory navicular
    d. Tarsal coalition

40. What clinical examination technique will establish whether an infant's hip is dislocated but reducible?
    a. Barlow test
    b. Ortolani's maneuver
    c. Hoffman test
    d. Galeazzi maneuver

41. All of the following may be part of the clinical picture of a child in the first 48 hours after onset of osteomyelitis EXCEPT
    a. Radiographs are positive for signs of infection and avascular necrosis.
    b. Needle aspiration may or may not be produce pus.
    c. The child does not appear sick and has no fever.
    d. High fever and refusal to walk.

42. In a child, the most common site of transient synovitis, slipped epiphysis and septic arthritis is the
    a. Shoulder
    b. Hip
    c. Knee
    d. Ankle

43. All of the following are common in children who have slipped capital femoral epiphysis EXCEPT
    a. Knee pain
    b. Obesity
    c. No history of trauma
    d. Negative findings on a frog lateral radiograph

44. Which of the following conditions are not implicated in overuse injuries in youth?
    a. Training errors
    b. Musculotendinous imbalances
    c. Anatomic malalignment of the lower extremity
    d. Constant practice on turf (grass)

45. The signs and symptoms of juvenile rheumatoid arthritis include all of the following except
    a. Swollen joints
    b. Neurologic impairments
    c. Stiffness
    d. Muscle weakness

46. Which of the following as an absolute contraindication to initiation of an outpatient cardiac rehabilitation program?
    a. Obesity
    b. Patient currently on dialysis 3 days a week because of renal failure
    c. Asthma
    d. Third-degree heart block

47. Fourteen weeks after surgical repair of the rotator cuff, a patient presents with significant deltoid weakness. Range of motion (ROM) is within normal limits and equal bilaterally. Internal and external rotation strength is equal bilaterally; flexion and abduction strength is significantly reduced. What is the most likely cause of this dysfunction?
    a. Poor compliance with a home exercise program
    b. Tightness of the inferior shoulder capsule
    c. Surgical damage to the musculocutaneous nerve
    d. Surgical damage to the axillary nerve

48. A patient has recently undergone an acromioplasty. What is the most important goal in early rehabilitation?
    a. Regaining muscle strength
    b. Return to activities of daily living (ADLs)
    c. Endurance and functional progression
    d. Return of normal ROM

49. A 35-year-old patient presents with complaints of pain and point tenderness slightly anterior to the temporomandibular joint. The tissue that likely is causing the pain is the
    a. Temporalis tendon
    b. Masseter
    c. Maxillary sinus
    d. Parotid gland

50. A 72-year-old female comes into the clinic complaining of new onset of sudden severe right temporal headache and pain with chewing. The likely cause of her headache is
    a. Migraine
    b. Subarachnoid hemorrhage
    c. Temporal arteritis
    d. Cervicogenic headache

51. A patient cannot open the jaw greater than 15 mm interincisal with active and passive opening. Lateral jaw movements are 8 mm bilaterally and protrusion is 6 mm. What type of disorder do these symptoms indicate?
    a. Anterior disc displacement with reduction
    b. Anterior disc displacement without reduction
    c. Trismus
    d. Capsulitis

52. A 15-year-old patient complains of acute jaw pain. The patient opens to 23 mm active and passive with deflection to the right. Right laterotrusion is 8 mm, left laterotrusion is 2 mm and protrusion is 3 mm with deflection to the right. Palpation is negative for crepitus. What type of disorder do these symptoms indicate?
    a. Right temporomandibular anterior disc displacement with reduction
    b. Right temporomandibular anterior disc displacement without reduction
    c. Trismus
    d. Left temporomandibular anterior disc displacement with reduction

53. What is a temporomandibular reciprocal click?
    a. Clicking that occurs during the end of opening
    b. Clicking that occurs during the beginning of opening
    c. Clicking that occurs during the middle of opening
    d. Clicking that occurs during opening and closing

54. A 28-year-old male complains of pain in his right jaw and his bite not touching on the right side after biting into beef jerky 5 days ago. What is the probable disorder?
    a. Right acute anterior disc displacement without reduction
    b. Right acute anterior disc displacement with reduction
    c. Right acute osteoarthritis
    d. Right acute capsulitis

55. What are signs and symptoms of an acute TMJ anterior displaced disc without reduction?
    a. Clicking and pain in the TMJ joint
    b. Absence of clicking and opening limited to 26 mm to 30 mm, lateral movements limited to contralateral side, deflection to same side with protrusion
    c. Crepitation and limitation to 26 mm
    d. Absence of clicking and opening is limited to 26 mm to 30 mm, lateral movements limited to ipsilateral side, deflection to same side with protrusion

56. A physical therapist is completing a manual muscle testing (MMT) examination of a patient with right lateral hip pain. The standing alignment reveals anterior pelvic tilt and associated hip flexion. During the MMT of the right posterior gluteus medius, which substitution is likely to occur?
   a. Increase in hip flexion angle to substitute with the tensor fascia latae
   b. Increase in lateral rotation to substitute with the tensor fascia latae
   c. Forward rotation of the pelvis to substitute with the gluteus minimus
   d. Knee flexion to substitute with the lateral hamstrings

57. Osgood-Schlatter's disease is primarily
   a. An inflammatory process
   b. An injury to apophyseal cartilage
   c. An injury in adolescent females
   d. Caused by tight calf muscles

58. A swollen knee immediately following trauma indicates
   a. Blood in the joint
   b. Blood or synovial fluid accumulation
   c. Possible gout
   d. Underlying arthritic degeneration

59. The most likely cause for a baseball pitcher to injure the throwing arm is
   a. Throwing side-arm
   b. High pitch counts
   c. Throwing curve balls
   d. "Dead arm" syndrome

60. The ulnar collateral ligament of the elbow is injured during which phase of the baseball pitch?
   a. Early cocking phase
   b. Late cocking phase
   c. Acceleration phase
   d. Deceleration phase

61. Anterior "black line" tibia stress fracture
   a. Is a failure in compression
   b. Heals predictably with rest and splinting
   c. Requires bone stimulation to heal
   d. May require intramedullary rodding to heal

62. Ankle pain anteriorly
   a. Is usually a bone bruise
   b. Is usually osteochondritis dissecans
   c. Is usually ligament pain following sprain
   d. Is usually soft tissue impingement

63. Swimmer's shoulder
    a. Occurs in all swimmers
    b. Is a rotator cuff tear
    c. Is worse with backstrokers
    d. Is an impingement syndrome

64. During manual muscle testing of knee flexion strength, the physical therapist wishes to differentiate between medial and lateral hamstrings. To test medial hamstrings, the therapist positions the patient in hip
    a. External rotation to test semimembranosis and biceps femoris
    b. Internal rotation to test semimembranosis and semitendinosis
    c. External rotation to test semimembranosis and semitendinosis
    d. Internal rotation to test biceps femoris

65. A patient is involved in a rear-end motor vehicle accident and now complains of neck pain, muscle spasm, and decreased cervical range of motion. After performing your subjective examination, the next thing you would most appropriately do is
    a. Ligamentous testing
    b. Muscle testing
    c. Active range of motion testing
    d. Passive motion testing

66. The piano key sign is a test used to assess the
    a. Glenoid labrum
    b. Long head of the biceps
    c. Acromioclavicular joint
    d. Anterior shoulder stability

67. Your patient is a 16 year-old-male who injured his left knee playing football. There was an onset of immediate swelling, a locking sensation, and restricted range of motion. You hypothesize the most likely structure involved is
    a. A collateral ligament
    b. A tear of the retinaculum
    c. A meniscal injury
    d. The cruciate ligament

68. You suspect that your patient has a torn rotator cuff. Which three tests would best confirm this diagnosis?
    a. The lift off test, the anterior apprehension test, and Speed's test
    b. The drop arm test, crank test, load and shift test
    c. The belly press test, drop arm test, and lift off test
    d. Internal rotation lag sign, drop arm test, crank test

69. A cause of a noncapsular pattern might be which of the following?
    a. Arthrosis in the knee
    b. Hemarthrosis of the shoulder
    c. Septic arthritis in the knee
    d. Loose body in the shoulder

70. In the single leg stance, when the contralateral hip drops because of weakness, it is considered
    a. A compensated hip varus
    b. An uncompensated Trendelenberg
    c. A compensated Trendelenberg
    d. An uncompensated hip varus

71. Your patient has sustained a fracture of the coronoid process. Which of the following is most true about these fractures?
    a. It is more commonly an isolated fracture.
    b. It is more often accompanied by avulsion of the biceps.
    c. Fractures of the coronoid process account for better than 50% of elbow fractures.
    d. Fractures of the coronoid process are usually accompanied by a radial head fracture.

72. A 45-year-old male electrician presents with a gradual onset of left shoulder pain. He notes it is most prominent with overhead activities and throwing. The position that hurts his shoulder the most is 90 degrees of flexion with internal rotation. This most likely indicates
    a. A SLAP lesion
    b. Anterior instability of the shoulder
    c. Impingement syndrome
    d. Posterior instability of the shoulder

73. Your patient presents with pain and tenderness over the distal radial forearm and pain with resistive thumb extension after using a screwdriver repeatedly for several days. Based on this history, the most likely diagnosis is
    a. Scaphoid instability
    b. Gout in the thumb
    c. De Quervain's syndrome
    d. Radial carpal syndrome

74. You find that a patient has a leg length discrepancy. Upon review of their radiographs, you notice that the angle of the neck of the femur to the femoral shaft is less than 120 degrees. You have determined that the apparent leg length difference is due to
    a. A pelvic obliquity
    b. A coxa varum
    c. A coxa valgum
    d. An acetabular tropism

75. Your patient presents with a non-contact injury from a quick stop. He reports an audible "pop" at the time of injury. He complains of pain on either side of his patella. He now complains of difficulty with cutting and pivoting when running. The patient did not have immediate swelling or joint line tenderness. The structure most likely involved is the
    a. Medial meniscus
    b. Medial collateral ligament
    c. Posterior cruciate ligament
    d. Anterior cruciate ligament

76. Your patient has been diagnosed as having pronator syndrome. You have determined that the structure involved is the lacertus fibrosis. The maneuver that would verify this is
    a. Elbow flexion of 120 to 135 degrees
    b. Resisted forearm supination
    c. Resisted forearm pronation
    d. Resisted long finger flexion

77. A patient reports to physical therapy with a referral from his primary care physician that reads "suspected partial biceps tear—evaluate and treat." The patient sustained the injury 2 days ago during soccer practice. Which of the following objective findings would be most consistent with the patient's condition during the physical examination?
    a. Pain with passive shoulder abduction
    b. Pain with resisted shoulder extension
    c. Pain with resisted forearm supination
    d. Pain with resisted elbow extension

78. During ambulation, a physical therapist notices that the patient is exhibiting genu recurvatum during the stance phase of the gait cycle. Of the choices listed below, the MOST LIKELY cause for the observed gait deviation is
    a. A tight gluteus maximus
    b. Tight hip flexors
    c. A tight gastrocnemius-soleus complex
    d. Tight ankle dorsiflexors

79. A physical therapist is performing a manual muscle test on a patient with reported lower extremity weakness. When examining the patient's ability to plantarflex the foot in a prone position, suspicion arises that the patient is using the tibialis posterior as a substitute for significant gastrocnemius-soleus weakness. The therapist's hypothesis is based on the following observation
    a. The foot moves into eversion and plantar flexion
    b. The foot moves into inversion and plantar flexion
    c. The forefoot moves into plantar flex
    d. The toes flex as the foot plantar flexes

80. A physical therapist is examining passive range of motion in a patient reporting hip pain. When measuring with a goniometer, the patient had 0 to 60 degrees of passive hip internal rotation. This finding is
   a. Normal
   b. Indicative of hypomobility
   c. Indicative of hypermobility
   d. Indicative of a capsular pattern

81. A physical therapist is treating a patient who has bilaterally "weak" knee and hip extensors. The patient is most likely to have the greatest difficulty performing which of the following functional activities?
   a. Transferring from a wheelchair to a mat
   b. Rolling from supine to side-lying
   c. Transferring from sitting to supine
   d. Transferring from sitting to standing

82. Your patient is a 21-year-old male who reports to you with complaints of low back pain and stiffness. This has been ongoing for the past several months. He has been experiencing difficulties breathing and has noticed a difficulty with cervical flexion. The stiffness is most prevalent in the morning. He has noticed a low grade fever over the past several weeks. What pathology is mostly likely the source of the patient's symptoms?
   a. Ankylosing spondylitis
   b. Rheumatoid arthritis
   c. Systemic lupus erythematosis
   d. Myasthenia gravis

83. A 16-year-old male basketball player complains of pain in lower back and notes that the pain increases after landing from a jump. After a supine-to-sit test, the therapist notes that the right lower extremity appears longer in supine and shorter in sitting. What is the most likely cause of this problem?
   a. Posterior rotation of the right innominate
   b. Anterior rotation of the left innominate
   c. Anterior rotation of the right innominate
   d. Inflare of right innominate

84. A patient with an upper motor neuron spinal cord lesion at C6 began receiving occupational therapy 2 weeks after the injury. During the third week, the therapist notices an increase in spasticity. The therapist should
   a. Conclude that symptoms are typical after spinal shock
   b. Conclude that the patient maybe in respiratory distress
   c. Suspect that a contracture is developing
   d. Look for signs of autonomic dysreflexia

85. At the caudal level of the medulla, what percentage of the fibers of the corticospinal tract cross at the pyramidal decussation?
    a. 90% to 100%
    b. 80% to 90%
    c. 70% to 80%
    d. 60% to 70%

86. This descending tract, the _____, originates in the superior colliculus and is involved with the orientation toward a stimulus in the environment by reflex turning of the head.
    a. Rubrospinal
    b. Reticulospinal
    c. Tectospinal
    d. Vestibulospinal

87. Which is the LEAST likely cause of dementia in the elderly?
    a. Stroke
    b. Alzheimer's disease
    c. Depression
    d. Cerebrovascular accident

88. Postinfectious ascending paralysis and radiculoneuropathy are characteristics of what condition?
    a. Guillain-Barré syndrome
    b. Myasthenia gravis
    c. Amyotrophic lateral sclerosis
    d. Multiple sclerosis

89. A 41-year-old woman presents with sudden onset of numbness and drooping of the left side of her face and pain directly behind her left ear. Further questioning and a general assessment of the patient revealed asymmetric facial expression lateralizing to the right side, mild slurring of speech, dysgeusia, hyperacusis, and difficulty drinking noted as the "dribbling" of a beverage. She was recently diagnosed with a viral upper respiratory infection 3 days ago and treatment consisted of rest and fluids. Ms. Ryan denies a traumatic episode, headache, vertigo, lightheadedness, tinnitus, use of oral contraceptives, and smoking of cigarettes. What is the most likely diagnosis?
    a. Guillain-Barré syndrome
    b. Bell's palsy
    c. Lyme disease
    d. Stroke

90. A 50-year-old man presents to your office with the following presentation: +2 muscle strength with left shoulder abduction and elbow flexion; +5 muscle strength of left elbow extension and the intrinsic muscles of the hand; bicipital reflex absent on the left and hypotonia of the biceps and deltoid muscles; triceps reflex +2 with normal triceps muscle tone; spasticity and hyperreflexia in the left lower extremity. Based upon this presentation, where is the MOST likely site of the lesion?
    a. Left side of the spinal cord at C5
    b. Left side of the spinal cord at C7
    c. Right side of the spinal cord at T1
    d. Right side of the spinal cord at C5

91. A patient recently diagnosed with multiple sclerosis presents to a physical therapy clinic. The patient asks the therapist what she needs to avoid with this condition. Which of the following should the patient avoid?
    a. Hot tubs
    b. Slightly increased intake of fluids
    c. Application of ice packs
    d. Strength training

92. The therapist is examining a patient with a diagnosis of cerebral palsy. The therapist notes that all of the extremities and the trunk are involved. Further assessment also reveals that the lower extremities are more involved than the upper extremities and that the right side is more involved than the left. This patient most likely has which classification of cerebral palsy?
    a. Spastic hemiplegia
    b. Spastic triplegia
    c. Spastic quadriplegia
    d. Spastic diplegia

93. The therapist receives an order to treat a 42-year-old man admitted to the hospital 3 days ago with a stab wound to the left lower thoracic spine. The patient is unable to move the left lower extremity and cannot feel pain or temperature differences in the right lower extremity. What is the most likely type of lesion?
    a. The patient most likely has an anterior cord syndrome.
    b. The patient most likely has a Brown-Sequard syndrome.
    c. The patient most likely has a central cord syndrome.
    d. The patient is equally as likely to have anterior cord syndrome as he is to have Brown-Sequard syndrome.

94. The therapist receives a referral to examine a patient with a boutonnière deformity. With this injury the involved finger usually presents in the position of
    a. Flexion of the proximal interphalangeal (PIP) joint and flexion of the distal interphalangeal (DIP) join
    b. Extension of the PIP joint and flexion of the DIP joint
    c. Flexion of the PIP joint and extension of the DIP joint
    d. Extension of the PIP joint and extension of the DIP joint

95. A therapist receives an order to examine and treat a 76-year-old woman who was involved in a motor vehicle accident 2 days ago. The patient's vehicle was struck in the rear by another vehicle. The patient has normal sensation and strength in bilateral lower extremities but paralysis and loss of sensation in bilateral upper extremities. Bowel and bladder function are normal. The patient most likely has what type of spinal cord injury?
    a. The patient most likely has an anterior cord syndrome.
    b. The patient most likely has a Brown-Sequard syndrome.
    c. The patient most likely has a central cord syndrome.
    d. There is no evidence of an incomplete spinal cord lesion.

96. A 31-year-old man has loss of vision in one eye, staggering gait, numbness in bilateral upper extremities, and decreased bowel and bladder control. The episodes of these symptoms have occurred every few weeks for the past 6 months. Each episode has been slightly worse than the last. What is the most likely condition?
    a. Parkinson's disease
    b. Guillain-Barré syndrome
    c. Multiple sclerosis
    d. Amyotrophic lateral sclerosis

97. A 35-year-old woman suffered brain injury in a motor vehicle accident and presents with an intention tremor, nystagmus, hypotonia, and dysdiadochokinesia. What is the most likely location of the lesion?
    a. Basal ganglia
    b. Dorsal columns
    c. Frontal lobe
    d. Cerebellum

98. A 42-year-old construction worker received a burst fracture in the cervical spine when struck by a falling cross-beam. Proprioception is intact in bilateral lower extremities. The patient has bilateral loss of motor function and sensitivity to pain and temperature below the level of the lesion. This type of lesion is most typical of which of the following syndromes?
    a. Central cord syndrome
    b. Brown-Sequard syndrome
    c. Anterior cord syndrome
    d. Conus medullaris syndrome

99. A 52-year-old man with sciatica presents to outpatient physical therapy. The patient indicates that he is experiencing paresthesia extending to the left ankle and severe lumbar pain. Straight leg raise test is positive with the left lower extremity. Of the following, which is the most likely source of pain?
    a. A lumbar disc with a left posterior herniation or protrusion
    b. A lumbar disc with a right posterior herniation or protrusion
    c. Piriformis syndrome
    d. Sacroiliac joint dysfunction

100. A patient who has suffered a recent fracture of the right tibia and fibula has developed foot drop of the right foot during gait. Which nerve is causing this loss of motor function?
    a. Posterior tibial
    b. Superficial peroneal
    c. Deep peroneal
    d. Anterior tibial

101. An infant with Erb's palsy presents with the involved upper extremity in which of the following positions?
    a. Hand supinated and wrist extended
    b. Hand supinated and wrist flexed
    c. Hand pronated and wrist extended
    d. Hand pronated and wrist flexed

102. When reviewing a patient's chart, the therapist determines that the patient has a condition in which the cauda equina is in a fluid-filled sac protruding from the back. What form of spina bifida does the patient most likely have?
    a. Meningocele
    b. Meningomyelocele
    c. Spina bifida occulta
    d. Lipoma

103. A physician is preparing a patient for an upcoming procedure. The physician explains that the procedure will provide a detailed image that appears to be a slice of the brain. This image is obtained with a highly concentrated x-ray beam. What procedure is the patient scheduled to undergo?
    a. Angiogram
    b. Magnetic resonance imaging (MRI)
    c. Positron emission tomography (PET)
    d. Computed tomography (CT)

104. A therapist is scheduled to treat a patient with cerebral palsy who has been classified as a spastic quadriplegic. What type of orthopedic deformity should the therapist expect to see in the patient's feet?
    a. Talipes equinovalgus
    b. Talipes equinovarus
    c. Hindfoot valgus
    d. Abnormally large calcaneous

105. A 32-year-old construction worker fell off a ladder. In his effort to prevent the fall, the worker reached for a beam with his right arm. This motion stretched the brachial plexus, resulting in decreased function in the right arm. Full function returned after 2½ weeks. What is the most likely type of injury?
    a. Axonotmesis
    b. Neurotmesis
    c. Neurapraxia
    d. Nerve root avulsion

106. A therapist is assessing a patient in an attempt to discover the source of her pain. She positions the patient's cervical spine in different directions in an attempt to elicit the patient's symptoms. In one such direction, the patient reports return of symptoms, including pain located at the right posterior scapular region, which extends down the posterior side of the right upper extremity to the ends of the fingers, and tingling in the second, third, and fourth digits. The patient also indicates that she often has a decrease in sensation on the dorsal side of the second and third digits. She also has noticeable weakness in the right triceps. Which nerve root is most likely involved?
    a. Fourth cervical root
    b. Fifth cervical root
    c. Sixth cervical root
    d. Seventh cervical root

107. A patient informs his therapist that his problem began 3 months after a bout of the flu. The patient originally experienced tingling in the hands and feet. He also reports progressive weakness to the point that he required a ventilator to breathe. He is now recovering rapidly and is expected to return to a normal functional level in 3 more months. From which of the following conditions is the patient most likely suffering?
    a. Parkinson's disease
    b. Guillain-Barré syndrome
    c. Multiple sclerosis
    d. Amyotrophic lateral sclerosis

108. A therapist is examining a patient in the intensive care unit. The therapist notices that the patient is moving his hands and fingers in slow, writhing motions. Which of the following terms best describes this type of movement?
    a. Lead-pipe rigidity
    b. Ballisms
    c. Chorea
    d. Athetosis

109. A 29-year-old woman who is 8 months pregnant presents to an outpatient clinic with complaints of "pain and tingling" over the lateral thigh. She also indicates no traumatic injury. The symptoms increase after she has been sitting for 30 minutes or longer, and the overall intensity of the symptoms has been increasing over the past 2 weeks. The therapist notes that repeated active lumbar flexion does not increase pain, and the patient's lumbar range of motion is normal for a pregnant woman. There is also no motor weakness in the hip or pelvis, and the sacroiliac joint is not abnormally rotated. What is the most probable diagnosis?
    a. L3 disc dysfunction
    b. Spondylolisthesis
    c. L4 disc dysfunction
    d. Meralgia paresthetica

110. A 14-year-old girl placed excessive valgus stress to the right elbow during a fall from a bicycle. Her forearm was in supination at the moment the valgus stress was applied. Which of the following is most likely involved in this type of injury?
    a. Ulnar nerve
    b. Extensor carpi radialus
    c. Brachioradialis
    d. Annular ligament

111. A patient presents to an outpatient clinic with an order to examine and treat the right forearm and wrist secondary to nerve compression. The patient has the following signs and symptoms: pain with manual muscle testing of pronation, decreased strength of the flexor pollicis longus and pronator quadrates, and pain with palpation of the pronator teres. What nerve is most likely compromised? What is the most likely area of compression?
    a. Median nerve, carpal tunnel
    b. Ulnar nerve, Guyon's canal
    c. Ulnar nerve, pronator quadratus
    d. Median nerve, pronator teres

112. The best predictor of ambulation in young children with cerebral palsy is
    a. Absence of primitive reflexes at 3months
    b. Absence of tonic neck reflexes
    c. Independent sitting by 24 months of age
    d. Independent standing by 1 year of age

113. Which complication of spinal cord injury is more likely to occur in children and teenagers than in adults?
    a. Hypercalcemia
    b. Autonomic dysreflexia
    c. Spasticity
    d. Deep venous thrombosis

114. Recovery from spinal cord injury occurring over several years is most likely with which syndrome
    a. Brown-Sequard
    b. Anterior cord
    c. Posterior cord
    d. Cauda equina

115. Which orthopedic complication is not probable in a child with tetraplegic spinal cord injury?
    a. Shoulder subluxation
    b. Scoliosis
    c. Heterotopic ossification
    d. Hip dislocation

116. All of the following are clinical signs of heterotopic ossification except
    a. Pressure sores
    b. Pain
    c. Decreased range of motion
    d. Joint swelling

117. The most common clinical signs of a cerebellar brain tumor may include all of the following except
    a. Hypotonia
    b. Ataxia
    c. Vomiting
    d. Low back pain

118. Areas that a physical therapist can address with a child with an acquired brain injury in terms of long-term health and well-being include all of the following except
    a. Neurologic sequelae
    b. Growth disturbance
    c. Obesity
    d. Arthritis

119. Based on recent studies in children with traumatic brain injury, you would expect to see recovery slow down after _____ in a child with a severe injury.
    a. 6 months
    b. 1 year
    c. 3 years
    d. 5 years

120. Research indicates there is a significant correlation between functional restrictions in children with juvenile rheumatoid arthritis and
    a. The number of tender joints
    b. Elbow flexion contractures of 10 to 20 degrees
    c. Loss of motion in the hips or shoulders
    d. Low back pain

121. What is necessary for an infant to have mastered before sitting independently on propped upper extremities can be achieved?
    a. Rolling prone to supine and supine to prone
    b. Translation of grasped objects from hand to hand
    c. Extending the head and neck in prone, and controlling the pelvis while using the upper extremities in supine
    d. Crawling and creeping

122. When should sport-specific drills begin for the athlete following surgical repair of the anterior shoulder capsule?
    a. When the involved upper extremity has 30% strength of the uninvolved upper extremity.
    b. When the involved upper extremity has 50% strength of the uninvolved upper extremity.
    c. When the involved upper extremity has 75% strength of the uninvolved upper extremity.
    d. When the involved upper extremity has 100% strength of the uninvolved upper extremity.

123. During examination of a patient with neck pain and left arm pain, the therapist is suspicious of a C6 nerve root irritation. Which of the findings below will help confirm that condition?
    a. Weakness in shoulder abduction of left arm
    b. Decreased triceps reflex on left compared to right
    c. Decreased biceps reflex on left compared to right
    d. Increased tone in left biceps

124. Your patient was in a car accident and now has a herniated nucleus pulposis at vertebral level C5-C6. She reports difficulty removing her shirt overhead. With nerve root injury at the level of C5-C6, what part of the motion will most likely be problematic for your patient and why?
    a. Grasping the shirt due to weakness of all finger flexors
    b. Internally rotating the shoulder due to weakness of teres minor
    c. Shoulder flexion due to weakness of deltoid
    d. Cervical flexion to remove shirt due to weakness of deep neck flexors

125. A 55-year-old man with type I diabetes mellitus reports double vision. On examination of his extraocular movements, he has limited adduction, elevation, and depression of his right eye. The pupils are equal and reactive. The patient most likely has a lesion of the following right side cranial nerve
    a. Abducens nerve VI
    b. Trochlear nerve IV
    c. Oculomotor nerve III
    d. Optic nerve II

126. An overweight patient presents with right lower thoracic and right shoulder pain. She noted that the pain began after eating fried chicken at a fast food restaurant. You suspect it is a visceral pain coming from the
    a. Gall bladder
    b. Pancreas
    c. Liver
    d. Heart

127. Your patient has an involvement of the 5th lumbar nerve root on the left secondary to a lumbar disc protrusion. Which of the following is true?
    a. The ankle jerk is diminished or absent.
    b. The patient has fatigueable weakness in the calf.
    c. Sensation was diminished between the first and second toe.
    d. Sensation was diminished on the plantar surface of the foot.

128. Your patient is a 65-year-old male who complains of pain radiating down both legs with static and dynamic standing, but with relief while sitting. In the absence of any serious disease he most likely has a
    a. Herniated disc
    b. Lateral stenosis
    c. Central stenosis
    d. Schmorl's node defect

129. The classification of a nerve injury that would produce pain, muscle wasting, complete motor and sympathetic function loss with a recovery time of months, with sensation restored before motor function best describes
    a. Neuropraxia
    b. Axonotmesis
    c. Neurotmesis
    d. Axonopraxia

130. When performing resistive testing to determine the integrity of the C5 myotome, the physical therapist should examine which of the following movements?
    a. Wrist radial deviation
    b. Elbow extension
    c. Thumb extension
    d. Elbow flexion

131. While performing an upper quarter screen, a physical therapist suspects neurologic system involvement. In examining the integrity of the C8 dermatome, the therapist should check sensation along the
    a. Thumb and index finger
    b. Ulnar border of the hand
    c. Middle three fingers
    d. Radial border of the hand

132. A patient has been referred to physical therapy for acute shoulder pain after shoveling snow in a driveway for 2 hours. Positive findings include pain and weakness with flexion of an extended upper extremity as well as scapular winging with greater than 90 degrees of abduction. The patient's problem is MOST LIKELY the result of
    a. Supraspinatus tendinitis
    b. Compression of the long thoracic nerve
    c. Compression of the suprascapular nerve
    d. Subdeltoid bursitis

133. A physical therapist is conducting a physical examination with a patient diagnosed with an American Spinal Injury Association (ASIA) A spinal cord injury at the level of C6. During manual muscle testing of the upper extremity, the patient should have function in all of the following muscles EXCEPT the
    a. Biceps
    b. Triceps
    c. Deltoid
    d. Diaphragm

134. A physical therapist is treating an 18-year-old male who had an ASIA T1 spinal cord injury (SCI) 6 months ago. Given the level and completeness of the lesion, what would be his EXPECTED functional capability for transfers?
    a. Dependent with all mat mobility
    b. Dependent with wheelchair to mat transfers
    c. Independent with wheelchair to mat transfers
    d. Independent with floor to wheelchair transfers

135. A physical therapist completes a developmental assessment and notes the child is able to crawl forward, pull to stand at furniture, and sits without hand support for extended periods of time. The most appropriate chronologic age of this child is
    a. 4 to 5 months
    b. 6 to 7 months
    c. 8 to 9 months
    d. 11 months

136. A physical therapist completes a developmental assessment and identifies that the infant is unable to roll from supine to side. Which of the following reflexes could interfere with the action of rolling?
    a. Asymmetric tonic neck reflex
    b. Moro Reflex
    c. Landau reflex
    d. Symmetric tonic neck reflex

137. An inpatient physical therapist is performing an examination of an 8-year-old female that sustained a traumatic brain injury because of a motor vehicle accident. Which of the following standardized instruments would be most appropriate to measure the child's level of consciousness?
    a. MRI
    b. Modified Ashworth Scale
    c. Glasgow Coma Scale
    d. Barthel Scale

138. A 12-year-old female with cerebral palsy is admitted to the hospital for a Baclofen test dose to determine if she is a candidate for a Baclofen pump. One hour postinjection, the physical therapist assesses the tone in the lower extremities. There is marked increase in muscle tone through most of the ROM, but it is easily moved. What level is the ankle on the Modified Ashworth Scale?
    a. 1+
    b. 0
    c. 4
    d. 2

139. You are performing an examination on a 36-month-old male who is able to ascend stairs with a step to pattern, jump off of a step and runs with decreased coordination. The patient is unable to maintain single limb stance. What do you determine from this observation?
    a. The patient is demonstrating age appropriate skills.
    b. The patient is demonstrating skills at approximately the 10- to 12-month level.
    c. The patient is demonstrating skills at approximately the 18- to 20-month level.
    d. The patient is demonstrating skills at approximately the 30- to 32-month level.

140. Recovery of the upper arm after a brachial plexus injury can occur for up to
    a. 2 years
    b. 1 year
    c. 6 months
    d. 9 months

141. What is the major concern of the physical therapist treating a patient with an acute deep partial-thickness burn covering 27% of the total body? The patient was admitted to the intensive care burn unit 2 days ago.
    a. Range of motion
    b. Fluid retention
    c. Helping the family cope with the injured patient
    d. Home modifications on discharge

142. A patient is referred to physical therapy services for care of a burn wound on the left foot. The majority of the wound is anesthetic. There is significant eschar formation over the dorsum of the involved foot, and moderate subcutaneous tissue damage is present. What is the most likely classification of this burn?
    a. Electrical
    b. Superficial partial thickness
    c. Deep partial thickness
    d. Full thickness

143. A therapist is examining a wound in a patient with the following signs: the right foot has a toe that is gangrenous, the skin on the dorsum of the foot is shiny in appearance, and no calluses are present. The patient has what type of ulcer?
    a. Venous insufficiency ulcer
    b. Arterial insufficiency ulcer
    c. Decubitus ulcer
    d. Trophic ulcer

144. The most common hand deformity following burn injury in children is
    a. Hyper-extension of fifth MCP
    b. Radial deviation of wrist
    c. Boutonniere deformity
    d. Palmar contracture

145. A physical therapist is assessing the skin integrity over the ischial tuberosities of a 17-year-old female with spastic cerebral palsy after being transferred out of the child's wheelchair. The therapist notes that the wound extends to the bone. The therapist would stage this pressure sore as
    a. Stage I
    b. Stage II
    c. Stage III
    d. Stage IV

146. A 21-year-old female has sustained a traumatic brain injury and is demonstrating significant neurologic impairments. The physical therapist notices on examination a blister with surrounding erythema on the patient's sacrum. The physical therapist should document the patient as having which of the following?
    a. Stage I pressure ulcer
    b. Stage II pressure ulcer
    c. Stage III pressure ulcer
    d. Stage IV pressure ulcer

147. A diabetic patient is exercising vigorously in an outpatient clinic. The patient informs the therapist that he or she received insulin immediately before the exercise session. Of the following symptoms which is an unlikely sign of hypoglycemic coma?
    a. Pallor
    b. Shallow respiration
    c. Bounding pulse
    d. Dry skin

148. After arriving at the home of a home health patient, the primary nurse informs the therapist that she has activated emergency medical services. The nurse found the patient in what appears to be a diabetic coma. Which of the following is most likely not one of the patient's signs?
    a. Skin flush
    b. Rapid pulse
    c. Weak pulse
    d. High blood pressure

149. A therapist is treating a new patient in an outpatient facility. The patient has recently been diagnosed with type 1 insulin-dependent diabetes mellitus. The patient asks the therapist the differences between type 1 insulin-dependent diabetes mellitus and type 2 non–insulin-dependent diabetes mellitus. Which of the following statements is true?
    a. There is usually some insulin present in the blood in type 1 and none in type 2.
    b. Ketoacidosis is a symptom of type 2.
    c. The age of diagnosis with type 1 is usually younger than the age of diagnosis with type 2.
    d. Both conditions can be managed with a strict diet only, without taking insulin.

150. A 65-year-old man presents to physical therapy with complaints of pain due to compression fractures of the C2 and C3 vertebrae. The patient has an unusually large cranium. He describes his condition by stating, "Much of my bone tissue is continually decreasing, then reforming." The patient also indicates that the condition has caused limb deformity. Which of the following diseases does he have?
    a. Paget's disease
    b. Achondroplastic dwarfism
    c. Osteogenesis imperfecta
    d. Osteopetrosis

151. Improved survival rates for cancer increase the likelihood that a physical therapist will be treating patients with a past medical history of cancer and cancer treatment. Which statement does not accurately describe presentation of potential side effects of cancer treatment?
    a. Increased risk of infections and bleeding due to bone marrow suppression
    b. Debilitating fatigue that may persist in spite of rest
    c. Demineralization and bone necrosis that increases risk of pathologic fractures
    d. Symptoms that are easily distinguishable from cancer recurrence

152. A physical therapist is discussing appropriate exercise parameters for a patient with type II diabetes. Which statement reflects inappropriate advice to the patient?
    a. Do not begin exercise if blood glucose is above 100 mg/dl.
    b. Be sure to stay adequately hydrated.
    c. Avoid insulin injections in the active extremities within 1 hour before exercise.
    d. Exercise at moderate intensity and use rate of perceived exertion to help determine response to exercise.

153. Which of the following statements about lymph node palpation is true?
    a. Normal lymph nodes are generally not visible or easily palpable.
    b. A nontender, immovable lymph node is not significant.
    c. Only tender lymph nodes are important in differential diagnosis.
    d. Lymph node palpation will confirm an infection.

154. A 5-year-old male diagnosed with medulloblastoma is currently receiving chemotherapy. The physical therapist is preparing to treat this patient in an inpatient hospital setting. What lab value must the therapist consider before initiating treatment?
    a. WBC
    b. Glucose
    c. HDL/LDL
    d. Platelets

155. Differentiation of the sources of pain is critical to the accurate diagnosis and appropriate treatment of patient conditions. Which of the following would not describe pain or symptoms from a visceral source?
    a. It can be produced by the heart and internal organs.
    b. The symptoms tend to be well localized.
    c. Hypersensitivity to touch or pressure often accompanies disease.
    d. Generally associated signs and symptoms are present.

156. Your patient has complaints of loss of urine as soon as she has the urge to urinate. She also complains of deep pressure (NOT PAIN) in her lower pelvis area with prolonged standing. What kind of incontinence do this patient's symptoms most likely mimic?
    a. Stress incontinence
    b. Urge incontinence
    c. Mixed incontinence
    d. Functional incontinence

157. A patient with fibromyalgia has performance deficits in ADLs, including lack of a daily routine because of a loss of energy and motivation to engage in daily occupations, depression and anxiety, and difficulty managing home and instrumental activities of daily living (IADL) because of fatigue and pain. Based on these performance deficits, the initial focus of treatment should be
    a. Completing IADL tasks independently
    b. Establishing a new daily routine that can be done within the patient's tolerance
    c. Referring to a support group to address depression and anxiety
    d. Energy conservation and activities for pain management

158. Which of the following is least likely in a woman in the eighth month of pregnancy?
    a. Center of gravity anteriorly displaced
    b. Heart rate decreased with rest and increased with activity (compared to heart rate before pregnancy)
    c. Edema in bilateral lower extremities
    d. Blood pressure increased by 5% (compared with blood pressure before pregnancy)

159. A physical therapist receives an order to evaluate a home health patient. The primary nurse states that the patient "may have suffered a stroke because she cannot move the right leg when she stands." The history that the therapist obtains from the patient and family members includes: (1) left total hip replacement 6 months ago, (2) inability to lift the right lower extremity off of the floor in a standing position, (3) recent fall at home 2 nights ago, (4) left lower extremity strength with manual muscle testing in supine is 2+/5 overall, (5) complaints of pain with resisted movement of the left lower extremity, (6) right lower extremity strength is 4+/5 overall, (7) no pain with resisted movements with the right lower extremity, (8) no difference in bilateral upper extremity strength, (9) no decreased sensation, (10) no facial droop, (11) history of dementia but no decreased cognitive ability or speech level as compared with the prior level of function, and (12) independence in ambulation with a standard walker before the recent fall. What should the therapist's recommendation to the nursing staff be?
    a. The patient should receive physical therapy for strengthening exercises to the right lower extremity with standing exercises and gait training.
    b. The patient should receive a physician's evaluation for a possible stroke.
    c. The patient should receive a physician's evaluation for a possible left hip fracture.
    d. The patient should receive physical therapy for strengthening the left lower extremity and gait training.

160. A patient has been diagnosed with systemic lupus erythematosus. Which of the following is not a sign of this autoimmune disease?
    a. Increased photosensitivity
    b. Oral ulcers
    c. Butterfly rash
    d. Increased number of white blood cells

161. Which of the following circumstances would normally decrease body temperature in a healthy person?
    a. Exercising on a treadmill
    b. Pregnancy
    c. Normal ovulation
    d. Reaching age of 65 years or older

162. A physical therapist is speaking to a group of pregnant women about maintaining fitness level during pregnancy. Which of the following statements contains incorrect information?
    a. Perform regular exercise routines at least three times per week.
    b. Perform daily at least 15 minutes of abdominal exercises in supine position during the second and third trimesters.
    c. Increase caloric intake by 300 kcal per day.
    d. Exercise decreases constipation during pregnancy.

163. A 30-year-old woman who had a full-term infant 4 weeks ago presents to physical therapy with diastasis recti. The separation was measured by the physician and found to be 3 cm. Which of the following exercises is most appropriate to minimize the separation?
    a. Sit-ups while using the upper extremities to bring the rectus abdominis to midline
    b. Bridges while using the upper extremities to bring the rectus abdominis to midline
    c. Dynamic lumbar stabilization exercises in quadraped position
    d. Gentle head lifts in supine position while using the upper extremities to bring the rectus abdominis to midline

164. Proper supportive positioning of an infant with osteogenesis imperfecta is important for all of the following reasons except
    a. Keeping extremities immobilized to prevent fractures
    b. Protection from fracturing
    c. Minimizing joint malalignment and deformities
    d. Promotion of muscle strengthening

165. A gross motor program for a school-aged child with osteogenesis imperfecta should not include
    a. Muscle strengthening
    b. Aerobic conditioning
    c. Protected ambulation
    d. Keeping extremities immobilized to prevent fractures

166. In a child who has sustained a submersion injury, the physical therapist needs to be aware of neurologic and _____ system changes before initiating treatment.
    a. Integumentary
    b. Orthopedic
    c. Cardiopulmonary
    d. Renal

167. Which of the following is the only appropriate exercise in the third
     trimester of pregnancy?
     a. One-legged balance activities
     b. Quadraped (crawling position) with hip extension
     c. Bilateral straight leg raise
     d. Bridging

168. A physical therapist is performing ultrasound over the lumbar paraspinals
     of a patient. Which of the following conditions would cause the therapist
     to use a lower intensity and shorter dosage of treatment?
     a. Diabetes
     b. Hypertension
     c. Hypothyroidism
     d. Parkinson's disease

169. A patient in the sixth month of pregnancy is in a physical therapy
     clinic for examination secondary to lumbar pain. Which of the
     following is incorrect advice to give to this patient?
     a. Sleep on the left with a pillow between the knees.
     b. Sleep on the right with a pillow between the knees.
     c. Sleep supine with a pillow under the knees.
     d. Sit with a lumbar support at all times.

170. Elderly patients often present with atypical signs and symptoms.
     Which of the following best explains the atypical presentation of
     symptoms in the elderly?
     a. The number of potential risk factors for disease may be greater.
     b. They fail to make connections between their signs and symptoms.
     c. The onset of new disease often presents in the most vulnerable
        systems.
     d. They utilize home remedies that alter their signs and symptoms.

171. In a direct access state, a physical therapist is examining a patient with
     joint pain complaints. The patient has had no diagnostic work-up before
     arrival at the clinic. Which finding below would raise suspicion of
     rheumatoid arthritis rather than just osteoarthritic complaints?
     a. Morning stiffness that resolves within 10 to 15 minutes after
        getting up
     b. Development of joint pain in more than one joint with onset
        between 20 to 40 years of age
     c. Unilateral joint pain in hip or knee
     d. Absence of associated symptoms such as fatigue, weight loss, or
        malaise

172. Which descriptors make you suspicious of a neuropathic pain source?
    a. Aching, sore, dull
    b. Dreadful, cruel, punishing
    c. Burning, shooting, pricking
    d. Throbbing, pulsing, pounding

173. Which of the following statements is true relative to differentiation of dementia from depression in older adults?
    a. Memory loss associated with dementia is often noticed by the patient.
    b. Disorientation is generally associated with dementia but not depression.
    c. Difficulty concentrating is more common with dementia.
    d. Writing, speaking, and motor impairments are more common with depression.

174. A patient is difficult to arouse and falls asleep without constant stimulation from the therapist. Even when the patient is aroused, he has difficulty interacting with the physical therapist. What would be the BEST description of the patient's level of arousal?
    a. Stupor
    b. Lethargic
    c. Obtunded
    d. Alert

175. Mrs. Brown is a patient on the acute rehabilitation unit. She is sleepy, but easily roused when you enter the room. She knows her name but thinks she is at home. She is unable to give the year. She tries to get out of bed when you approach, and doesn't seem to realize she has weakness on the left side. Briefly describe Mrs. Brown's arousal, orientation, and cognition.
    a. Alert, oriented ×2, confused
    b. Obtunded, oriented ×1, confused
    c. Lethargic, oriented ×1, confused
    d. Sleepy, oriented ×3, confused

176. A physical therapist is testing a patient with diagnosis of vestibular impairment. Which of the following is most likely to be true?
    a. The vestibulo-ocular reflex (VOR) is normal so you can rule out posterior canal benign paroxysmal positional vertigo (BPPV).
    b. The VOR is delayed so you suspect a unilateral hypofunction.
    c. The dynamic visual acuity test shows a two-line loss so you suspect a unilateral hypofunction.
    d. The dynamic visual acuity test shows a four-line loss so you suspect posterior canal BPPV.

177.   Individuals with impaired vestibular system function are most likely
        to experience a loss of balance on the foam and dome test, or the
        Clinical Test of Sensory Integration and Balance (CTSIB), when
        information from the _____ is/are altered during testing.
        a. Spinal reticular system
        b. Visual system
        c. Somatosensory system
        d. Somatosensory and visual systems

178.   Your patient is a 45-year-old female with complaints of right
        shoulder pain and paresthesias running down her right arm. No
        specific dermatome. Symptoms have been increasing in the past
        3 months and now are continuous in nature. She has a history of
        smoking but quit 3 years ago. Her shoulder pain increases at night, as
        do her arm symptoms. She reports that in recent months she has been
        feeling tired more frequently and has been losing weight. What
        pathology is mostly likely the source of the patient's symptoms?
        a. Cancer
        b. Rotator cuff tear
        c. Cervical radiculopathy
        d. Thoracic outlet syndrome

179.   An 18-year-old male was involved in a motorcycle accident and has
        sustained a traumatic brain injury. The patient is starting to squeeze
        the therapist's hand upon command, beginning to recognize his
        mother, and withdraws to pain. The patient is at what stage on the
        Rancho Los Amigos Levels of Cognitive Functioning?
        a. II—generalized response
        b. III—localized response
        c. IV—confused-agitated
        d. V—confused-inappropriate, nonagitated

180.   You will be performing an examination on a 20-week-old female
        and will be completing the Peabody Developmental Motor Scale to
        determine the severity of developmental delay. In order to accurately
        score the patient, you must determine if the patient was born premature.
        During your examination, you learn that the patient was born at
        32 weeks' gestation. What is the patient's corrected/adjusted age?
        a. No adjustment is needed for this patient.
        b. The patient's corrected/adjusted age 10 weeks.
        c. The patient's corrected/adjusted age 12 weeks.
        d. The patient's corrected/adjusted age 14 weeks.

181. A patient requires examination 4 months following treatment for
      breast cancer and mastectomy. She is complaining of chest, arm,
      and shoulder pain with overhead activities. Which of the following
      conditions is most likely the source of her pain?
      a. Torn rotator cuff
      b. Adhesive capsulitis
      c. Cervical pathology
      d. Recurrence of the breast cancer

182. You observe that your patient walks with the spine in extension
      (increased lumbar lordosis). This could be due to all of the following
      except
      a. Tight semitendinosis
      b. Tight rectus femoris
      c. Tight psoas major
      d. Weak gluteus maximus

183. During normal gait, in single-limb stance,
      a. The center of mass is at its highest point
      b. Potential energy is at a low point
      c. Kinetic energy is at its highest point
      d. The magnitude of the ground reaction force is always greater than
          body weight

184. Which of the following is false regarding osteoarthritis?
      a. The initial biochemical changes include loss of proteoglycan and
          loosening of the collagen matrix.
      b. In severe cases, ulnar deviation of the metacarpophalangeal joints
          is observed.
      c. Later changes include cartilage thinning and joint space narrowing.
      d. In severe cases, total joint replacements are a realistic treatment
          option.

Answers

1. b. Thromboembolus formation is a common complication of thrombophlebitis in lower leg veins. Thrombi can pass through the heart and obstruct major pulmonary arteries.

2. d. These are signs and symptoms of a patient with bronchiectasis.

3. a. Claudication is a lack of blood flow. This test is performed by having a patient walk on a treadmill and recording how long the patient can walk before the onset of claudication. Homan's sign is a test performed to see whether a patient may have a deep vein thrombosis. The percussion test is designed to assess the integrity of the greater saphenous vein. Hoffa's test checks the integrity of the Achilles tendon.

4. b. A decreased tidal volume is caused by a restrictive lung dysfunction. An increased tidal volume is caused by an obstructive lung dysfunction. Choices C and D are in the family of obstructive pulmonary disease.

5. a. These signs are consistent with restrictive lung dysfunction. All other choices are obstructive lung dysfunctions.

6. d. Hypertension is a risk factor in atherosclerosis.

7. c. Patients with congestive heart failure often develop an enlarged heart because of the burden of an increased preload and afterload.

8. d. Apneusis can be described as an inspiratory cramp. Orthopnea is difficulty with breathing in a lying position. Eupnea is normal breathing. Apnea is the absence of breathing.

9. c. Mucoid sputum is clear or white and is not usually associated with infection. Thick sputum is referred to as tenacious. Foul-smelling sputum is called fetid and is often associated with infection.

10. b. Frothy sputum is thin and white or has a slight pink color. This type of sputum is commonly present with pulmonary edema. Purulent sputum resembles pus, with a yellow or green color. Mucopurulent sputum is yellow to light green in color. Rusty sputum is a rust-colored sputum often associated with pneumonia.

11.   c.   All exercises for this population should avoid the possibility of joint bleeding. High velocity isokinetics or high weight, low repetition exercises are a contraindication. Provided there is no active bleeding, exercise to any joint is indicated.

12.   d.   In cryoglobulinemia, ischemia can be caused by abnormal blood proteins gelling at low temperatures. Moist heat will not affect this condition.

13.   a.   The Six Minute Walk Test is used to determine a patient's functional exercise capacity.

14.   a.   An infant with a congenital heart defect often has a labored breathing pattern, increased respiratory rate, diaphoresis, tachycardia, edema, and feeding difficulties.

15.   b.   The pelvic diaphragm is composed of the levator ani and coccygeus muscles. This pelvic diaphragm assists in forced expiration, coughing, sneezing, vomiting, urinating, defecating, and fixation of the trunk during strong movements of the upper limb.

16.   b.   All four muscles are hamstring muscles of the posterior thigh. All four muscles extend the hip. Only the hamstring portion of adductor magnus does not cross the knee. It inserts on the adductor tubercle of the femur. The other three muscles cross the knee posteriorly and therefore flex the knee.

17.   c.   Adductor longus, rectus femoris, and iliopsoas are the muscles typically involved in hip muscle strain/tendonitis/tendinosis. Pain is aggravated by activity or in resistance testing. Adductor strains arise in horseback riders, skiers, and skaters.

18.   a.   History and type/site of pain are the most important features to direct the examination. Piriformis irritation often presents as dull posterior hip pain radiating down the leg, mimicking radicular symptoms. Limping, pain aggravated by active external rotation, or passive internal rotation on palpation of sciatic notch is a salient feature.

19.   c.   While direct visualization of articular cartilage is possible with both MRI and CT, MRI gives better resolution and detail. Neither bone scan nor plain film radiography will show the cartilage.

20.   a.   MRI does not provide any form of radiation to the patient.

21. a. Ortolani's test is used to detect a congenitally dislocated hip in an infant. Choices B and C are common meniscus damage tests for the knee. Choice D is performed by placing the infant in supine position with the hip at 90 degrees of flexion and slight abduction and the knee flexed to 90 degrees. The examiner then moves the infant's hip anterior and posterior in an effort to detect abnormal joint mobility.

22. c. Osgood-Schlatter disease is severe tendinitis of the patellar tendon. It is characterized by pronounced tibial tubercles. The increased size of the tubercles is attributed to the patella tendon pulling away from its insertion. Jumper's knees (or normal patella tendinitis) does not necessarily present with tubercle enlargement. Sever's disease involves the Achilles tendon pulling away from its insertion on the calcaneus.

23. a. Choice A describes rheumatoid arthritis, a systemic condition. All of the other choices are signs and symptoms of osteoarthritis (OA). Sometimes OA can involve symmetric joints, but it is not systemic.

24. c. Dupuytren's contracture is a progressive thickening of the palmar aponeurosis of the hand. The progression is gradual, and the interphalangeal joints are pulled into flexion.

25. a. The screw home mechanism that is present in the last few degrees of terminal knee extension stresses the MCL. Side-lying hip adduction also places the MCL in a position of stretch.

26. d. A positive Tinel's sign screens for carpal tunnel syndrome when the tapping force is performed over the carpal tunnel itself. In Phalen's test, the therapist places the patient's wrists in maximal flexion and holds for 1 minute. The test is positive if there is paresthesia in the median nerve distribution. The Finkelstein test screens for de Quervain's disease by allowing the patient to make a fist with the thumb wrapped in the fingers. The test is positive if there is pain over the adbuctor pollicis longus and extensor pollicis brevis tendons.

27. d. The hip strategy is used to compensate for large movements in the center of mass, and the ankle strategy is used to compensate for small movements.

28. c. This scenario describes a greenstick fracture, which is common in young people. In a comminuted fracture, the bone is broken into pieces. An example of an avulsion fracture is when the tibial tuberosity is pulled off the tibia. A bone that has a segmental fracture is fractured in two places.

29. b. Nursemaid's elbow is defined as dissociation of the radial head from the annular ligament. Choices A and D are usually to the result of a fall on an extended elbow. Erb's palsy is due to cervical trauma.

30. d. Sever's disease is traction apophysitis of the gastrocnemius tendon in children. In other words, the gastrocnemius attempts to pull away from the calcaneus, causing an inflammatory condition.

31. c. The signs and symptoms are most consistent with a slipped capital epiphysis. Bursitis presents with pain located over the bursa and is associated with overuse or rheumatoid arthritis. Avascular necrosis most frequently involves men 30 to 50 years of age. Septic arthritis is usually present in children 2 years of age or younger and often is due to steroid use or fever.

32. a. The anterior cruciate ligament prevents excessive posterior roll of the femoral condyles during flexion of the femur at the knee joint.

33. b. The extensor carpi radialis brevis absorbs most of the stress placed on the involved upper extremity in the position of wrist flexion, ulnar deviation, forearm pronation, and elbow extension (as with a backhand swing in tennis).

34. c. Swan-neck deformity involves hyperextension of the proximal interphalangeal (PIP) joint and flexion of the distal interphalangeal (DIP) joint. Splinting to avoid this deformity is the treatment of choice. Boutonnière deformity involves flexion of the PIP joint and DIP joint hyperextension. Dupuytren's contracture is contracture of the palmar aponeurosis. Claw hand is the result of laceration of the ulnar nerve.

35. b. The extensor carpi ulnaris is frequently subluxed after rupture of the triangular fibrocartilage complex. Subluxation leads to many mechanical changes in the wrist that are common in patients with rheumatoid arthritis.

36. d. A patient with hammer toes exhibits hyperextension of the distal interphalangeal joints and metatarsophalangeal joints and flexion of the proximal interphalangeal joints.

37. c. Race has no role in progression of scoliosis, idiopathic or congenital.

38. d. In clubfoot, the calcaneus is small, the hindfoot is in varus, and there is equinas of the ankle. There is typically no tibial involvement.

39. a. In calcaneovalgus, the forefoot is lateral, the hind foot is in valgus, and the foot is in full dorsiflexion. This results simply from a large infant in too small of a space, and the condition improves spontaneously. Calcaneovalgus should not be confused with a vertical talus. A vertical talus is a serious deformity involving malalignment of the talus and navicular. The forefoot is dorsiflexed, the hind foot is plantar flexed, and the foot bends at the instep.

40. b. Ortolani's maneuver involves dislocation of the hip in flexion and adduction. Gentle flexion, abduction, and traction reduce the hip. Ortolani's maneuver indicates a more unstable hip than the Barlow test.

41. a. Osteomyelitis is a rapid infection of the bone in adolescents often in the distal femur or proximal tibia. Radiographic changes are not seen until 7 to 14 days after onset.

42. b. Although these diagnoses can occur in most joints, the hip is the most common site of occurrence.

43. d. Hip pain is common with this diagnosis, as is a traumatic history; However, a slipped capital femoral epiphysis can have a chronic onset as well. Because a standard anterior or posterior view can miss the slip, the frog leg radiograph will need to be viewed to determine the correct diagnosis.

44. d. Training errors are common if the correct techniques are not taught vigorously. Musculotendinous imbalances can occur if training overemphasizes a certain muscle group over its antagonist. Malalignment of the lower extremities is seen with muscular imbalances over a period of time. Grass or turf has not been shown to increase risk of overuse injury.

45. b. Since juvenile rheumatoid arthritis attacks the joint as in adult rheumatoid arthritis, there are no neurologic signs or symptoms.

46. d. A third-degree heart block can appear as dizziness and fatigue and may require a pacemaker. Patients with asthma and obesity should be monitored closely but should be permitted to exercise. Dialysis should be scheduled on non-dialysis days.

47. d. The axillary nerve is in close proximity to the surgical field in this patient. ROM is normal so choice B is incorrect; poor compliance would lead to a multitude of problems rather than just deltoid weakness. The musculocutaneous nerve is not involved with this procedure, and it innervates muscles involved in elbow flexion.

48. d. The other choices will be important later in the rehabilitation of this diagnosis. ROM is important early to reduce abnormal scar tissue formation.

49. b. The masseter muscle (deep portion) is likely the cause of the pain. The temporalis tendon is located anterior to the masseter on the coronoid process, the maxillary sinuses are located under the cheeks, and the parotid glands are located on the masseter. Parotid infection involves swelling and problems producing saliva.

50. c. The likely cause of her headache is temporal arteritis. Giant cell arteritis can affect the temporal artery. It is an inflammatory vascular condition of the temporal arteries and can cause intermittent claudication of the masseter with pain on chewing. The age, new onset of headache, and acute severity of temporal headache are a red flag the patient should see the physician because of possible progressive blindness.

51. c. The disorder has to be muscular because of the normal mobility of lateral and protrusive movements. If it were a joint dysfunction, both joints would be involved and there would be diminished mobility of lateral and protrusive movements.

52. b. The right TMJ is hypomobile, and the left is moving normally. An anterior disc displacement with reduction should display clicking, and the passive opening will increase with overpressure. Trismus would display normal range of motion of laterotrusion and protrusion.

53. d. Temporomandibular reciprocal click is clicking that occurs during opening and closing. Reciprocal clicking is caused by the disc being displaced partially anteriorly. The condyle slides under the disc and clicks into its normal position during opening then slips back out during closing.

54. d. If the right TMJ is inflamed, swelling may cause the bite to change and shift to the opposite side.

55. b. For example: the right joint is locked. Anterior translation primarily occurs after 26 mm; therefore, opening will be restricted at 26 mm and deflection will occur to the right (same side). Lateral movement to the opposite side (movement to the left, or contralateral side) will be restricted because the right joint cannot translate; protrusion will deflect to the hypomobile side (right) and be restricted.

56. a. Patients tend to posteriorly rotate the pelvis to substitute with the tensor fascia latae or the gluteus minimus. These muscles are medial rotators not lateral rotators like the posterior gluteus medius. The lateral hamstrings are not hip abductors.

57. b. Osgood-Schlatter's is an injury to apophyseal cartilage. It is not an inflammatory condition and occurs mainly in young boys.

58. a. An immediate knee effusion after trauma always indicates bleeding from fracture, ligament tear, meniscus tear, or patella dislocation.

59. c. High pitch counts have been shown in several studies to be responsible for the majority of shoulder problems in pitchers.

60. c. The acceleration phase is the phase where maximum valgus stress is placed on the elbow and ulnar collateral ligament.

61. d. Black line tibial stress fractures occur on the anterior cortex and form because of stress in tension. They can be extremely difficult to heal and require intrameddulary rodding to achieve union.

62. d. Soft tissue ankle impingement is recognized as a common source of anterior ankle pain following injury. It is more common than bone injury.

63. d. Swimmer's shoulder is an impingement of the greater tuberosity against the anterior acromial arch and coracoacromial ligament.

64. c. Obtunded. This patient requires continual stimulus to stay awake. The patient in a stupor is not interactive, while a lethargic patient stays interactive with stimulation during a session.

65. c. Based on the history of trauma you must first test AROM before you touch the patient. If there happens to be something serious such as a fracture in the upper cervical spine then motion will be restricted. You will need to send the patient back to a physician before risking injury.

66. c. The piano key sign is used specifically for testing for an acromio-clavicular separation. Pushing down on the distal clavicle that is elevated from injury will cause it to come back up once the force is released.

67. c. Based on the symptoms, the most likely cause of the injury is a torn meniscus. There is immediate swelling with blood in the joint, and locking of the joint with restricted range. A and B are extraarticular and will not cause bleeding inside the joint. You will not typically find joint locking with this injury. Cruciate ligament injuries do not usually get immediate swelling unless accompanied by a meniscal injury.

68. c. The only correct answer is C. The load and shift test assesses anterior instability. The crank test in answers B and D is a test for stability of the labrum. Speed's test assesses the long head of the biceps and the anterior apprehension tests for shoulder instability.

69. d. A, B, and C will present with the typical capsular patterns in their respective joint. A loose body in the shoulder will inhibit one plane of motion but will not limit any other motions. Hence, it would not be a capsular pattern.

70. b. The only possible correct answer is B. It is the typical pattern one sees with a Trendelenberg gait, where because of weakness of the gluteus medius on the weight-bearing leg, the hip on the contralateral side lowers.

71. d. Coronoid fractures seldom are isolated fractures. They are usually accompanied by radial head fractures. The brachialis is the muscle usually avulsed. Coronoid fractures only account for 1% to 2% of all elbow fractures.

72. c. This is a classic sign of an impingement. The position of 90 degrees of flexion with internal rotation is actually the position for a Hawkins Kennedy test. A patient with instability will present with a loose joint that feels like it is going to sublux. Patients with SLAP lesions will complain of intermittent painful popping, clunking, or clicking in the shoulder with occasional catches. An impingement will be most painful in certain positions such as extreme overhead reaches and with the test position just described.

73. c. This is a classical description of a De Quirvain's syndrome, which is a tendinitis of the abductor pollicus longus and extensor pollicus brevis. Gout will cause the thumb to be painful, but will not respond to stretch because it affects the joint and not the surrounding musculature. A scaphoid instability will be painful to certain movements accompanied by pops and cracks. It is an inert tissue and will not respond to stretch or resistance. Radial carpal syndrome is an impingement syndrome that takes place at the wrist.

74. b. This is classic description of a coxa varum, first described radiographically by Hofmeister in 1894. A coxa valgum has an angle of above 140 degrees. An acetabular tropism describes changes in the acetabular surface. Pelvic obliquity describes angulation of the pelvis from the horizontal in the frontal plane, possibly secondary to a contraction below the pelvis (e.g., of the hip joint).

75. d. The anterior cruciate is one of the most commonly injured ligaments without contact. Injuries to the posterior collateral ligament (PCL) do not usually feel the "pop" that the ACL does. They are usually injured from hitting a dash board or falling on a bent knee in sports. The meniscus injury will present with popping, catching, locking, and immediate joint swelling. The medial collateral ligament usually is exquisitely tender over the ligament and usually is torn with a lateral force.

76. b. There are four structures that are responsible for the pronator syndrome: the flexor digitorum arcade, the lacertus fibrosis, the pronator teres, and supraconcylar process. The lacertus fibrosis is tested by resisted supination.

77. c. Resisting forearm supination should place stress on the biceps brachii which functions as both an elbow flexor and forearm supinator. Resisting the action of the muscles, which is suspected of have a lesion, is one way to implicate or verify involvement of the tissue structure. Any decision is based on the pattern of pain elicited by both active and passive movements. The findings in the clinical case presented in the question begin to implicate or verifies involvement of the biceps.

78. c. Tightness of the gastrocsoleus muscle complex can cause a loss of dorsiflexion at the ankle. Having adequate ankle dorsiflexion throughout the stance phases of gait is important to the kinematics of tibial movement. When there is inadequate ankle dorsiflexion, which can occur due to gastrocsoleus tightness, one common finding is knee hyperextension or genu recurvatum.

79. b. The observed action of the foot would be consistent with motion produced by the tibialis posterior. The tibialis posterior plantar flexes and inverts the foot.

80. b. Based on the values provided by the American Academy of Orthopedic Surgeons, the clinical finding exceeds the expected normal range of motion for hip internal rotation, which is 0 to 45 degrees.

81. d. Transferring from a sitting to a standing position will pose the greatest challenge because of the need to generate force in the extensor muscles. Going from sitting to standing requires the recruitment of the hip and knee extensors.

82. a. Classic symptoms of anklylosing spondylitis include insidious onset of worsening, dull, lumbosacral back pain; progressive morning stiffness; pain in the sacroiliac region; prolonged stiffness with inactivity; absence of neurologic signs; tenderness at the sacral ligaments; and chest pain with deep breathing.

83. c. The supine to sit test demonstrates a functional left length difference resulting from a pelvic dysfunction caused by pelvic torsion or rotation.

84. a. An initial spinal cord lesion results in spinal shock, which lasts for 1 week to 3 months. During spinal shock, the spinal cord may function as though it is alive both above and below the level. The problem is one of communication; the brain cannot receive sensory information beyond the lesion site and cannot volitionally control motor function below that point. Eventually, this subsides, and in upper motor neuron lesion, spasticity normally increases.

85. b. Most anatomists agree that 80% to 90% of the fibers of the corticospinal tract cross over.

86. c. The rubrospinal tract originates in the red nucleus; the reticulospinal tract originates in the medullary and pontine reticular formation; and the vestibulospinal tract originates in the lateral vestibular nucleus.

87. c. Alzheimer's and stroke (cerebrovascular accident) are the two most common causes of dementia in the elderly. Depression may coincide with dementia but is not a cause.

88. a. About two thirds of the cases of Guillain-Barré syndrome are preceded by an acute influenza-like illness. It is also characterized by weakness beginning in the distal limb and advancing to affect the proximal muscles and inflammation and demyelination of spinal nerve roots and peripheral nerves.

89. b. Bell's palsy is a disease process affecting the seventh cranial nerve leading to abrupt facial paralysis/weakness and the symptoms presented in the case study; it is usually unilateral and self-remitting within a few months to a year. Several possible causes have been linked to the onset or recurrence of the disease process, one of which is a recent viral infection. Obvious physical examination findings involve those structures innervated by the seventh cranial nerve. Other areas of the body are not affected with Bell's palsy, as would be evident with Lyme disease, Guillain-Barré syndrome, and stroke. In stroke, the patient is able to wrinkle the forehead.

90. a. Spinal cord lesions usually present with upper motor neuron signs below the level of the lesion; however, if the lesion involves the anterior horn cells, there will also be lower motor neuron signs at the site of the lesion. Therefore, based on the information provided in the question, the lesion must be located at C5 on the left side of the spinal cord and involving the anterior horn cells.

91. a. The danger in using a hot tub for a person with multiple sclerosis is that it may cause extreme fatigue. There is no need to avoid the other activities listed.

92. d. A child with spastic diplegia most often presents with the lower extremities and trunk more involved than the upper extremities. Also one side is often more involved than the other side.

93. b. The question describes a hemisection of the spinal cord, which is classified as a Brown-Sequard lesion. Anterior spinal cord injuries present with loss of motor function and insensitivity to pain and temperature bilaterally. Central cord injuries are characterized by loss of function in the upper extremities and normal function in the trunk and lower extremities.

94. c. Choice B describes a swan-neck deformity.

95. c. This scenario describes a central cord lesion. It is common in the geriatric population after cervical extension injuries (such as whiplash).

96. c. This set of signs and symptoms most likely points to multiple sclerosis. The other conditions listed are progressive, but the best answer is multiple sclerosis.

97. d. These signs and symptoms are most likely associated with damage to the cerebellum. Injuries to the basal ganglia can present with: rigidity, resting tremor, choreiform movements (jerky movements), and difficulty with initiating movement. Frontal lobe lesions lead to a change in mood or overall personality. The dorsal columns are involved in proprioception and awareness of movement.

98. c. A burst fracture causes damage to the spinal cord because bony fragments are pushed posteriorly into the spinal canal. This type of fracture is often accompanied with anterior cord syndrome.

99. a. The symptoms involving the left lower extremity are an indication that a disc is herniated or protruding onto a nerve root on the left side. A positive straight leg-raise test is also often an indication of a disc herniation or protrusion.

100. c. The foot drop is caused by a lack of active dorsiflexion. The tibialis anterior is responsible for this motion and is innervated by the deep peroneal nerve.

101. d. The involved upper extremity is in this position because of damage to the C5 and C6 spinal roots.

102. b. This form of spina bifida is associated with direct involvement with the cauda equina. The muscles that are innervated by the cauda equina usually present with flaccid paralysis.

103. d. This is a description of a CT scan. A PET scan is performed by injecting a radioactive compound into the person being tested and then forming a picture of the brain with a computer that picks up the compound that reaches the brain tissue. An MRI picks up radiofrequency waves that are emitted by atomic particles displaced by radio waves in a magnetic field. An angiogram uses a high contrast dye that reveals the vessels of the brain by x-ray.

104. d. A person with spastic quadriplegia presents with talipes equinovarus. This term is synonymous with clubfoot. The hindfoot will be in varus and the calcaneous will be abnormally small.

105. c. Neurapraxia is not associated with axon degeneration; it is associated instead with demyelination and complete recovery. With axonotmesis there is wallerian degeneration below the site of the lesion. In neurotmesis the damage is so severe that full function may not be regained.

106. d. Dermatome charts in distribution vary from source to source, but one common aspect of C7 innervation is the middle finger. The triceps muscles are also innervated by C7.

107. b. This patient is suffering from Guillain-Barré syndrome. Some permanent damage can result, with loss of sensory or motor function, but most patients make a full recovery in approximately 6 months. The syndrome often starts after a person has had a bout of the flu or a respiratory infection.

108. d. This type of movement, known as athetosis, also can involve the feet, proximal parts of the extremities, and face. Chorea is rapid movements of the hands, wrist, or face. Ballism refers to forceful and uncontrollable throwing of the extremities outward. Lead-pipe rigidity is increasing resistance of an extremity to passive ranging. All of the aforementioned can result from damage to the basal ganglia.

109. d. Meralgia paresthetica is the compression of the lateral femoral cutaneous nerve of the thigh as it passes under the inguinal ligament near the anterior superior iliac spine. Examples of the source of this problem include periods of obesity, postural changes, and tight clothing. Lumbar disc involvement and spondylolisthesis are less likely choices because the question indicates normal range of motion, lack of motor weakness, and no change with repeated active lumbar flexion.

110. a. A valgus stress is most likely to injure any medial elbow structures, such as the ulnar nerve. The structures on the lateral side are likely to be injured with a varus stress. Choice C originates on the lateral supracondylar ridge.

111. d. These signs and symptoms are common with median nerve compression as it travels through the two heads of the pronator teres. Carpal tunnel syndrome usually presents with a positive Tinel's sign, a positive Phalen's test, and decreased strength and sensation over the median nerve distribution. Ulnar nerve compression at Guyon's canal typically presents with numbness, pain, and tingling along the ulnar nerve distribution.

112. c. Cerebral palsy children are slow to reach motor milestones. This is the most accurate choice. Studies show that his group of children will walk by age 8.

113. a. While all of the choices do occur in children with a spinal cord injury, choice A is the most appropriate. During the first year of spinal cord injury, 40% of bone mineral density is lost through calcium excreted in the urine.

114. d. Cauda equine syndrome is the most likely of the choices to regrow damaged axons, since it is essentially damage to the peripheral nerves. All other choices are damage to the spinal cord itself.

115. a. The other choices are more probable in a tetraplegic child.

116. a. Since heterotopic ossification involves pathologic bone formation around joints, pressure sores are not an indication of the presence of heterotopic ossification.

117. d. Low back pain is not an indicator of a brain lesion.

118. b. A physical therapist can provide intervention for all of the other choices listed regardless of the presence of a brain injury. Growth disturbances are out of the control of the therapist.

119. b. Progress will slow to a halt 1 year after a severe injury. The actual length of recovery varies according to many factors such as area of the brain injured, type of injury, treatment after injury, and so on.

120. b. Choice B involves the larger joints. Loss of motion in these joints is more likely to impact daily function. Low back pain is common, but not debilitating, as is a minimal elbow flexion contracture.

121. c. Choice C is the most appropriate. Some of the other choices may be mastered, but C is the most necessary. Choice B is achieved around 3 months of age, and D around 9 months of age.

122. c. Choice C is appropriate. This level of strength would allow normal ROM throughout the specific skill involved. Less than this level of strength would risk damage to the joint or surgical repair.

123. c. Examination of root irritation can be conducted by myotome, dermatome, or reflexes. The bicep brachii reflex is indicative of a C6 lesion. Increased tone is associated with upper motor lesions. Shoulder abduction tests the C5 nerve root, while the tricep brachii reflex is involves the C7 nerve root.

124. c. A herniation at C5-6 results in nerve root compression of C5. This corresponds to the axillary nerve supplying the deltoid. The teres minor is also innervated by the axillary nerve; however it is an external rotator. Cervical flexion is innervated by the cervical spinal nerves C1-C4. Finger flexors are innervated by the ulnar nerve arising from nerve root levels C7, C8 and T1.

125. c. Oculomotor nerve III. The occulomotor nerve innervates muscles that produce eye adduction, elevation, and depression.

126. a. The answer that is most true is that the gall bladder and liver both can refer pain to the right shoulder area. However, the liver is usually not affected by eating but rather lack of eating and alcohol. The pancreas refers pain to the middle of the back and left upper abdominal quadrant. The heart refers pain mostly to the chest and left side of the face, neck, and arm. Occasionally it can refer to the opposite side. However, there would be other symptoms accompanying the pain such as clamminess and a change in vital signs. The gallbladder, if involved, responds poorly when fatty foods are ingested.

127. c. The most consistent area of L5 sensation loss is between the first and second toe. The ankle jerk tests the S1 level. The nerve that comes out of L5-S1 interspace is S1. Sensation loss on the bottom of the foot could be S1 or S2 involvement. Weakness in the calf incriminates S1.

128. c. The narrowing of the central canal can produce bilateral leg symptoms as can a large central disc dysfunction. However, pain from a disc dysfunction will increase with sitting because of a flexed posture. Backward bending will increase lateral stenosis and central stenosis pain, but typically but it is unilateral and may only affect one dermatome or motor area, whereas central stenosis may affect several dermatomes. Sitting will provide relief with a central stenosis.

129. b. According to Sunderland's and Seddon's classification of nerve injuries, the description provided best describes axonotmesis. Neurotmesis involves complete disruption of the nerve while neuropraxia is only transient, and there is little or no muscle wasting. Axonopraxia is a similar term for neuropraxia.

130. d. Myotome testing can be important in localizing central and peripheral lesions. A lesion involving the C5 myotome will affect the client/patient's ability to flex the elbow. Key muscles innervated at this level include the biceps brachii and the deltoid.

131. d. Several dermatomes, C6-C8, are responsible for sensory innervation of the hand. The dorsum and palmer surfaces of the thumb, first finger and thenar eminence receive their sensory component from C6. Dermatome C7 is responsible for the palmar and dorsal surfaces of the third and fourth fingers and middle portion of the palm. The C8 dermatome specifically provides sensation along the ulnar boarder of the hand, including the fifth finger and is part of the screen for peripheral or central nervous system impairment.

132. b. Compression of the long thoracic nerve will result in serratus anterior weakness, which has associated postural and motor disturbances. In terms of posture, weakness of the serratus anterior will result in scapular winging. Motor disturbances can also occur because of the action of the serratus anterior on the scapula during overhead reaching.

133. b. In a complete ASIA A C6 lesion, muscle function impairments would be expected below the indicated level of the identified lesion. The triceps is innervated by the radial nerve, which arises from spinal levels C7-C8. Spinal levels C3-C5 give rise to the phrenic nerve, which innervates the diaphragm. The biceps is innervated by spinal levels C5-C6. The axillary nerve, which runs to the deltoid, arises from the C5-C6 spinal levels.

134. c. Achieving independence for wheelchair to mat transfers is a realistic expected level of function given the lesion. According to Somers (Spinal Cord Injury: Functional Rehabilitation) and Sisto, Druin and Sliwinski (Spinal Cord Injuries: Management and Rehabilitation), achieving independence is a realistic goal for the level and type of lesion. Upper extremity function is present, which allows independence for most transfers; thus, that patient is not likely to be dependent for mat mobility and wheelchair to mat transfers. Transferring from the floor to wheelchair may require assistance.

135. c. Between 8 and 9 months the patient is able to obtain quadruped from a prone position, sit without support, pivot in sitting, crawl forward, and cruise along furniture.

136. a. Asymmetric tonic neck reflex occurs when an infant's head is positioned to one side with flexion of the contralateral upper extremity extension of the other. This would interfere with rolling.

137. c. The Glasgow Coma scale is used to assess the child's ability to respond to various stimuli (eye opening, verbal responses, and motor responses).

138.　d.　A 2 on the Modified Ashworth Scale is defined by more marked increase in muscle tone through most of the ROM, but affected limbs easily moved.

139.　c.　The 18- to 20-month-old toddler will be able to ascend stairs with a step to pattern, run, and jump off of a bottom step.

140.　a.　Continued recovery can occur for up to 2 years in the upper arm and 4 years in the lower arm.

141.　a.　A therapist's main responsibility with this patient is to maintain range of motion. Fluid retention is an important concern but for other medical staff. Choices C and D will be addressed later in the patient's course of therapy.

142.　d.　A superficial partial-thickness burn and a deep partial-thickness burn are not deep enough to involve the subcutaneous tissue. An electrical burn is complete destruction of the subcutaneous tissue. A full-thickness burn produces moderate subcutaneous tissue damage and little pain.

143.　b.　These signs are characteristic of an arterial insufficiency ulcer. A venous ulcer often presents with the following symptoms: no pain around the wound, no gangrene, location typically on the medial ankle, pigmented skin around the ulcer, and significant edema. A trophic ulcer (also known as a pressure or decubitus ulcer) presents with decreased sensation, callused skin, and no pain and is located over bony prominences.

144.　d.　The relative weakness of the musculature of a child will allow scar tissue to contract the palmar aponeurosis. Careful splinting of this area should be considered.

145.　d.　A stage IV pressure sore is a full-thickness skin loss with extensive destruction, tissue necrosis or damage to muscle, bone or supporting structures.

146.　b.　A stage II pressure sore results in partial-thickness skin loss involving the epidermis, dermis, or both. The ulcer is superficial and presents clinically as an abrasion, blister, or shallow crater.

147.　d.　Dry skin is a sign of a diabetic coma.

148.　d.　A person in a diabetic coma has low blood pressure.

149.   c.   A person is usually diagnosed with type1 at 25 years of age or younger. A person is usually 40 years of age or older when diagnosed with type 2. Ketoacidosis is a symptom of type 1. Metabolism of free fatty acids in the liver causes this condition, which is an excess of ketones. A type 2 diabetic may be able to control his or her condition with diet only (depending on the severity of the condition), but a type I diabetic needs insulin.

150.   a.   In Paget's disease (also known as osteitis deformans), bone is resorped and deposited at different rates during different stages of the disease. One of the deformities sometimes present is an enlarged cranium. This increased weight can result in compression fractures of the more superior cervical vertebrae. The origin of this condition is not exactly known. It usually involves people over 60 years of age.

151.   d.   It is not always possible to determine side effects of cancer treatment versus cancer recurrence. Therapists must therefore be aware of immediate and long-term effects of cancer treatment.

152.   a.   Blood glucose levels should be between 100 to 250 mg/dl. The other instructions are all appropriate for the diabetic patient.

153.   a.   Normal lymph nodes are generally not palpable or visible. Current guidelines suggest any suspicious lymph node should be evaluated by a physician. Hard, immobile lymph nodes tend to raise suspicion of cancer. Tender, moveable nodes are associated with infections, allergies, or food intolerance. Lymph node palpation will not confirm a diagnosis, which is why medical referral is necessary.

154.   d.   A low platelet count or thrombocytopenia is a common side effect of chemotherapy. A low platelet count places the patient at risk for bleeding and therefore needs to be considered before intervention.

155.   b.   Visceral sources of pain are not well localized because of multisegmental innervation and lack of receptors in the structures. The other statements are all correct.

156.   b.   Though this patient may also have some pelvic organ descension, her symptoms are most likely matching urge incontinence, which is defined as "involuntary loss of urine occurring for no apparent reason while suddenly feeling the need or urge to urinate. The most common cause of urge incontinence is involuntary and inappropriate detrusor muscle contractions."

157. d. An initial short-term goal is to instruct in energy conservation and assist the patient in dealing with fatigue and pain. Because energy level and pain are more tolerable, the patient can establish a new daily routine. Creating a sense of control over the daily routine can lead to a feeling of success and may have an impact on anxiety and depression.

158. b. During pregnancy a woman normally experiences an increase in resting heart rate and a decrease in heart rate during exercise. This change is compared with the heart rate of the particular woman before pregnancy. The other answers about pregnancy are true.

159. c. The right lower extremity is still strong, and there is no facial droop or diminished sensation. Although these signs are not always present after a stroke, the other signs and symptoms, such as a history of a recent fall and the past total hip replacement, should lead the therapist to choice C. The patient cannot lift the right lower extremity in the standing position because it increases weight bearing on the fractured left lower extremity. The left leg also shows a definite strength loss as graded with manual muscle testing.

160. d. The white cell count in a patient with this diagnosis would decrease. Lupus affects mostly young women.

161. d. The geriatric population usually has a decreased body temperature due to poor diet, decreased cardiovascular status, and decreased metabolic rates.

162. b. Supine positioning after the first trimester is associated with decreased cardiac output.

163. d. With a separation of this size, the therapist should use gentle abdominal strengthening while binding the abdominal region.

164. a. Immobilizing the extremities would not allow for normal growth and development. Care must be taken for proper positioning and management of possible fractures, but immobilizing the extremities would not allow for motor milestones to be reached. Proper positioning will also promote muscle strengthening and bone mineralization.

165. d. Children with osteogenesis imperfecta should be allowed to mature at the same rate as other children. Social skill development may be compromised if the child is not allowed to participate in some activities. Keeping the extremities immobilized will not allow for more normal growth and development.

166. c. After the neurologic system is compromised, the cardiovascular system will shut down, causing irreparable damage. Although all systems are important, the cardiovascular is the most important.

167. d. Choice A may result in undue stress to the pubic symphysis, or SI, and can be dangerous secondary to center of gravity changes. Hip extension in a quadraped position may cause abnormal hyperextension of the lumbar spine, and bilateral straight leg raises could cause a diastasis recti because of the additional stress to the abdominal muscle group.

168. a. Ultrasound treatments performed on a diabetic may cause a reduction in blood sugar. All the other choices are not affected by ultrasound.

169. c. At this stage of pregnancy, the weight of the uterus can compromise the vena cava. The supine position should only be assumed for 5 minutes at a time.

170. c. Although the elderly often use home remedies and have additional co-morbidities, the onset of a new disease generally presents with symptoms in the most vulnerable systems. This explains the atypical presentation of disease in these individuals. The elderly are not different from other patients in terms of failure to make connections between signs and symptoms.

171. b. The onset of RA is most common in persons between the ages of 20 and 40 years. Morning stiffness usually lasts 45 minutes or longer. RA tends to involve more than one joint, and frequently has associated signs and symptoms such as fatigue and malaise.

172. c. Pain descriptors provide clues to the source of the pain. Choice C is a typical description for neuropathic pain. Choice A describes musculoskeletal symptoms. Choice B is a group of emotional complaints. Choice D communicates vascular patterns.

173. b. Disorientation is present only with dementia. Dementia patients do not tend to notice memory losses and do usually have trouble concentrating. They will also have writing, speaking, and motor impairments.

174   c. Obtunded. This patient requires continual stimulus to stay awake. The patient in a stupor is not interactive, while a lethargic patient stays interactive with stimulation during a session.

175. c. Lethargic, oriented ×1, confused. The patient is best described in this way. Sleepy is not a proper clinical description. She is easily roused so obtunded does not apply. She is oriented to name only.

176. b. The VOR is delayed so you suspect a unilateral hypofunction. This question looks at several vestibular tests and interpretation of findings. The VOR is the vestibular ocular reflex. A normal reflex remains intact with BPPV. A delayed VOR indicates unilateral vestibular hypofunction. The dynamic visual acuity tests horizontal canal function in upright. A two-line loss in visual acuity is normal. A four-line loss is positive for unilateral vestibular hypofunction, not BPPV. Positive findings for posterior canal BPPV are with head positional changes only. The gold standard test for posterior canal BPPV is the Dix-Hallpike test.

177. d. The foam and dome test, also known as the Clinical Test of Sensory Integration and Balance, is an easy to use clinical test that attempts to identify the source of balance loss. In the presence of vestibular system dysfunction, altering information from two systems simultaneously can result in an immediate loss of the balance. While all three systems contribute to balance, the vestibular system has a roll in resolving visual-somatosensory conflicts that can lead to destabilization and falling. The CTSIB induces visual-somatosensory conflict that can only be resolved through effective function of the vestibular system.

178. a. Although the other answers could be potential sources of the patient's symptoms, cancer is the answer that fulfills the most of the patient's symptoms. Classic signs of cancer are continuous pain, fatigue, and weight loss. The history of smoking and paresthesias makes one suspect pancoast tumor to the right lung.

179. b. A patient functioning at Level III (localized response) demonstrates withdrawal to painful stimuli, turns toward or away from auditory stimuli, begins to recognize family members, follows simple commands such as "Look at me" or "squeeze my hand," reacts slowly and inconsistently, and begins to respond inconsistently to simple questions.

180. c. A full-term pregnancy is 40 weeks. However, a patient is not considered premature and his/her age does not need to be adjusted unless delivered earlier than 37 weeks. This patient was born 8 weeks early (40 − 32) and therefore is considered premature. This patient's age needs to be corrected in order to accurately determine the degree of developmental delay using a standardized test. This patient's corrected age is 12 weeks (20 − 8).

181. b. Forty percent of women with post-breast-therapy-pain-syndrome present with frozen shoulder/adhesive capsulitis symptoms. These symptoms coincide with neuropathic pain in the upper quarter of the surgical side of the breast cancer. Symptoms are defined as lasting longer than 3 months.

182. a. The correct choice is tight semitendinosis. Based on their attachment to the pelvis, increased lumbar lordosis may be related to tightness of the anterior musculature (psoas, rectus femoris) or weakness of the posterior musculature (gluteals, hamstrings).

183. a. The correct answer is the center of mass is at its highest point. The center of mass is at its highest during singlelimb support.

184. b. In severe cases, ulnar deviation of the metacarpophalangeal joints is observed. Osteoarthritis is characterized by joint space narrowing. Ulnar deviation of metacarpophalangeal joints is commonly seen in rheumatoid arthritis as the joint fills with panus.

CHAPTER 4

Interventions

1. During a home health visit, the physical therapist observed several items that require modification in the home of an elderly patient. In terms of priority, the environmental hazard that needs the most immediate attention is
   a. The cracked toilet seat
   b. A malfunctioning thermostat
   c. A throw rug
   d. A cluttered kitchen

2. A 55-year-old patient sees a physical therapist for an examination of upper extremity function 1 week after Botox to the patient's finger flexors in the right upper extremity. The patient had a stroke 1 year ago and is continuing to work on increasing function. During your examination you find that you are unable to fully extend the wrist and the fingers. One of the goals you establish with the patient is to increase ROM in this area. The best way to achieve this goal is by
   a. AROM
   b. PROM
   c. Splinting to provide low load prolonged stretch
   d. Stretching and weight bearing

3. A physical therapist is treating a patient with a Colles fracture. The patient's forearm has been immobilized for 3 weeks and will require 4 additional weeks in the cast before the patient can begin functional tasks. An initial focus of treatment should be
   a. Passive ROM (PROM)
   b. Placement of the extremity in a sling
   c. Movement of the joints surrounding the fracture
   d. To avoid treatment until the cast is removed

4. During a treatment session, the physical therapist observes that the patient can flex the affected shoulder through its full ROM in a side-lying position. The PT should progress to activities that place the extremity in
   a. A gravity-assisted position
   b. A gravity-eliminated position
   c. A neutral position
   d. An antigravity position

5. Which activity of daily living (ADL) activity would the PT caution a patient with a recent hip replacement to avoid?
   a. Tying shoes
   b. Pulling up pants
   c. Putting on shirt
   d. Bathing the back

6. During a treatment session, the PT simulates the need for the client to walk up stairs to a kitchen with a painful/weak left leg. The patient should be instructed to move the
   a. Left leg up to the next step with the cane
   b. Right leg up to the next step with the cane
   c. Right leg up and then his left leg/cane
   d. Left leg up and then his right leg/cane

7. You are working with a 53-year-old client who has had a right CVA. The patient is lying on a therapy mat, and you are performing passive ROM to her left arm. Once you have the patient's arm in 90 degrees of flexion, the patient complains of some discomfort and pain. The best course of action would be to
   a. Continue as tolerated, because passive ROM must be maintained
   b. Begin the ROM again and make sure the scapula is gliding
   c. Continue and do not go past the point of pain
   d. Consult an orthopedic specialist

8. The BEST strategy to use with a contracted joint that has a soft end field is to
   a. Perform tendon gliding exercises
   b. Apply low-load, long duration stretch
   c. Use a quick stretch technique
   d. Perform active ROM

9. Which of the following is considered an absolute contraindication to manipulation?
   a. Smoking and hypertension
   b. Whiplash injury
   c. Birth control pills and smoking
   d. Acute myelopathy

10. Which of the following disc herniations would you expect to respond MOST favorably to traction therapy?
    a. Medial to the nerve root
    b. Lateral to the nerve root
    c. Anterior to the nerve root
    d. Posterior to the nerve root

11. For the best protection of lumbar mechanics, the driver's car seat should be positioned
    a. As far from the steering wheel as possible
    b. With the front of the seat lower than the back of the seat
    c. With the entire seat bottom level with the floor of the car
    d. As close to the steering wheel as practical

12. A pitcher is exercising in a clinic with a sports cord mounted behind and above his head. The pitcher simulates the pitching motion using the sports cord as resistance. Which proprioceptive neuromuscular facilitation (PNF) diagonal is the pitcher using to strengthen the muscles involved in pitching a baseball?
    a. D1 extension
    b. D1 flexion
    c. D2 extension
    d. D2 flexion

13. A therapist is mobilizing a patient's right shoulder. The movement taking place at the joint capsule is not completely to end range. It is a large-amplitude movement from near the beginning of available range to near the end of available range. What grade mobilization, according to Maitland, is being performed?
    a. Grade I
    b. Grade II
    c. Grade III
    d. Grade IV

14. A 29-year-old woman is referred to a therapist with a diagnosis of recurrent ankle sprains. The patient has a history of several inversion ankle sprains within the past year. No edema or redness is noted at this time. Which of the following is the best treatment plan?
    a. Gastrocnemius stretching, ankle strengthening, and ice
    b. Rest, ice, compression, elevation, and ankle strengthening
    c. Ankle strengthening and a proprioception program
    d. Rest, ice, compression, elevation, and gastrocnemius stretching

15. The therapist is treating a male patient for a second-degree acromioclavicular sprain. The patient has just finished the doctor's prescription of 3 sessions/week for 4 weeks. The therapist is treating the patient with iontophoresis (driving dexamethasone), deltoid-strengthening exercises, pectoral-strengthening exercises, and ice. The patient reports no decline in pain level since the initial examination. Which of the following is the best course of action for the therapist?
    a. Phone the doctor and request continued physical therapy.
    b. Tell the patient to go back to the doctor because he is not making appropriate progress.
    c. Discharge the patient because he will improve on his own.
    d. Take the problem to the supervisor of the facility.

16. A therapist working in an outpatient physical therapy clinic examines a patient with a diagnosis of rotator cuff bursitis. The physician's order is to examine and treat. During the examination the following facts are revealed:
    - Active shoulder flexion = 85 degrees with pain
    - Passive shoulder flexion = 177 degrees
    - Active shoulder abduction = 93 degrees with pain
    - Passive shoulder abduction = 181 degrees
    - Active external rotation = 13 degrees with pain
    - Passive eternal rotation = 87 degrees
    - Drop arm test = positive
    - Impingement test = negative
    - Biceps tendon subluxation test = negative
    - Sulcus sign = negative

    Of the following, which is the best course of action?
    a. Treat the patient for 1 week with moist heat application, joint mobilization, and strengthening. Then suggest to the patient that he or she return to the physician if there are no positive results.
    b. Treat the patient for 1 week with ultrasound, strengthening, and ice. Then suggest to the patient that he or she return to the physician if there are no positive results.
    c. Treat the patient for 1 week with a home exercise program, strengthening, passive range of motion by the therapist, and ice. Then suggest to the patient that he or she return to the physician if there are no positive results.
    d. Treat the patient for 1 week with strengthening, a home exercise program, and ice. Then suggest to the patient that he or she return to the physician if there are no positive results.

17. The therapist is crutch training a 26-year-old man who underwent right knee arthroscopy 10 hours ago. The patient's weight-bearing status is toe-touch weight-bearing on the right lower extremity. If the patient is going up steps, which of the following is the correct sequence of verbal instructions?
    a. "Have someone stand below you while going up, bring the left leg up first, then the crutches and the right leg."
    b. "Have someone stand above you while going up, bring the left leg up first, then the crutches and the right leg."
    c. "Have someone stand below you while going up, bring the right leg up first, then the crutches and the left leg."
    d. "Have someone stand above you while going up, bring the right leg up first, then the crutches and the right leg."

18. What is the best way to first exercise the postural (or extensor) musculature when it is extremely weak to facilitate muscle control?
    a. Isometrically
    b. Concentrically
    c. Eccentrically
    d. Isokinetically

19. A 42-year-old receptionist presents to an outpatient physical therapy clinic complaining of low back pain. The therapist decides that postural modification needs to be part of the treatment plan. What is the best position for the lower extremities while the patient is sitting?
    a. 90 degrees of hip flexion, 90 degrees of knee flexion, and 10 degrees of dorsiflexion
    b. 60 degrees of hip flexion, 90 degrees of knee flexion, and 0 degrees of dorsiflexion
    c. 110 degrees of hip flexion, 80 degrees of knee flexion, and 10 degrees of dorsiflexion
    d. 90 degrees of hip flexion, 90 degrees of knee flexion, and 0 degrees of dorsiflexion

20. A 67-year-old woman presents to an outpatient facility with a diagnosis of right adhesive capsulitis. The therapist plans to focus mostly on gaining abduction range of motion. In which direction should the therapist mobilize the shoulder to gain abduction range of motion?
    a. Posteriorly
    b. Anteriorly
    c. Inferiorly
    d. Superiorly

21. A patient is positioned in the supine position. The involved left upper extremity is positioned by the therapist in 90 degrees of shoulder flexion. The therapist applies resistance into shoulder flexion, then extension. No movement takes place. The therapist instructs the patient to "hold" when resistance is applied in both directions. Which of the following proprioceptive neuromuscular facilitation techniques is being used?
    a. Repeated contractions
    b. Hold-relax
    c. Rhythmic stabilization
    d. Contract-relax

22. The therapist is treating a patient who recently received a below-knee amputation. The therapist notices in the patient's chart that a psychiatrist has stated that the patient is in the second stage of the grieving process. Which stage of the grieving process is this patient most likely exhibiting?
    a. Denial
    b. Acceptance
    c. Depression
    d. Anger

23. A 32-year-old man is referred to physical therapy with the diagnosis of a recent complete anterior cruciate ligament tear. The patient and the physician have decided to avoid surgery as long as possible. The therapist provides the patient with a home exercise program and instructions about activities that will be limited secondary to this diagnosis. Which of the following is the best advice?
    a. There are no precautions.
    b. The patient should avoid all athletic activity for 1 year.
    c. The patient should avoid all athletic activity until there is a minimum of 20% difference in the bilateral quadriceps muscle as measured isokinetically.
    d. The patient should wear a brace and compete in only light athletic events.

24. A physician has ordered a physical therapist to treat a patient with chronic low back pain. The order is to "increase gluteal muscle function by decreasing trigger points in the quadratus lumborum." What is the first technique that should be used by the physical therapist?
    a. Isometric gluteal strengthening
    b. Posture program
    c. Soft tissue massage
    d. Muscle reeducation

25. A 60-year-old woman is referred to outpatient physical therapy services for rehabilitation after receiving a left total knee replacement 4 weeks ago. The patient is currently ambulating with a standard walker with a severely antalgic gait pattern. Before the recent surgery the patient was ambulating independently without an assistive device. Left knee flexion was measured in the initial examination and found to be 85 degrees actively and 94 degrees passively. The patient also lacked 10 degrees of full passive extension and 17 degrees of full active extension. Which of the following does the therapist need to first address?
    a. Lack of passive left knee flexion
    b. Lack of passive left knee extension
    c. Lack of active left knee extension
    d. Ability to ambulate with a lesser assistive device

26. A home health physical therapist is sent to examine a 56-year-old man who has suffered a recent stroke. The patient is sitting in a lift chair, accompanied by his 14-year-old nephew. He seems confused several times throughout the examination. The nephew is unable to assist in clarifying much of the subjective history. The patient reports to the therapist that he is independent in ambulation with a standard walker as an assistive device and in all transfers without an assistive device. Based on the above information, which of the following sequence of events, chosen by the therapist, is in the correct order?
    a. Ambulate with the standard walker with the wheelchair in close proximity; transfer sit to stand in front of the wheelchair; transfer wheelchair to bed; assess range of motion and strength of all extremities in supine position
    b. Ambulate with the standard walker with the wheelchair in close proximity; transfer wheelchair to bed; assess range of motion and strength of all extremities in supine position; transfer sit to stand at bedside
    c. Assess range of motion and strength of all extremities in the lift chair; transfer sit to stand in front of the lift chair; ambulate with the standard walker with the wheelchair in close proximity; transfer wheelchair to bed
    d. Assess range of motion and strength of all extremities in the lift chair; ambulate with the standard walker with the wheelchair in close proximity; transfer sit to stand in front of the wheelchair; transfer wheelchair to bed

27. A patient is receiving crutch training 1 day after a right knee arthroscopic surgery. The patient's weight-bearing status is toe-touch weight-bearing on the right lower extremity. The therapist first chooses to instruct the patient how to perform a correct sit-to-stand transfer. Which of the following is the most correct set of instructions?

a. (1) Slide forward to the edge of the chair; (2) put both the crutches in front of you and hold both grips together with the right hand; (3) press on the left arm rest with the left hand and the grips with the right hand; (4) lean forward; (5) stand up, placing your weight on the left lower extremity; (6) place one crutch slowly under the left arm, then under the right arm.

b. (1) Slide forward; (2) put one crutch in each hand, holding the grips; (3) place crutches in a vertical position; (4) press down on the grips; (5) stand up, placing more weight on the left lower extremity.

c. (1) Slide forward to the edge of the chair; (2) put both the crutches in front of you and hold both grips together with the left hand; (3) press on the right arm rest with the right hand and the grips with the left hand; (4) lean forward; (5) stand up, placing your weight on the left lower extremity; (6) place one crutch slowly under the right arm, then under the left arm.

d. (1) Place crutches in close proximity; (2) slide forward; (3) place hands on the arm rests; (4) press down and stand up; (5) place weight on the left lower extremity; (6) reach slowly for the crutches and place under the axilla.

28. A 20-year-old man with anterior cruciate ligament reconstruction with allograft presents to an outpatient physical therapy clinic. The patient's surgery was 5 days ago. The patient is independent in ambulation with crutches. He also currently has 53 degrees of active knee flexion and 67 degrees of passive knee flexion and lacks 10 degrees of full knee extension actively and 5 degrees passively. What is the most significant deficit on which the physical therapist should focus treatment?

a. Lack of active knee extension
b. Lack of passive knee extension
c. Lack of active knee flexion
d. Lack of passive knee flexion

29. A physical therapist is ordered to examine and treat in the acute setting a patient who received a left total knee replacement 1 day ago. Before surgery, the patient was independent in all activities of daily living, transfers, and ambulation with an assistive device. The family reports that ambulation was slow and guarded because of knee pain. The physician's orders are to ambulate with partial weight bearing on the left lower extremity and to increase strength/range of motion. At this point, bed-to-wheelchair transfers, sit-to-stand transfers, and wheelchair-to-toilet transfers require the minimal assistance of one person. The left knee has 63 degrees of active flexion and 77 degrees of passive flexion. The left knee also lacks 7 degrees of full extension actively and 3 degrees passively. Right hip strength is recorded as follows: hip flexion and abduction = 4+/5, hip adduction and extension = 5/5, knee flexion = 4+/5, knee extension = 5/5, ankle plantar flexion = 4+/5, and dorsiflexion = 5/5. Left lower extremity strength is recorded as follows: hip flexion = 3/5, hip abduction and adduction = 3+/5, hip extension =3/5, knee flexion and extension = 3-/5, ankle dorsiflexion = 3+/5, and plantar flexion = 3+/5. The patient is currently able to ambulate 30 feet × 2 with a standard walker and minimal assistance of one person on level surfaces. She also ambulates with a flexed knee throughout the gait cycle. According to the physician, she most likely will be discharged home (with home health services), where she lives alone, within the next 2 to 3 days. Of the choices below, which is the most important long-term goal in the acute setting?
    a. In 3 days the patient will be independent in all transfers.
    b. In 3 days the patient will ambulate with a quad cane independently, with no gait deviations, on level surfaces 50 feet × 3.
    c. In 3 days the patient will increase all left lower extremity manual muscle testing grades by one half grade.
    d. In 3 days the patient will have active left knee range of motion from 0 to 90 degrees and passive range of motion from 0 to 95 degrees.

30. A patient presents to therapy with poor motor control of the lower extremities. The therapist determines that to work efficiently toward the goal of returning the patient to his prior level of ambulation, he must work in the following order regarding stages of control
    a. Mobility, controlled mobility, stability, skill
    b. Stability, controlled stability, mobility, skill
    c. Skill, controlled stability, controlled mobility
    d. Mobility, stability, controlled mobility, skill

31. A 23-year-old woman arrives at an outpatient physical therapy clinic with a prescription to examine and treat the right hand. One week earlier the patient underwent surgical repair of the flexor tendons of the right hand at zone 2. She also had her cast removed at the physician's office a few minutes before coming to physical therapy. What is the best course of treatment for this patient?
   a. Ultrasound to decrease scarring
   b. Gentle grip strengthening with putty
   c. Splinting the distal interphalangeal joint and proximal interphalangeal joints at neutral
   d. Splinting with the use of rubber bands to passively flex the fingers

32. A 67-year-old man with a below-knee amputation presents to an outpatient clinic. His surgical amputation was 3 weeks ago, and his scars are well healed. Which of the following is incorrect information about stump care?
   a. Use a light lotion on the stump after bathing each night.
   b. Continue with use of a shrinker 12 hours per day.
   c. Wash the stump with mild soap and water.
   d. Use scar massage techniques.

33. A physical therapist is teaching a class in geriatric fitness/strengthening at a local gym. Which of the following is not a general guideline for exercise prescription in this patient population?
   a. To increase exercise intensity, increase treadmill speed rather than the grade.
   b. Start at a low intensity (2 to 3 METs).
   c. Use machines for strength training rather than free weights.
   d. Set weight resistance so that the patient can perform more than 8 repetitions before fatigue.

34. A 76-year-old woman received a cemented right total hip arthroplasty (THA) 24 hours ago. The surgeon documented that he used a posterolateral incision. Which of the following suggestions is inappropriate for the next 24 hours?
   a. Avoid hip flexion above 30 degrees.
   b. Avoid hip adduction past midline.
   c. Avoid any internal rotation.
   d. Avoid abduction past 15 degrees.

35. The therapist is examining a 38-year-old man who complains of right sacroiliac joint pain. The therapist decides to assess leg length discrepancy in supine versus sitting position. When the patient is in supine position, leg lengths are equal; however, when the patient rises to the sitting position, the right lower extremity appears 2 cm shorter. Which of the following should be a part of the treatment plan?
   a. Right posterior SI mobilization
   b. Right anterior SI mobilization
   c. Left posterior SI mobilization
   d. Left anterior SI mobilization

36. In taping an athlete's ankle prophylactically before a football game, in what position should the ankle be slightly positioned before taping to provide the most protection against an ankle sprain?
   a. Inversion, dorsiflexion, abduction
   b. Eversion, plantar flexion, adduction
   c. Eversion, dorsiflexion, abduction
   d. Inversion, plantar flexion, adduction

37. A physical therapist is treating a 35-year-old man with traumatic injury to the right hand. The patient has several surgical scars from a tendon repair performed 6 weeks ago. What is the appropriate type of massage for the patient's scars?
   a. Massage should be transverse and longitudinal.
   b. Massage should be circular and longitudinal.
   c. Massage should be transverse and circular.
   d. Massage is contraindicated after a tendon repair.

38. A patient is being treated in an outpatient facility after receiving a meniscus repair to the right knee 1 week ago. The patient has full passive extension of the involved knee but lacks 4 degrees of full extension when performing a straight leg raise. The patient's active flexion is 110 degrees and passive flexion is 119 degrees. What is a common term used to describe the patient's most significant range of motion deficit? What is a possible source of this problem?
   a. Flexion contracture, quadricep atrophy
   b. Extension lag, joint effusion
   c. Flexion lag, weak quadriceps
   d. Extension contracture, tight hamstrings

39. A physical therapist is attempting to increase a patient's functional mobility in a seated position. To treat the patient most effectively and efficiently, the following should be performed in what order?
   1. Weight shifting of the pelvis
   2. Isometric contractions of the lower extremity
   3. Trunk range of motion exercises
   4. Isotonic resistance to the quadriceps
   a. 1, 2, 3, 4
   b. 2, 3, 1, 4
   c. 4, 3, 2, 1
   d. 3, 2, 1, 4

40. A physical therapist is speaking to a group of avid tennis players. The group asks how to prevent tennis elbow (lateral epicondylitis). Which of the following is incorrect information?
   a. Primarily use the wrist and elbow extensors during a backhand stroke.
   b. Begin the backhand stroke in shoulder adduction and internal rotation.
   c. Use a racket that has a large grip.
   d. Use a light racket.

41. A physical therapist is fabricating a splint for a patient who received four metacarpophalangeal joint replacements. The surgical joint replacement was necessary because of severe rheumatoid arthritis. Which of the following is the correct placement of the metacarpophalangeal joints in the splint?
   a. Full flexion and slight radial pull
   b. Full flexion and slight ulnar pull
   c. Full extension and slight radial pull
   d. Full extension and slight ulnar pull

42. A therapist is ordered to fabricate a splint for a 2-month-old infant with congenital hip dislocation. In what position should the hip be placed while in the splint?
   a. Flexion and adduction
   b. Extension and adduction
   c. Extension and abduction
   d. Flexion and abduction

43. A physical therapist is discharging a 32-year-old man from outpatient physical therapy. The patient received therapy for a traumatic ankle injury that occurred several months earlier. The surgery performed on the patient's ankle required placement of plates and screws, which resulted in a permanent range of motion deficit of 10 degrees of active and passive dorsiflexion. Strength in the ankle is 5/5 with manual muscle testing. Of the following, which is the highest functional outcome that the patient can expect?
    a. Independent ambulation with no gait deviations
    b. Ambulation with a cane with minimal gait deviations
    c. Running with no gait deviations
    d. Ascending or descending stairs with no gait deviations

44. A physical therapist is performing passive range of motion on the shoulder of a 43-year-old woman who received a rotator cuff repair 5 weeks ago. During passive range of motion, the therapist notes a capsular end feel at 95 degrees of shoulder flexion. What should the therapist do?
    a. Begin isokinetic exercise at 180 degrees per second.
    b. Begin joint mobilization.
    c. Schedule the patient an appointment with the physician immediately.
    d. Begin aggressive supraspinatus activity.

45. In which of the following situations should the therapist be most concerned about the complications resulting from grade IV joint mobilization techniques?
    a. A 37-year-old man with a Colles fracture suffered 10 weeks ago
    b. A 23-year-old woman with a boxer's fracture suffered 10 weeks ago
    c. A 34-year-old man with a scaphoid fracture suffered 12 weeks ago
    d. A 53-year-man with a Bennett's fracture suffered 12 weeks ago

46. Which of the following is an inappropriate exercise for a patient who received an anterior cruciate ligament reconstruction with a patella tendon autograft 2 weeks ago?
    a. Lateral step-ups
    b. Heel slides
    c. Stationary bike
    d. Pool walking

47. A physical therapist is speaking to a group of receptionists about correct posture. Which of the following is incorrect information?
    a. Position computer monitors at eye level.
    b. Position seats so that the feet are flat on the floor while sitting.
    c. Position keyboards so that the wrists are in approximately 20 degrees of extension.
    d. Take frequent stretching breaks.

48. A physical therapist is treating an automobile mechanic. The patient asks for tips on preventing upper extremity repetitive motion injuries. Which of the following is incorrect advice?
    a. Use your entire hand rather than just the fingers when holding an object.
    b. Position tasks so that they are performed below shoulder height.
    c. Use tools with small straight handles when possible.
    d. When performing a forceful task, keep the materials slightly lower than the elbow.

49. A patient presents to physical therapy with a long-standing diagnosis of bilateral pes planus. The therapist has given the patient custom-fit orthotics. After using the orthotics for 1 week, the patient complains of pain along the first metatarsal. The therapist decides to use joint mobilization techniques to decrease the patient's pain. In which direction should the therapist mobilize the first metatarsal?
    a. Inferiorly
    b. Superiorly
    c. Laterally
    d. Medially

50. A 14-year-old boy with a diagnosis of osteosarcoma of his right distal femur underwent resection of the distal third of his femur and implantation of an expandable endoprosthetic device 2 months ago. He is now referred to outpatient physical therapy with no restrictions except PWB gait with crutches. What impairment would you expect to most interfere with function at the time of the examination?
    a. Leg length discrepancy
    b. Limited right knee ROM
    c. Limited right hip ROM
    d. Pain at the site of surgical intervention

51. A 4-year-old-child diagnosed with osteosarcoma of the distal femur, is scheduled for resection of the distal third of the femur. What surgical intervention would provide the best long term functional outcome?
    a. Allograft
    b. Endoprosthetic implant
    c. Hip disarticulation
    d. Rotationplasty

52. A 6-month-old infant with acetabular dysplasia of the right hip diagnosed by radiograph, with a history of a dislocatable hip at birth, would usually be treated with
    a. Arthrogram and closed reduction
    b. Spica cast
    c. Pavlik harness
    d. Open reduction

53. Which degree of strain in the following joints would normally take the longest amount of time to rehabilitate?
    a. Grade I medial collateral ligament of the knee injury
    b. Grade I anterior cruciate ligament injury
    c. Grade II ulnar collateral ligament of the elbow injury
    d. Grade III anterior talofibular ligament injury

54. It is 6 weeks after acromioplasty and a patient is showing difficulty performing shoulder flexion and scaption exercises correctly. The patient shows shoulder "hike" above 70 degrees of shoulder flexion. Which of the following interventions would most quickly improve this problem?
    a. Eccentric elbow flexion
    b. Heavy resistance supraspinatus exercise
    c. Gravity resistance supraspinatus exercise
    d. Upper trapezius strengthening

55. Shoulder ROM is restricted in a patient 8 weeks after rotator cuff repair. Internal rotation and horizontal adduction are the most restricted motions. Which portion of the shoulder capsule should be stretched or mobilized?
    a. Anterior
    b. Posterior
    c. Inferior
    d. Superior

56. A patient who underwent an acromioplasty 8 weeks ago presents with complaints of pain when reaching overhead and during the last 30 degrees of shoulder flexion. End range pain is also felt when using PROM into horizontal adduction, shoulder flexion, and shoulder abduction. Which of the following treatments would be most helpful for this patient?
    a. Shoulder mobilizations for the anterior shoulder capsule
    b. Shoulder mobilizations for the superior shoulder capsule
    c. Acromioclavicular joint mobilization with the upper extremity in 20 degrees of shoulder flexion
    d. Acromioclavicular joint mobilization with the upper extremity in 140 degrees of shoulder flexion

57. A patient who underwent shoulder acromioplasty 6 days ago presents with pain and limited use for the involved upper extremity during ADLs. What is the most appropriate advice to decrease this patient's pain while at home?
    a. Discontinue use of sling and ice at home.
    b. Use a sling during waking hours and ice throughout the day.
    c. Begin progressive resistance exercises at home.
    d. Discontinue use of a sling and use a moist heat pad at home.

58. Considering a patient with recent anterior capsulolabral reconstruction, when can active range of motion (AROM) of the shoulder be initiated?
    a. As soon as 1 to 2 days after surgery
    b. 2 to 3 weeks postoperatively
    c. 4 to 6 weeks postoperatively
    d. 6 to 8 weeks postoperatively

59. In an outpatient physical therapy clinic, a patient presents with complaints of pain with elbow flexion at the anterior shoulder. He underwent anterior capsulolabral reconstruction 10 weeks ago. Shoulder ROM is restricted in internal rotation, but all other motions are normal. Elbow ROM is normal, but painful at 90 to 100 degrees of elbow flexion. What is the most appropriate course of action by the physical therapist?
    a. Shoulder posterior mobilization, and treatment for biceps tendonitis
    b. Shoulder anterior mobilization, and treatment for biceps tendonitis
    c. Shoulder posterior mobilization only
    d. Shoulder anterior mobilization only

60. During an intervention session, a patient with recent (1 week ago) rotator cuff repair complains of cervical pain. His complaints are in the upper trapezius and medial scapular area of the involved upper extremity. What is the most appropriate course of action by the physical therapist?
    a. Apply ice to the area of complaint.
    b. Assure the patient this is normal and continue with PROM treatments.
    c. Call the physician immediately.
    d. Examine the cervical spine.

61. A baseball pitcher underwent rotator cuff repair 8 weeks ago. Which portion of the shoulder capsule does not need to be mobilized under normal conditions?
    a. Anterior
    b. Posterior
    c. Superior
    d. Inferior

62. A patient complains of pain in the ear, what structure does not refer to the ear?
    a. Sternocleidomastoid trigger point
    b. Deep masseter trigger point
    c. Anterior digastric trigger point
    d. Temporomandibular joint

63. What symptoms are indicative of a temporomandibular dysfunction problem?
    a. Limited range of motion or altered mechanics
    b. Tinnitus and hyperacousia
    c. Dizziness and spinning
    d. Retro-orbital headache and sinus pain

64. What is a reasonable rehabilitation goal for active opening after arthroscopy of the TMJ for an anterior disc displacement without reduction?
    a. Opening to 58mm
    b. Opening to 28 mm
    c. Opening to 38mm
    d. Opening to 48mm

65. What is the best evidence based intervention for a painful anterior displaced disc with reduction in the TMJ?
    a. Exercises that avoid painful click such as hinge axis and midline opening
    b. Aggressive mobilization to reduce the clicking
    c. Wide opening exercises to reduce the clicking
    d. Ice and no exercise

66. When is a dental splint not indicated for a TMJ patient?
    a. Aggressive bruxers when exercises are not enough to decrease the clench/grind habit
    b. Osteoarthritic joints, bite changes
    c. Muscle incoordination, bite changes, cannot find a position to rest the jaw
    d. Anterior disc displacement without reduction

67. What is the long-term prognosis for an anterior disc displacement without reduction without surgery of the TMJ?
    a. Osteoarthritis will develop.
    b. The range of motion will be limited to a 30 mm opening.
    c. Clicking and pain will be persistent.
    d. With or without surgery, the joint will adapt and have functional opening with little or no pain.

68. What is the best intervention for an acute anterior displaced disc without reduction?
    a. Ultrasound and heat to calm the joint pain and no exercises
    b. Aggressive PT to manipulate joint to unlock in 3 to 4 visits
    c. Referral to the dentist for splint therapy
    d. Exercises to limit opening

69. Distal radius fractures
    a. Are always best treated surgically
    b. Are always best treated in a cast
    c. Can be allowed to heal with some deformity
    d. Are a "solved" problem in orthopedics

70. Stiffness at the MCP joints following casting
    a. Is caused by tightness of the saggital bands
    b. Can always be avoided by proper casting
    c. Is unavoidable
    d. Requires surgical correction

71. A patient sustained a Colles fracture of the wrist. Her cast was removed and she now lacks wrist extension. To increase her passive closed chain wrist extension, mobilize the
    a. Distal concave radius on the convex ulna
    b. Concave distal radius on the convex proximal carpals
    c. Convex distal radius on the concave distal carpals
    d. Concave distal ulna on the convex proximal carpals

72. A pediatric patient is referred to physical therapy with a diagnosis of right torticollis. The physical therapist is developing a home program. What position does the patient need to move his head to correct his posture?
    a. Right cervical rotation and left lateral cervical flexion
    b. Right cervical rotation and right lateral cervical flexion
    c. Left cervical rotation and right lateral cervical flexion
    d. Cervical flexion and scapular retraction

73. How much cervical spine rotation will your patient have after a complete cervical spine fusion at level C1-C2?
    a. Complete loss of cervical rotation
    b. 25% loss of cervical rotation
    c. 50% loss of cervical rotation
    d. No loss of cervical rotation

74. Your patient has limited knee flexion in the preswing phase of gait. You suspect the following
    a. Hamstring weakness
    b. Plantar flexor spasticity
    c. Plantar flexor weakness
    d. Dorsiflexor weakness

75. A patient demonstrates excessive hip adduction in the swing phase of gait. What are the hypothesized causes for this deviation?
   a. Adductor hypertonicity of the swing leg
   b. Quadriceps weakness of the swing leg
   c. Plantar flexor weakness of the swing leg
   d. Gluteus medius hypertonicity of the swing leg

76. Your patient is recovering from ACL surgery and is 8 weeks post operative. They have difficulty with flexion beyond 10 degrees. You have determined that the most appropriate way to restore extension would be to mobilize the
   a. Tibia posteriorly on the femur
   b. Femur anteriorly on the tibia
   c. Tibia anteriorly on the femur
   d. The patella distally in the trochlear groove

77. Your patient has been diagnosed as having thoracic outlet syndrome. You perform the Adson's maneuver and it is positive. As a result you have determined that the best way to address this problem is to stretch the
   a. Pectoralis minor
   b. Clavopectoral fascia
   c. Anterior scalenes
   d. Sternocleidomastoids

78. A physical therapist is providing intervention to a 6-month-old infant diagnosed with right torticollis. The therapist instructs the family in a home exercise program that stretches the patient's neck into
   a. Left side bend and left rotation
   b. Left side bend and right rotation
   c. Right side bend and right rotation
   d. Right side bend and left rotation

79. You are performing an examination on a 2-year-old patient diagnosed with leukemia who has been hospitalized for 1 month and is currently undergoing chemotherapy. Upon observation, you notice that the patient has difficulty with transitioning from low to high kneel. You would suspect which primary muscle is weak?
   a. Biceps Femoris
   b. Gastrocnemius
   c. Gluteus maximus
   d. Iliopsoas

80. The physical therapist is treating a patient with a history of coronary artery disease. During the treatment, the patient complains of recurring angina that increases when performing activities in standing. The MOST appropriate course of action by the PT is to
    a. Stop treatment and contact the physician
    b. Stop treatment until symptoms subside
    c. Assist patient in taking medication for chest pain
    d. Perform treatment in a sitting position

81. A patient who sustained a severe heart attack was categorized at a metabolic equivalent table (MET) level of 2 to 3. The patient has completed the goal of doing homemaking activities, such as washing dishes and ironing. The physical therapist should progress intervention to include the occupational task of
    a. Driving an automobile
    b. Performing upper and lower extremity dressing
    c. Gardening in the yard
    d. Preparing 1 to 2 meals per day

82. A patient with emphysema complains of shortness of breath and generalized weakness in the upper extremities when performing daily chores. The physical therapist should encourage
    a. Pursed-lip breathing when working
    b. Gravity assisted exercises before performing chores
    c. Use of oxygen with daily activities
    d. Avoidance of activities that consume a lot of energy

83. Persuading a sedentary patient to become more active, the therapist explains the benefits of exercise. Which of the following is an inappropriate list of benefits?
    a. Increased efficiency of the myocardium to obtain oxygen, decreased high-density lipoprotein (HDL) cholesterol, and decreased cholesterol
    b. Decreased low-density lipoprotein (LDL) cholesterol, decreased triglycerides, and decreased resting blood pressure
    c. Increased efficiency of the myocardium to obtain oxygen, decreased cholesterol, and decreased LDL
    d. Decreased resting blood pressure, decreased LDL, increased HDL

84. The therapist is working in an outpatient cardiac rehabilitation facility. A 50-year-old healthy man inquires about the correct exercise parameters for increasing aerobic efficiency. Which of the following is the most correct information to convey to this individual?
    a. Exercise at 80% to 90% of maximal volume of oxygen utilization (Vo_2)
    b. Exercise with heart rate between 111 and 153 beats/minute
    c. Exercise at approximately 170 beats/minute
    d. Exercise at level 17 to 18 on the Borg rating of perceived exertion (RPE) scale

85. What lobe of the lungs is the therapist attempting to drain if the patient is in the following position? Resting on the left side, rolled one quarter turn back, supported with pillows, and the foot of the bed raised 12 to 16 inches.
    a. Right middle lobe-lingular segment
    b. Left upper lobe-lingular segment
    c. Right upper lobe-posterior segment
    d. Left upper lobe-posterior segment

86. The therapist works in a cardiac rehabilitation setting. Which of the following types of exercises are most likely to be harmful to a 64-year-old man with a history of myocardial infarction?
    a. Concentric
    b. Eccentric
    c. Aerobic
    d. Isometric

87. The patient is referred by a physician to begin outpatient cardiac rehabilitation. Which of the following is not a contraindication to enter an outpatient program?
    a. Resting systolic blood pressure of 210 mm Hg
    b. Third-degree atrioventricular block
    c. Resting ST displacement less than 1 mm
    d. Acute fever

88. In order to determine if an exercise session should be terminated, the patient is asked to assess the level of exertion using the Borg Rating of Perceived Exertion Scale (RPE). The patient rates the level of exertion as 9 on the 6 to 19 scale. A rating of 9 corresponds to which of the following?
    a. Very, very light
    b. Very light
    c. Somewhat hard
    d. Hard

89. A physician orders stage II cardiac rehabilitation for a patient. The orders are to exercise the patient below 7 metabolic equivalents (METs). Which of the following is a contraindicated activity?
    a. Riding a stationary bike at approximately 5.5 mph
    b. Descending a flight of stairs independently
    c. Ironing
    d. Ambulate independently at 5 to 6 mph

90. A therapist is treating a patient with cystic fibrosis who has just walked 75 feet before experiencing significant breathing difficulties. In an effort to assist the patient in regaining her normal breathing rate, the therapist gives a set of instructions. Which of the following set of instructions is appropriate?
    a. "Take a slow deep breath through pursed lips, and exhale slowly through your nose only."
    b. "Take small breaths through your nose only, and exhale quickly through pursed lips."
    c. "Breath in through your nose, and exhale slowly through pursed lips."
    d. "Breath in through pursed lips, and breath out slowly through pursed lips."

91. A physical therapist is treating a 65-year-old man with COPD. The patient questions the benefits of the flow incentive spirometer left in the room by the respiratory therapist a few minutes ago. Which of the following is an appropriate response to the patient's question?
    a. "It gives visual feedback on lung performance."
    b. "You should use this for the rest of your life."
    c. "You need to ask the respiratory therapist this question."
    d. "It really doesn't do anything useful."

92. Which of the following is not an indication for pulmonary suctioning?
    a. Unproductive coughs
    b. Breath sounds of wet rales
    c. Respiratory distress
    d. Hyperoxygenation

93. Which of the following exercises does not increase strength of the muscles of forceful inspiration?
    a. Active cervical flexion exercises
    b. Active glenohumeral extension exercises
    c. Shoulder shrugs
    d. Crunches

94. A 63-year-old man presents to an outpatient physical therapy clinic with a diagnosis of sciatica. The MRI report is negative for lumbar disc involvement. During the examination the physical therapist cannot reproduce the symptoms of radiculopathy with any test. Lower extremity strength is equal bilaterally and is not weak in any particular pattern. The patient informs the therapist that the pain is bilateral, located in the gastrocnemius area, and increases with prolonged ambulation. The pain stops soon after resting in a seated position. What is the most likely source of this patient's pain?
    a. Impingement of the L5 dorsal root
    b. Multiple sclerosis
    c. Compartment syndrome
    d. Intermittent claudication

95. An 81-year-old woman with right-side hemiparesis due to stroke is being treated by a physical therapist through home health services. The therapist is attempting to increase the functional reach of the right upper extremity. The patient currently has 120 degrees of active flexion. The therapist decides to use trunk mobility/stability facilitation techniques to help achieve the patient's functional goals. Which of the following skills need to be mastered by the patient to attain the ability to reach 2 feet in front of her wheelchair and 2 feet to the right of mid-line at 125 degrees of shoulder flexion with the right upper extremity?
    a. Weight shifting to the left buttock and right-side trunk elongation
    b. Weight shifting to the left buttock and left-side trunk elongation
    c. Weight shifting to the right buttock and right-side trunk elongation
    d. Weight shifting to the right buttock and left-side trunk elongation

96. The physical therapist in beginning examination of a patient in an outpatient cardiac rehabilitation facility. A chart review shows that this patient has active atrial fibrillation with a controlled ventricular rate. What is the most appropriate intervention for this patient?
    a. Low intensity aerobic exercise
    b. High intensity aerobic exercise
    c. High intensity lower extremity exercise only
    d. Low intensity lower extremity exercise only

97. Which of the following is incorrect advice to give to a patient with a diagnosis of congestive heart failure who complains of shortness of breath and "smothering" while attempting to sleep?
    a. Sleep with the head on 2 to 3 pillows.
    b. Sleep without any pillows.
    c. Sleep in a recliner during exacerbations.
    d. During exacerbations, come to a standing position for short-term relief.

98. A physical therapist is working with a patient who has a history of coronary artery disease and a reported history of chest pain. Which of the following from the medical interview is NOT a reason to refer a patient back to their physician for further follow-up?
    a. Reported anginal pain is not relieved by rest.
    b. Chest pain is reported lasting 20 minutes or longer.
    c. There is a reported change in the pattern of angina.
    d. Nitroglycerine tablets are reported to relieve the angina.

99. All of the following cardiopulmonary function variables will increase in children in response to training except
    a. Heart volume
    b. Respiratory rate
    c. Stroke volume
    d. Tidal volume

100. You are performing an examination and providing intervention to a patient diagnosed with hemophilia. You have confirmed that hemostasis has been achieved after an acute bleed in the right knee. During the objective examination, you determine that the knee has 100 degrees of knee flexion and there is a 5 degrees knee flexion contracture. All are appropriate therapeutic interventions except
    a. Passive ROM of the right knee
    b. Instruct patient and family in a home exercise program consisting of AROM and strengthening
    c. Active resisted exercises
    d. Isometrics of the quadriceps muscle

101. A patient with reflex sympathetic dystrophy syndrome (RSDS), or complex regional pain syndrome (CRPS), has severe edema and increased pain while performing simple grooming activities such as face washing. The initial care plan should focus on
    a. Pain management
    b. Using the uninvolved extremity
    c. Gentle mobilization
    d. Light activities, such as brushing teeth

102. A 45-year-old patient is in the first stage of RSDS or CRPS with the classic signs of hand edema, fear of ROM, and pain in the shoulder and hand of the involved extremity. What is the FIRST priority of treatment?
    a. Reduction of edema
    b. Aggressive PROM
    c. Instruct in self-ROM
    d. Perform grip strength test

103. A patient with a spinal cord injury at the level of C8 would like to be independent in mobility. Based on the expected functional outcomes, the physical therapist would recommend the following piece(s) of adapted equipment
    a. Manual wheelchair
    b. A motorized wheelchair
    c. A manual wheelchair and sliding board
    d. A walker and wheelchair

104. A PT working in early intervention is helping a parent to get the baby to hold and drink from a bottle. Based on typical development, the therapist should begin to introduce this skill between
    a. 12 to 14 months
    b. 10 to 12 months
    c. 8 to 10 months
    d. 6 to 8 months

105. After 3 months of intervention, the physical therapist notices that the child is beginning to integrate the reflex that turns the head toward the child's extended arm while in prone. This reflex is
    a. Asymmetric tonic neck reflex
    b. Symmetric tonic neck reflex
    c. Moro reflex
    d. Tonic labyrinthine reflex

106. A physical therapist arrives at a child's home to begin a treatment session. When the therapist enters the home, the child is running through the house screeching. The PT determines that the first step in the intervention session will be
    a. Sitting still on a therapy ball
    b. Placing the child in a high chair
    c. Rhythmic linear swinging
    d. Rapidly brushing extremities

107. A child has poor ability to maintain trunk and neck extension. The PT uses which of the following as the best technique to facilitate increased strength and control
    a. Have child prone on a therapy ball and play with toys
    b. Have child supine on a platform swing while playing with toys
    c. Have child in side lying on a mat shield playing with toys
    d. Have child sit on physioball while playing with toys

108. A PT is working with a child who has cerebral palsy. The child has limited range of motion (ROM) in bilateral upper extremities and is unable to reach out for objects. The PT provides intervention that focuses on allowing the child to participate in play activities. The best position to place the child in is
   a. Side-lying
   b. Prone
   c. Supine
   d. Sitting

109. A child diagnosed with cerebral palsy has severe spasticity in the bilateral upper extremities. The occupational therapy referral states "fabricate splints to prevent hand deformities." The theoretical approach for splinting should emphasize placement of the hands in the
   a. Intrinsic minus position
   b. Anticlaw position
   c. Resting hand position
   d. Reflex inhibiting position

110. A spinal cord injury patient who can breathe on his own, uses a sip and puff switch to operate his power wheelchair and environmental control unit, and a mouth stick for writing, table games, and the computer would MOST likely have a spinal cord injury at this level.
   a. C3
   b. C4
   c. C5
   d. C6

111. The highest level of spinal cord injury at which you would expect a client to become independent in all self-care and driving with equipment would be
   a. C7
   b. C8
   c. C5
   d. C6

112. You are treating a client that recently had a spinal cord injury at C5. The BEST piece of equipment to help the client with feeding, hygiene, grooming, writing, and driving a power wheelchair would be
   a. Deltoid assist
   b. Weighted pulley
   c. Mobile arm supports
   d. Suspension sling

113. The MOST beneficial piece of adaptive equipment to aid a client with C6 tetraplegia to work toward independence with lower extremity dressing is
    a. A trigger reacher to get the pants over the feet
    b. Loops to manipulate the lower extremities
    c. A universal cuff to assist with grip and closures
    d. A standard dressing stick

114. As a home health therapist, you are treating a 55-year-old who has a very supportive spouse and a caregiver during the day who helps with self-care and other tasks needed in the home. The patient enjoys their children and grandchildren who live in the immediate area. The patient is currently in stage 3 of amyotrophic lateral sclerosis, with severe weakness of the ankles, wrists, and hands. The patient minimally ambulates and fatigues easily. An appropriate intervention would be
    a. Light strengthening program
    b. Help prioritize activities and provide work simplification
    c. Learning how to cook three-course meals
    d. Worksite assessment

115. A 3-year-old has spina bifida and needs mobility augmentation to be able to move outdoors, in hallways, and in corridors. A mobility device that could be recommended would be a(n)
    a. Hand-propelled tricycle model
    b. Supine scooter
    c. Aeroplane mobility device
    d. Crocodile posterior walker

116. You are visiting the home of a client recently diagnosed with Alzheimer's. The environment is terribly cluttered and seems to add to the patient's current level of confusion. You decide to
    a. Clean up the place by yourself, throw away a lot, and put everything else away properly to help organize the environment for the client
    b. Leave it alone and just recognize that this is how the person will be living
    c. Engage family members in helping the client to sort through some of the cluttered items and make some choices about what to and what not to keep
    d. Encourage the family to hire a housekeeper, who will make sure that the environment is clean and tidy all the time

117. Which of the following is the most important to assess first during an examination of a patient with a recent stroke?
    a. Sensory status
    b. Motor control
    c. Mental status
    d. Ambulation potential

118.   A therapist receives an order to examine a 72-year-old woman who has suffered a recent stroke. The therapist needs to focus on pregait activities. Which of the proprioceptive neuromuscular facilitation (PNF) diagonals best encourages normal gait?
    a.   D1
    b.   D2
    c.   PNF is contraindicated
    d.   Pelvic PNF patterns only

119.   The following is a long-term goal for a patient with a spinal cord injury: independence in performing a manual cough without applying pressure to the abdomen. This goal is the most challenging and obtainable for a patient with a complete lesion at which of the following spinal cord levels?
    a.   C5
    b.   C7
    c.   T2
    d.   T10

120.   To treat effectively most patients with Parkinson's disease, the therapist should emphasize which proprioceptive neuromuscular facilitation (PNF) pattern for the upper extremities?
    a.   D2 extension
    b.   D2 flexion
    c.   D1 extension
    d.   D1 flexion

121.   Which of the following is the most energy efficient and allows a T1 complete paraplegic the most functional mobility during locomotion?
    a.   Manual wheelchair
    b.   Electric wheelchair
    c.   Bilateral knee-ankle orthoses and crutches
    d.   Bilateral ankle-foot orthoses and crutches

122.   To facilitate development of a functional tenodesis grip in a patient with a spinal cord injury, the treatment plan should include
    a.   Stretching of the finger flexors and finger extensors
    b.   Stretching of the finger flexors
    c.   Allowing the finger flexors and finger extensors to shorten
    d.   Allowing the finger flexors to shorten

123. A therapist is treating a patient with an injury at the T8 level and compromised function of the diaphragm. If no abdominal binder is available, what is the most likely position of comfort to allow him to breathe most efficiently?
    a. Sitting position
    b. Semi-Fowler's position
    c. Upright standing position using a tilt table
    d. Supine

124. A therapist is assisting a patient with an injury at the C5 level in performing an effective cough. The patient has experienced significant neurologic damage and is unable to perform an independent, effective cough. If the patient is in a supine position, which of the following methods is most likely to produce an effective cough?
    a. The therapist places the heel of one hand just above the xiphoid process, instructs the patient to take a deep breath while pressing down moderately on the sternum, and instructs the patient to cough.
    b. The therapist places the heel of one hand, reinforced with the other hand, just above the xiphoid process, instructs the patient to take a deep breath, instructs the patient to hold the breath, and presses moderately as the patient coughs.
    c. The therapist places the heel of one hand on the area just above the umbilicus, instructs the patient to take a deep breath, applies moderate pressure, and releases pressure just before the patient attempts to cough.
    d. The therapist places the heel of one hand just above the umbilicus, instructs the patient to take a deep breath, and applies moderate pressure as the patient is instructed to cough.

125. A physical therapist is ordered to examine a 65-year-old woman who has suffered a recent stroke. The occupational therapist informs the physical therapist that the patient has apraxia. She cannot brush her teeth on command. However, she can point out the toothbrush and verbalize the purpose of the brush. From this information, what sort of apraxia does this patient have? How should the physical therapist approach treatment?
    a. Ideomotor apraxia; The physical therapist should speak in short, concise sentences.
    b. Ideational apraxia; The physical therapist should always give the patient 3-step commands.
    c. Ideomotor apraxia; The physical therapist should always give the patient 3-step commands.
    d. Ideational apraxia; The physical therapist should speak in short, concise sentences.

126. A 60-year-old woman who has suffered a recent stroke has right-side homonymous hemianopsia. Which of the following statements is true about placement of eating utensils in early rehabilitation?
    a. The utensils should be placed on the left side of the plate
    b. The utensils should be placed on the right side of the plate.
    c. The utensils should be placed on both sides of the plate.
    d. The plate and utensils should be placed slightly to the right.

127. A 25-year-old man suffered C4 quadriplegia in a motor vehicle accident. The injury is acute, and the patient is beginning to work on increasing upright tolerance in the sitting position with an abdominal binder. He is looking to the therapist for encouragement. The therapist is attempting to convey realistic long-term goals for self-care ability and overall mobility. Of the below listed goals, what can this patient reasonably expect at his highest level of function in the future?
    a. Transfer from wheelchair to bed independently with a sliding board
    b. Use of a power wheelchair
    c. Independent feeding without an assistive device
    d. Donning a shirt independently and pants with minimal assistance

128. A 17-year-old boy presents to therapy after being involved in a motor vehicle accident resulting in C7 quadriplegia. The therapist is setting long-term goals for the patient. Which of the following goals represents the most reasonable and highest level of function that the patient should achieve?
    a. Use of a wheelchair with power hand controls on even terrain
    b. Negotiation of uneven terrain with a manual wheelchair
    c. Ambulation for short distances on level surfaces with knee-ankle-foot orthoses
    d. Use of a power wheelchair with head or chin controls on even surfaces

129. A therapist is treating a patient with a spinal cord injury. The therapist is discharging the patient after completion of all physical therapy goals. One of the completed long-term goals involved the ability to dress and bathe independently with assistive devices. This would be a most challenging but obtainable goal for which of the following?
    a. C5 quadriplegia
    b. C7 quadriplegia
    c. T1 paraplegia
    d. C4 quadriplegia

130. A physical therapist is examining a 5-day-old infant with cerebral palsy. The infant has an abnormal amount of extensor tone. Which of the following is incorrect positioning advice for the family and nursing staff?
    a. Keep the infant in a supine position.
    b. Keep the infant in a prone position.
    c. Keep the infant in a right side-lying position.
    d. Keep the infant in left side-lying position.

131. A physical therapist is treating a 76-year-old woman with left lower extremity hypotonia secondary to a recent stroke. Which of the following is an incorrect method to normalize tone?
    a. Rapid irregular movements
    b. Approximation
    c. Prolonged stretch
    d. Tactile cues

132. A therapist is attempting to open the spastic and flexed hand of a patient who has suffered a recent stroke. Which of the following does not inhibit hand opening?
    a. Avoid touching the interossei.
    b. Apply direct pressure to the thenar eminence.
    c. Hyperextend the metacarpophalangeal joint.
    d. Apply direct pressure to the hypothenar eminence.

133. Which of the following is inappropriate for a physical therapist to include in the treatment plan of an infant with a gestational age of 27 weeks and Down's syndrome?
    a. Bottle feeding
    b. Encourage sidlying position
    c. Tactile stimulation with the entire hand rather than the fingertips of the examiner
    d. Prone positioning

134. Which of the following sources of stimulation is least effective in obtaining functional goals when treating an infant with decreased muscular tone?
    a. Vestibular
    b. Weight bearing
    c. Cutaneous
    d. Vibratory

135. Which of the following is the most important goal in treating pediatric patients with postural reaction deficits?
    a. Age-appropriate responses
    b. Automatic responses
    c. Conscious responses
    d. Lower extremity control before upper extremity control

136. A physical therapist is treating an 81-year-old man with Parkinson's disease. The patient has been ambulating with a cane. He was referred to physical therapy because of a fall at home. The family reports a decrease in gait ability during the past several months. The therapist decides to begin gait training with a rolling walker. Which of the following is incorrect for the treatment of this patient?
    a. Strengthening of the hip flexors, and stretching of the gluteals
    b. Slow, rhythmical rocking techniques
    c. Biofeedback during ambulation
    d. Prolonged passive stretching of the gastrocnemius muscle group bilaterally

137. A patient who has suffered a recent stroke is being treated by a physical therapist. The patient exhibits increased extensor tone in the supine position along with an exaggerated symmetric tonic labyrinthine reflex (STLR). What position should be avoided if the therapist is attempting to initiate flexion movements of the lower extremity?
    a. Prone position
    b. Right side-lying position
    c. Supine position
    d. Left side-lying position

138. A patient presents to outpatient physical therapy with tarsal tunnel syndrome. What nerve is involved? Where should the therapist concentrate treatment?
    a. Superficial peroneal nerve, inferior to the medial malleolus
    b. Posterior tibial nerve, inferior to the medial malleolus
    c. Superficial peroneal nerve, inferior to the lateral malleolus
    d. Posterior tibial nerve, inferior to the lateral malleolus

139. Which of the following positions should be avoided in the right upper extremity with a patient who has a diagnosis of right hemiplegia secondary to a stroke?
    a. Prolonged shoulder adduction, internal rotation, elbow flexion
    b. Prolonged shoulder abduction, internal rotation, elbow flexion
    c. Prolonged finger and thumb flexion
    d. Prolonged wrist flexion and finger adduction

140. A 35-year-old male patient has a diagnosis of right C5-C6 cervical nerve root compression. He is being seen in physical therapy for gentle manual cervical traction. What position is ideal for traction with this patient?
    a. Upper cervical flexion and lower cervical extension
    b. Cervical lateral flexion to right
    c. Cervical extension
    d. Cervical flexion

141. During physical therapy sessions, the physical therapist protects tenodesis of the patient with diagnosis of C6 tetraplegia. What position must be maintained during upper extremity weight bearing and why?
    a. Maintain finger flexion with wrist extension to protect extrinsic wrist extensors.
    b. Maintain wrist flexion to protect intrinsic finger extensors.
    c. Maintain finger flexion to protect extrinsic finger flexors.
    d. Maintain wrist extension to protect intrinsic finger flexors.

142. A patient on the acute rehabilitation unit was diagnosed with traumatic closed head injury. He is functioning at a Rancho Cognitive Level of Function IV. He has no significant muscle weakness or gait impairments and walks without assistance. The team needs physical therapy's input on recommendations for safety and supervision. The physical therapist recommends
    a. No supervision is needed as the patient walks safely
    b. Constant supervision is needed because of confusion and possible agitation
    c. Intermittent supervision is needed to monitor his ability to follow a schedule
    d. Occasional supervision is needed when faced with new situations or schedule changes

143. Which is not a typical clinical finding of a patient with a brachial plexus injury?
    a. Decreased ROM/contractures
    b. Decreased muscle strength
    c. Spasticity
    d. Altered sensation

144. All are appropriate physical therapy goals for a 6-month-old patient with a brachial plexus injury except
    a. Able to creep forward 5 cycles
    b. Able to demonstrate protective reactions to each side in sitting
    c. Able to prop on forearms in a prone position with the head elevated 90 degrees
    d. Family independent with a home exercise program consisting of ROM and positioning

145. What would be the most appropriate intervention to include in the physical therapy plan of care for a 7-year-old female diagnosed with myelomeningocele at the T10-T11 level?
    a. Aggressive ROM of the lower extremities
    b. Gait training with a HKAFO and walker
    c. Gait training with a KAFO and forearm crutches
    d. Gait training with a reciprocating gait orthosis

146. An appropriate physical therapy program for an infant with a brachial plexus injury during the second week of life would include
    a. Teaching the parents how to support the arm while dressing and moving the infant to prevent further injury
    b. Daily PROM exercises including full shoulder abduction and elevation
    c. Daily AROM exercises including full shoulder abduction and elevation
    d. Splinting the shoulder in abduction and internal rotation

147. Which of the following exercise programs is most appropriate for a 62-year-old, postmenopausal female patient with MS who has poor balance and decreased strength?
    a. Stretching, posture, and balance program, with strengthening exercises as tolerated
    b. Stretching and progressive hill training on treadmill
    c. Warm water aquatic therapy
    d. Progressive hill training on treadmill with plyometric training

148. A therapist is instructed to provide electrical stimulation to a patient with a venous stasis ulcer on the right lower extremity. What is the correct type of electrical stimulation to promote wound healing?
    a. Biphasic pulsed current
    b. Direct current
    c. Interferential current
    d. Transcutaneous electrical stimulation

149. Which of the following is the best and first treatment for a wound with black eschar over 90% of the wound bed?
    a. Lidocaine
    b. Dexamethasone
    c. Silvadene
    d. Elase

150. A therapist is treating an acute full-thickness burn on the entire right lower extremity of a 27-year-old man. What movements need to be stressed with splinting, positioning, and exercise to avoid contractures?
    a. Hip flexion, knee extension, and ankle dorsiflexion
    b. Hip extension, knee flexion, and ankle plantar flexion
    c. Hip extension, knee extension, and ankle dorsiflexion
    d. Hip flexion, knee extension, and ankle plantar flexion

151. A therapist is teaching a family how to care for a family member at home. The patient is totally bed-bound. To prevent pressure ulcers most effectively, what should be the maximal amount of time between position changes?
    a. 1 hour
    b. 2 hours
    c. 6 hours
    d. 8 hours

152. Which of the following does not facilitate ambulation when the feet are burned?
    a. Constant movement, avoiding standing still
    b. Loosening or removing the bandages/wraps
    c. Establishing a clear goal for walking (e.g., to a favorite person/place)
    d. Exercise before standing upright

153. In which of the following wounds would the physical therapist consider using enzymatic debridement?
    a. Black eschar over the wound
    b. Clean wound
    c. A dry ischemic wound
    d. A dry wound with active infection

154. What is the most correct ambient temperature for a room that normally has a predominant population of burn patients?
    a. 65° F
    b. 72° F
    c. 78° F
    d. 85° F

155. A 47-year-old man with end-stage renal disease arrives at an outpatient facility. He has a physician's order to examine and treat 3 times/week for 4 weeks secondary to lower extremity weakness. The patient also attends dialysis 3 times a week. If the clinic is open Monday through Friday, which of the following schedules is appropriate?
    a. On the days that the patient has dialysis, schedule the therapy session before the dialysis appointment.
    b. On the days that the patient has dialysis, schedule the therapy session after the dialysis appointment.
    c. Contact the physician and obtain a new order to decrease the frequency to 2 times/week.
    d. Contact the physician and recommend home health physical therapy because outpatient therapy may be too aggressive.

156. Though relapses associated with multiple sclerosis (MS) tend to decrease during pregnancy, postpartum they increase. As physical therapists we are concerned with these patients' _____, _____ _____, and _____ to care for their new baby.
    a. sleeping patterns, strength, and attention
    b. vision, strength, and financing
    c. balance, fatigue, and ability
    d. balance, posture, and attention

157. Which is NOT a maternal response to mild-to-moderate exercise?
    a. Increased cardiac output
    b. Increased stroke volume
    c. Normal to increased heart rate
    d. Decreased respiratory rate

158. You are working in home health and visit a woman who is 8 months pregnant. The doctor has just placed her on strict bed rest; she is only allowed up to go to the bathroom. In what position will you have the patient do most of her exercise?
    a. Standing
    b. Supine
    c. Prone
    d. Side-lying

159. Three weeks earlier, your patient delivered via C-section a healthy baby girl who weighed in at 8 pounds, 6 ounces. This was her first pregnancy/delivery. Besides the incisional pain, she is having trouble "making it to the bathroom" and is very nervous of reaching over to pick up the baby. Which combination of activities is appropriate to do/complete on her first visit?
    a. MMT abdominals, education of abdominal exercises to help restore abdominal strength
    b. Education of pelvic floor exercises to help restore appropriate urinary frequency, body mechanics education
    c. MMT pelvic floor, weight training exercises to help patient lift the baby and gear
    d. ROM tests, electrical stimulation to help restore appropriate urinary frequency

160. In developing the plan of care for a 28-year-old pregnant woman, which of the following muscles should be the focus of the strengthening exercises to maintain a strong pelvic floor?
    a. Piriformis, obturator internus, and pubococcygeus
    b. Obturator internus, pubococcygeus, and coccygeus
    c. Rectus abdominis, iliococcygeus, and piriformis
    d. Iliococcygeus, pubococcygeus, and coccygeus

161. You ask your patient to extend her knee. She lacks 10 degrees of reaching full extension. In order for the knee to extend fully in this situation (sitting), the
    a. Tibia must rotate medially on the femur
    b. Tibia must rotate laterally on the femur
    c. Femur must rotate medially on the tibia
    d. Femur must rotate laterally on the tibia

162. Your 40-year-old male patient was playing basketball and describes hearing a pop and feeling as though someone kicked him in the back of the leg, followed by pain and weakness in the lower leg. The most common injury and special test to assess the problem is
    a. Anterior cruciate ligament tear, Lachman's test
    b. Achilles tendon rupture, Ober's test
    c. Anterior cruciate ligament tear, Thomas test
    d. Achilles tendon rupture, Thompson test

Answers

1. c. The presence of a throw rug could result in a fall, which would be far more hazardous to the health of an elderly client than the other objects in the environment. In the elderly, falls are the major cause of fractures.

2. c. If soft tissue shortening has occurred over time, low load prolonged stretch splinting would be ideal. This technique is very different from stretching and weight bearing, which typically position the patient into the greatest amount of stretch tolerated. AROM and PROM will have significantly less effect on the structures.

3. c. Fractured sites should remain stable to promote healing and realignment of the bones. However, the PT should encourage the movement of adjacent joints to assist in maintaining muscle strength and lengthening of tendons and muscles.

4. d. If grading shoulder flexion, the next step after achieving full shoulder flexion in a side-lying position is to begin to work or perform activities against gravity to begin increasing strength. Shoulder flexion against gravity is achieved with the individual in the sitting or standing position.

5. a. A person with a hip replacement should avoid any activity, such as shoe tying, which could potentially cause hip flexion to 90 degrees or greater. Such a position could actually undo the benefits of the surgical procedure.

6. c. When ascending or descending stairs, the cane should move with the painful/weak leg. Specifically, when ascending the stairs the leg without the cane should move first, allowing the weak leg and cane to bear the weight for only a short amount of time until the strong leg is able to provide the needed stability.

7. b. Discomfort and damage can occur if the scapula is not gliding with the humerus during movement. Passive ROM can cause damage if the structures are not moving properly. An orthopedic specialist may be beneficial if therapy interventions have not been successful.

8. b. The term "soft end field" is a spongy quality at end range of a joint contracture. It usually indicates that the joint has the potential to remodel. A low-load, long duration stretch may yield the best results.

9.   d.   Acute myelopathy is considered an absolute contraindication to manipulation. This may be seen in cervical spondylotic myelopathy. Smoking, hypertension, and use of birth control pills are considered risks for vertebrobasilar insufficiency.

10.   b.   When the disc is in the axilla of the nerve root (medial), axial traction may irritate the problem.

11.   d.   With the seat close to the pedals, the lumbopelvic region is flexed, separating the posterior facets and disc space at L5-S1. Adding a lumbar pillow supports the lumbar curve at the same time.

12.   c.   The pitcher is moving into D2 extension with the throwing motion. He is strengthening the muscles involved in shoulder internal rotation, adduction, and forearm pronation.

13.   b.   Grade I is a small oscillating movement at the beginning of range. Grade III is a large movement up to the end of available range. Grade IV is a small movement at the end of available range.

14.   c.   Patients with recurrent ankle sprains benefit from proprioceptive exercises. Choices B and D are not indicated because of the lack of acute signs and symptoms. Choice A is a good plan, but not the most correct because there is no mention of proprioception.

15.   b.   The patient should have made adequate progress in this period with this protocol. Because of the lack of progress, the patient needs further evaluation by the physician.

16.   d.   The patient most likely has a rotator cuff tear. Choices A and B are incorrect because there is no need for heating modalities. Choice C is wrong because the patient has full passive range of motion.

17.   a.   Choice A is the correct gait sequence for ascending stairs in the given scenario. A caregiver should stand below the patient because the patient is most likely to fall down the stairs. This same rule holds true for descending stairs.

18.   a.   Isometric exercises in the shortest range of the extensor muscle are used to begin strengthening. In contrast, weak flexor muscles should be strengthened in the middle-to-lengthened range, because they most often work near their end range.

19.   d.   This position places the least amount of stress on the lumbar spine in the sitting position.

20. c. The therapist must stretch the inferior portion of the capsule in an effort to gain abduction of the involved shoulder. This principle is supported by the convex-concave rule.

21. c. Rhythmic stabilization involves a series of isometric contractions of the agonist then the antagonist.

22. d. The five stages of grieving are (in order from first to last) are denial, anger, bargaining, depression, and acceptance.

23. d. The ACL-deficient patient has a significant rotatory instability. Bracing may prevent some of this instability. Sports that are especially difficult on the knees (e.g., skiing, competitive tennis) are contraindicated.

24. c. Trigger points are often treated with soft tissue massage. Other techniques include strain/counterstrain, myofascial release, and muscle energy techniques.

25. b. Choice B is correct because the patient has to achieve passive knee extension before she can gain full active knee extension. Full active knee extension and full flexion are important and should be a major focus of the patient's session, but the question asks for the most serious deficit. Ambulating with a lesser assistive device should be the focus at a later time because the patient's gait is still severely antalgic and obvious instability is still present. Usually a patient is advanced to a lesser assistive device when he or she can ambulate without large gait deviations with the current assistive device.

26. c. Because of the unreliable history obtained in the evaluation, the therapist at least should make a quick assessment of range of motion and strength before the patient attempts to stand. Sit-to-stand transfer should then be assessed in front of the lift chair before the patient attempts to ambulate.

27. a. The method used in Choice A is the safest. The method used in Choice C is too unstable.

28. b. Passive extension is the most important motion to gain after an anterior cruciate ligament reconstruction, regardless of the graft type. Active extension can be achieved once passive extension is full (or equal bilaterally).

29. a. Because the patient lives alone, independent transfer is the most important goal listed. Functional ambulation is an important goal, but choice B is an unrealistic goal for the patient to accomplish in a 2- or 3-day period.

30. d. This choice lists the stages of control in the correct order.

31. d. Choice D is the correct treatment. Strengthening is not indicated at this time, and splinting as described in Choice C places too much stretch on the tendons. In addition, static splinting does not allow tendon gliding. Ultrasound is contraindicated over a healing tendon repair.

32. b. The shrinker should be removed only for bathing. Because the surgical scars are healed, the stump can be immersed in water.

33. a. Because of poor balance, geriatric patients should increase the treadmill grade rather than the speed. Use of machines allows better posture and low intensities and limits the exercise within the patient's safe range of motion.

34. d. Movements that stress the posterolateral hip joint capsule should be avoided. Sources vary on the exact amount of flexion that should be avoided. Passive hip abduction should be maintained after surgery with a wedge.

35. a. This patient most likely has a right anterior rotation of the right innominate and thus needs right posterior mobilization of the right innominate.

36. c. This position, which limits inversion, plantar flexion, and adduction, is the most common position for ankle sprains.

37. c. Transverse (perpendicular to the scar) or circular massage assists in mobilization of scar tissue.

38. b. The patient has an extension lag, which may be due to any source that has inhibited the quadriceps and results in an inability to fully extend the knee actively.

39. d. The treatment techniques should be performed in the order of mobility, stability, controlled mobility, and skill.

40. a. Tennis elbow results from overuse of the wrist extensors. The shoulder external rotators should be used to power a backhand.

41. c. The radial pull component is designed to allow tightening of the radial side of the capsule.

42. d. This is the most stable position of the hip, which allows for more normal growth.

43. a. Normally, the ankle requires 20 degrees or more of dorsiflexion for a patient to run or ascend/descend stairs properly. Independent ambulation with a normal gait pattern requires 10 degrees of dorsiflexion.

44. b. Because of the length of the time since the surgical procedure, the patient may have adhesive capsulitis. The capsule should continue to be stretched to increase range of motion. The patient should visit the physician if the range of motion deficits continue. Active exercise may be necessary at this stage of recovery, but it will not help to relieve a capsular dysfunction.

45. c. Because the scaphoid has a poor vascular supply, aggressive therapy should be avoided until the bone is fully healed (12 to 24 weeks). A Colles fracture (fracture of the distal radius with dorsal movement of the fixed segment) should heal in 6 to 8 weeks. A boxer's fracture (fracture of the fifth metacarpal) requires 4 to 6 weeks. A Bennett's fracture (fracture of the proximal first metacarpal) usually requires 6 to 8 weeks. The length of healing time given in the above examples obviously depends on the individual patient and the type of surgical fixation (if any).

46. a. Lateral step-ups are probably too difficult for a patient who received an anterior ligament reconstruction with a patella tendon autograft 2 weeks ago.

47. c. The wrists should be in neutral position when the fingers are on the middle row of the keyboard.

48. c. Tools with small handles require more grip strength. Tasks below shoulder height reduce the risk of impingement, and more force can be applied to tasks if they are kept below elbow height.

49. a. In response to a pronated subtalar joint, the forefoot undergoes a supination twist and the first ray dorsiflexes. Because the distal first cuneiform is convex and the proximal first metatarsal is concave, inferior mobilization of the first metatarsal is required.

50. b. The leg length discrepancy would have been resolved by the surgical procedure, and pain at the surgical site will have diminished by 2 months postoperatively. Knee ROM will be more limited than hip because the procedure involved the distal femur.

51. d. An endoprosthetic implant is limited in the amount of growth that can be accommodated. Allografts are only appropriate for children nearing skeletal maturity, and a hip disarticulation would not allow for normal active play even with a prosthesis. Rotationplasty is a radical surgery, but it is the best option in this case.

52. c. The Pavlik harness allows the hips to be maintained in flexion and abduction by limiting extension and adduction. This position limits avascular necrosis common with this diagnosis.

53. d. Grade III injuries are complete ruptures of the ligament involved. Grade I injuries are considered minor, while grade II injuries will have associated edema, pain, and some loss of joint stability.

54. c. Upper trapezius strengthening will only exacerbate this dysfunction, and the elbow exercise is irrelevant to this type of biomechanical problem. The supraspinatus responds best to gravity-resisted exercise early and a slow progression of resistance not to exceed 3 to 5 pounds.

55. b. The arthrokinematics of the shoulder joint would lead one to believe that the posterior capsule is the most in need of mobilization.

56. d. Since the motion restriction occurs in the upper ranges of flexion, mobilizations should focus on this portion of ROM. Arguments could be made for glenohumeral mobilization for the posterior and inferior capsule, but those choices do not exist.

57. b. The shoulder is still early in rehabilitation at 6 days postoperatively. Protection by the sling (along with ice for pain control) is a good suggestion. It is too early for aggressive exercise, and heat should never be used at this stage of recovery.

58. a. Since no trauma to the shoulder musculature is involved with this procedure, AROM can begin immediately (within painful limits and surgical guidelines).

59. a. Posterior mobilization would release any restriction on ROM into internal rotation. Lack of treatment for the biceps tendonitis symptoms would possibly delay strengthening of the upper extremity.

60.   d.   Although these complaints are very common after this particular procedure, the cervical spine should be examined. A cervical condition may have been masked by shoulder pain. Often there is abnormal muscle tone in this area as a response to the surgery.

61.   a.   The anterior capsule in the overhead throwing athlete should not be mobilized or stretched. Typically these athletes already have hypermobilty in this area. Treatment should focus on the posterior capsule.

62.   c.   Anterior digastric trigger point refers to the incisors of the mandible.

63.   a.   Other symptoms may include pain and tenderness located at the joint, clicking, and crepitation. Although tinnitus, headache, and dizziness may be associated with a temporomandibular joint disorder, they are not caused by the disorder.

64.   c.   Thirty-eight millimeters is a reasonable opening range for function: eating, placing food in the mouth, brushing teeth, singing and yawning

65.   a.   Add stabilization exercises within the click free range. These patients may need anterior stabilization splinting if painful clicking and catching persists.

66.   d.   A locked joint will not "unlock" by using a splint. A "locked joint" is represented by choice D

67.   d.   Arthroscopy has not been found to be better than physical therapy in the treatment of reduced jaw ROM and pain due to intra-articular disease.

68.   b.   To alleviate an acute closed lock disorder (anterior disc displacement without reduction), aggressive PT may mobilize the joint to unlock in 3 to 4 visits. The disc may not have permanent deformation changes or adhesions form, if the patient is young and the mobilization is done early. If unsuccessful, additional less aggressive PT would be indicated to decrease joint inflammation, or a surgical consult may be necessary.

69.   c.   Distal radius fractures are common and controversial. The current trend is to treat them surgically, but many patients heal with some deformity and acceptable function.

70.   a.   Saggital band tightness can be difficult to resolve, but nonoperative treatment remains the treatment of choice.

71. b. The concave distal radius on the convex proximal carpals should be mobilized. The wrist joint consists of the concave distal radius, an articular disc and the relatively convex proximal row of carpal bones. All other choices include the wrong bony surfaces.

72. a. Right cervical rotation and left lateral cervical flexion is the correct choice. To correct the right torticollis the patient needs to move into right rotation and left lateral flexion to stretch his right sternocleidomastiod (SCM).

73. c. The patient will have 50% loss of cervical rotation. The C1-C2 level produces approximately 50% of the cervical rotation allowed in the entire cervical spine.

74. b. Plantar flexor spasticity. Spastic plantar flexors will produce excessive plantar flexion, and also knee extension throughout the stance phase, and prevent adequate passive knee flexion in preswing. The hamstrings are not responsible for knee flexion in preswing phase of gait. Plantar flexor weakness would cause tibial forward collapse and therefore excess knee flexion. Dorsiflexors are not responsible for knee flexion in preswing.

75. a. Adductor hypertonicity of the swing leg. The swing leg is adducting because of hypertonicity. The quadriceps does not play a key role during swing. The plantar flexors are not active in swing; weakness is not going to create a significant problem in this phase. Plantar flexor weakness impacts terminal stance. A person with plantar flexor weakness would demonstrate excessive hip flexion in swing, not adduction. Gluteus medius hypertonicity would cause excess hip abduction, NOT adduction.

76. c. Based on the convex concave rule concept, moving the concave surface of the tibia anteriorly onto the convex surface of the femur will increase extension. Roll and glide will occur in the same direction. Choices A and B will both increase flexion while mobilization of the patella will be more advantages in helping with flexion of the knee because of its attachment to the quadricep muscle.

77. c. The Adson's maneuver tests the patency of the subclavian artery as it passes from beneath the anterior scalene and middle. If that muscle is tight, then the result will be a diminished radial pulse. Choice B would be tested by the costoclavicular test, and the pectoralis minor is assessed with the hyperabduction test. The sternocleidomastiods do not affect the thoracic outlet.

78. b. Right torticollis involves the right sternocleidomastoid and results in cervical right side bend and left rotation. In order to stretch the muscle, the cervical spine must be placed in left side bend and right rotation.

79. c. To transition from low to high kneel requires active hip extension; therefore, the gluteus maximus needs to be activated.

80. a. Angina is recurring chest pain and is an indication of coronary artery disease. An onset of angina during treatment should be considered an emergency because of the possibility of a heart attack and will need to be addressed by the physician.

81. d. MET refers to the amount of energy consumed at rest that is equal to the approximately equivalent to 3.5 milliliters of oxygen per kilogram of body weight per minute. Various tasks or activities require a certain amount of energy to perform. After performing homemaking activities, such as washing dishes and ironing, the next progression in homemaking tasks from the choices listed would be preparing a meal (MET level 3 to 4). Driving and dressing qualify as a MET level of 2 to 3; gardening has an MET level of 4 to 5.

82. a. Pursed-lip breathing technique is helpful when shortness of breath occurs. Technique: the person inhales deeply through the nose, purses the lips as though whistling, and very slowly exhales through the lips.

83. a. Exercise has many benefits. Decreased HDL in choice A makes this an inappropriate list of the benefits of exercise. HDL is considered "good" cholesterol. Exercise decreases LDL and increases HDL in the bloodstream.

84. b. Choice B has the patient exercising at 65% to 90% of his age-adjusted maximal heart rate. Choice C is the patient's age-adjusted maximal heart rate. Choice A is much too high a parameter. Exercise in the 65% to 90% of maximal Vo_2 is much more appropriate. Patients should exercise at level 12 to 15 on the RPE scale.

85. a. Choice A is the correct postural drainage. Choice B is drained by resting on the right, one quarter turn to the back, and foot of the bed elevated 12 to 16 inches. Choices C and D are drained with patient in long sitting position or leaning forward over the pillow in sitting position.

86. d. Performing isometric exercises places too much load on the left ventricle of the heart for many cardiac patients.

87. c. ST-segment displacement greater than 3 mm is a contraindication. Resting systolic pressure above 200 mm Hg is a contraindication.

88. b. A rating of 9 corresponds with "very light." A rating of 7 is "very, very light." A rating of 13 is "somewhat hard." A rating of 15 is "hard." A rating of 17 is "very hard." A rating of 19 is "very, very hard."

89   d. Riding a stationary bike at 5.5 mph is approximately 3.5 METs. Descending a flight of stairs is approximately 4 to 5 METs. Ironing is approximately 3.5 METs. Ambulating 5 to 6 mph is approximately 8.6 METs.

90. c. Patients with chronic obstructive airway disease are often given this set of instructions, which is known as the method of pursed-lip breathing. This method helps a patient regain control of his or her breathing rate and increase tidal volume and amount of oxygen absorbed.

91. a. The incentive spirometer provides visual feedback of maximal inspiratory efforts. The physical therapist is qualified to answer the patient's question. Incentive spirometry should only be used in acute episodes of COPD. There is a risk of air trapping with long-term use.

92. d. Suctioning also can be performed in patients with significant hypoxemia. All other choices are valid indications for suctioning. Patients should be supplied with 100% oxygen before suctioning to prevent hypoxemia.

93. d. Choice A increases strength of the scalenes and sternocleidomastoid. Choice B strengthens the latissimus dorsi. Choice C increases the strength of the upper trapezius. All of these are accessory inspiratory muscles. Choice D strengthens the abdominals, which are muscles of forceful expiration.

94. d. Intermittent claudication is a sign of chronic arterial disease. Choice A is incorrect because it produces unilateral signs and symptoms. Choice B is incorrect because, although the signs and symptoms may be present in a patient with multiple sclerosis, this scenario paints a more accurate picture of a patient who has intermittent claudication. A compartment syndrome usually involves the anterior tibialis. In addition, patients with compartment syndrome require a longer rest time than this question implies before pain subsides.

95. c.   To reach as described in the question, the patient must shift weight to the right buttock and elongate the right side of the trunk. With the same circumstances given in the question, but to the left side, the patient would shift weight to the left buttock and elongate the left side of the trunk.

96. a.   Atrial fibrillation is a relative contraindication for therapy. Exercise should start at a lower intensity and be progressed slowly if the ventricular rate remains controlled. There is no contraindication against upper extremity exercise.

97. b.   In complete supine, patients with this diagnosis will have excess fluid move from the lower body to the chest cavity. This causes a decrease in heart and lung function and efficiency.

98. d.   According to Goodman and Snyder (Differential Diagnosis in Physical Therapy, 3rd edition), Choices A through C are red flags and indicate the need for immediate referral and follow-up for patients with a history of cardiac dysfunction. There is a concern that the patient is not medically stable or there is an expansion of the infarction. Exercise at present is contraindicated. Chest pain that is managed effectively with nitroglycerin is not an immediate cause for concern.

99. b.   Training effects usually include increases in myocardial mass, stroke volume, ventilation, and respiratory muscular endurance.

100. a.   Once hemostasis has been achieved after an acute hemorrhage, the physical therapy program should include instruction of a home exercise program consisting of active ROM and strengthening exercises, isometrics, knee extension exercises in supine and sitting, and active resistive exercises may be initiated if the knee has at least 90 degrees of flexion and less than 15 degrees flexion contracture. Passive ROM is contraindicated.

101. a.   The PT should work to control pain before using the involved extremity for functional activities, such as grooming and basic ADLs. Although gentle mobilization may be used, pain management techniques should be the immediate focus. Pain management spans a wide array of techniques, including relaxation, massage, biofeedback, and positioning.

102. a.   The first priority is to reduce edema because other symptoms may be somewhat relieved and motion can be enhanced with a reduction in swelling.

103.   c.   If there are no other complications, a person with a spinal cord injury at the level of C8 would most likely be independent in mobility with the use of either a manual or motorized wheelchair and a sliding board for transfers

104.   d.   The skill of holding and drinking from a bottle typically emerges around 6 months of age.

105.   a.   The asymmetric tonic neck reflex (ATNR) is present in utero through 6 to 8 months while the child is awake and up to 42 months while the child is sleeping. Because of the ATNR reflex, the child's head turns toward the extended arm and leg and the opposite arm and leg bend. This reflex may help in the birth process, assist in the development of visual motor integration, and protect the airway while the child is in the prone position.

106.   c.   Rhythmic swinging calms the child while maintaining a level of alertness. This is an effective use of sensory preparation for activity. Combine this with rhythmic vocalization and deep pressure to help calm the child before engaging in an activity. The therapist must watch the child for response to the sensory preparation and gear input accordingly.

107.   a.   The prone position is the best for facilitating neck and trunk extension whether on a ball, bolster, or wedge.

108.   d.   The most common and effective position to place a child in is sitting, with attention given to head and neck control, visual regard, and visual tracking. Although the child can be placed in the supine and side-lying positions, sitting is the most commonly used position.

109.   d.   The NDT approach advocates the use of the reflex-inhibiting patterns to inhibit spasticity. Finger and thumb abduction are key to controlling spasticity by facilitating extensor muscle tone and inhibiting flexor tone.

110.   b.   A client with a C4 injury would have innervation of the muscles controlling the head, neck, and diaphragm and would be the most appropriate choice for these activities.

111.   d.   A client with a C6 injury would have control of the head, neck, diaphragm, deltoids, biceps, and wrist extensors, giving the client enough function to complete the activities.

112.   c.   Mobile arm supports would be the best choice because they can be mounted to the wheelchair and will allow for the most ease of movement in a safe manner.

113.   b.   The loops would be the best. The client would be unable to use a trigger reacher and the standard dressing stick because the client does not have a functional grasp. The universal cuff would be of no benefit to grip and don pants and could only be used for closure with an additional device (button hook/zipper pull).

114.   b.   Amyotrophic lateral sclerosis is a degenerative disease without a cure that results in death. Stage 3 is characterized by moderate dependence in self-care ADLs and IADLs along with severe weakness of the arms and legs. At this stage of the disease, conserving energy and quality of life are paramount.

115.   a.   Hand-propelled tricycle models are available for children who do not have the ability to pedal with their legs. These can provide mobility outdoors, in hallways, and in corridors.

116.   c.   Alzheimer's patients often have difficulty with change. The family members can contribute information about what items are valuable and should be retained and can also assist the client in gradually changing in the environment to reduce stress and allow time to adjust.

117.   c.   Mental status is the first item to assess. A therapist must first determine whether the patient is able to provide a reliable subjective history. It is also important to know whether the patient can follow a 1- or 2-step command before beginning a formal evaluation. The other choices should be assessed later in the evaluation.

118.   a.   The therapist would use a PNF D1 diagonal to encourage the combined movements of hip flexion, adduction, and knee flexion. The diagonal also encourages the combined movements of hip adduction and extension. This is the combination of muscle activity most needed for gait.

119.   b.   A patient with a spinal cord injury at the C5 level would apply pressure to the abdomen to perform a cough. A patient with an injury at the T2 level and T10 level should be able to perform a cough independently, but this goal would be most challenging and obtainable for a patient with an injury at the level of C7.

120. b. D2 flexion patterns support upper trunk extension, which is important for patients with Parkinson's disease who tend to develop excessive kyphosis.

121. a. An electric wheelchair definitely uses less energy but does not require the physical effort needed by this patient to maintain functional mobility. Ambulation with a knee-ankle-foot orthosis is probably possible but requires much more energy than locomotion with a manual wheelchair. Ankle-foot orthoses alone do not provide enough support for the patient to attempt ambulation.

122. d. To assist a patient in developing a tenodesis grip, the therapist should allow the patient's finger flexors to tighten. This grip functions with active extension of the wrist, which allows flexion of the fingers because of shortened flexor tendons.

123. d. Choice D is the correct answer because in the supine position the abdominal contents are located more superiorly than in the other positions. This places the diaphragm in a more elevated resting position, which allows greater excursion of the diaphragm. Semi-Fowler's position resembles a reclining position, with the knees bent and the upper trunk slightly elevated. Semi-Fowler's position, without an abdominal binder, allows gravity to pull the abdominal contents downward, which does not put the diaphragm in an optimal resting position. Semi-Fowler's position is, however, the position of choice for patients with uncompromised innervation of the diaphragm who have chronic respiratory difficulty. The standing and sitting positions present the same problem, but to a greater extent, as semi-Fowler's position.

124. d. The pressure applied by the therapist should be applied as the patient coughs to assist in a forceful exhalation. Placing the heel of one hand approximately one inch above the umbilicus applies pressure immediately inferior to the diaphragm.

125. a. Patients with ideomotor apraxia often can identify objects but cannot use them correctly on command. Such patients often can perform the activity spontaneously. Patients with ideational apraxia often cannot identify objects or use them. Both situations call for short one-step commands.

126. a. As perception improves, objects should be moved into the area of the deficit (the right side in this case), but initially they should be placed in plain view of the patient (the left side in this case).

127. b. A person with C4 quadriplegia can be reasonably expected to use a power wheelchair for locomotion with mouth, chin, breath, or sip-and-puff controls. A person with C5 quadriplegia may be reasonably expected to be able to transfer independently from wheelchair to bed with a sliding board. A person with C4 quadriplegia may be able to feed independently but will need some type of assistive device. A person with C5 quadriplegia may be able to don a shirt with assistance. Sources vary significantly on this subject.

128. b. A person with C7 quadriplegia should be able to use a wheelchair without power controls. The goals set in Choices A and D do not represent the maximal functional potential for this patient. The goal in Choice C is set too high for this patient.

129. b. This goal should be most challenging and obtainable for a patient with C7 quadriplegia. A person with C4 or C5 quadriplegia probably needs assistance from another person to dress and bathe. A person with C7 quadriplegia would find this goal more challenging than a person with T1 paraplegia.

130. a. Prone and side-lying positions would encourage flexion of the extremities with this patient. In this population, prone positioning allows more efficient cardiovascular function. The right or left side of side-lying does not make any difference in this situation.

131. c. A prolonged stretch assists in decreasing tone.

132. a. Avoiding the interossei helps to inhibit tone. Direct pressure to any hand musculature may increase tone. Hyperextension of the MCP joints also may cause an increase in tone.

133. a. Bottle or breastfeeding is rarely performed successfully before 34 weeks of gestational age. Side-lying position allows the infant to move the hands toward the mouth. The prone position encourages flexion. Full contact with the hand is more comforting to the infant.

134. d. Although vibration often elicits a muscle contraction, a therapist should first choose stimuli that are more likely to occur naturally.

135. b. Postural reactions are automatic unconscious reactions to changes in center of mass. Choice A is an appropriate goal but not always the most important.

136. a. Patients with Parkinson's disease usually ambulate with the trunk
          in flexion. Increased trunk flexion causes a festinating gait to be
          more pronounced. Therapy should strengthen extensor muscles
          while stretching the flexors. Slow rocking has been shown to
          decrease tone, and biofeedback can improve a gait with shorter
          step and stride length by placement of markers on the floor for
          the feet.

137. c. When an exaggerated symmetric tonic labyrinthine reflex is
          present, supine positioning increases extensor tone and prone
          positioning increases flexor tone. Side-lying also provides an
          opportunity for the physical therapist to stimulate flexion. Right
          of left side-lying makes no difference in this case.

138. b. Tarsal tunnel syndrome is caused by compression of the posterior
          tibial nerve as it travels through the tarsal tunnel. The tarsal tunnel
          is formed by the medial malleolus, medial collateral ligament,
          talus, and calcaneus.

139. b. Flexed postures should be avoided with this patient population.
          Positions of shoulder adduction, internal rotation, and wrist
          flexion are contraindicated. As well as wrist, finger, thumb
          flexion, and finger thumb adduction.

140. d. Cervical flexion. Cervical flexion opens up the cervical
          intervertebral joint spaces. Any extension or lateral flexion
          towards the impingement will result in nerve root compression.

141. c. Maintain finger flexion to protect extrinsic finger flexors.
          Tenodesis is passive insufficiency of the extrinsic finger flexors.
          After SCI lesion at C6, people can use preserved wrist extension
          combined with passive finger flexion to grip objects. Preserving
          extrinsic finger flexor tightness is essential to maintaining passive
          insufficiency.

142. b. Constant supervision is needed due to confusion and possible
          agitation. Rancho Los Amigos Cognitive Level of Function IV is
          confused-agitated and will need constant supervision.

143. c. A brachial plexus injury is a lower motor neuron injury; and
          therefore, it does not cause spasticity, an upper motor neuron sign.

144. a. All are appropriate goals and gross motor skills for a 6-month-old
          with a brachial plexus injury except creeping forward, which is
          more appropriate for an 8 to 9 month old.

145. d. A patient with myelomeningocele at the T10-T11 level would have innervation of the abdominals but not of the lower extremities. Therefore, the patient would require a reciprocating gait orthosis in order to ambulate. In addition, aggressive ROM of the lower extremities would be contraindicated for a patient with this diagnosis because of possible osteoporosis and risk for fracture.

146. a. The physical therapy program should focus on preserving function and minimizing further injury to the affected extremity. Nursing staff and parents need to be taught how to handle the patient during dressing and transfers to reduce stress and pain in the arm. Passive ROM is important and should be initiated around week 1 but no later than 3 weeks. Shoulder abduction and elevation is limited to 90 degrees for the first 3 weeks. It is no longer recommended that the arm be splinted in abduction and external rotation position because of the risk of causing shoulder dislocations.

147. a. Activities that unduly increase body temperature are not recommended for patients with MS. Keep in mind that spasticity is a significant complication of MS and can adversely affect gait parameters. If the patient is presenting with poor balance and decreased strength, hill training and plyometric training may be too aggressive for this particular patient. At this age, improving balance, strength, and coordination are paramount to preventing falls and future injury.

148. b. Direct current is shown to have the greatest benefit in wound healing. Monophasic pulsed current has also been shown to have wound healing benefits.

149. d. The correct treatment involves debridement of the eschar over the wound. Elase is an enzymatic wound debridement ointment. Lidocaine is an anesthetic. Dexamethasone is a steroid used mainly with iontophoresis. Silvadene is an antimicrobial used to prevent infection.

150. c. This answer is correct because the most common deformity after a severe burn such as this is hip flexion, hip adduction, knee flexion, and ankle plantar flexion.

151. b. To prevent pressure (decubitis) ulcers effectively, patients should be turned every 2 hours.

152. b. Choices A, C and D are key to early ambulation after a burn. Bandages should not be loosened unless they are painful. Loose bandages might cause edema.

153. a. Enzymatic debridement is only appropriate in wounds that have thick black eschar. The enzymes have no effect on infections.

154. d. Burn patients lose heat more rapidly than other individuals. It is advisable to keep room temperatures at a higher than normal level.

155. a. Dialysis leads to a change in blood chemistry and volume, often causing extreme fatigue, treatments should be before dialysis. There is no need to decrease frequency or recommend home health.

156. c. Most women experience relief of most, if not all MS symptoms during pregnancy. However, relapse rate postpartum is considered to be 20% to 40%. It is recommended that patients with MS have a contingency plan in place to plan for changes in the ability to take care of the baby.

157. d. As pregnancy advances, oxygen and carbon dioxide have more challenge transferring from the air to cells. Though there is increased cardiac output, there is also increased demand. Pregnant women compensate for this by breathing more deeply and with increased frequency.

158. d. Usually assigned to allow improved uterine blood flow, bed rest can have devastating effects on a mother's body and mind. It is recommended to do exercise in side-lying to limit stress/pressure on the inferior vena cava possibly achieved in supine positioning; prone positioning at this stage in pregnancy is impractical, standing may be too stressful on the cervix and uterus.

159. b. Reassurance and education are key components to helping a new mother understand how to best take care of herself and her baby. Three weeks is too early to initiate an abdominal training program (or manually muscle test them), and usual recommendations following C-section include not lifting anything heavier than the baby during early recovery.

160. d. One of the main reasons that pelvic floor exercises are beneficial for a pregnant woman is the extra weight of the viscera.

161. b. The tibia must rotate laterally on the femur. Choice B describes the screw home mechanism in which the tibia rotates around the femur.

162. d. Achilles tendon rupture, Thompson test is the correct choice. The injury mechanism described is a classic Achilles rupture. The Thompson test assesses the integrity of the Achilles tendon. The Thompson test involves the patient in the prone position. The calf muscle complex is squeezed by the therapist. A positive test results in no movement of the ankle. If the ankle plantar flexes slightly, the Achilles tendon is considered intact.

CHAPTER 5

Equipment and Devices

1. Which of the following is a contraindication to ultrasound at 1.5 watts/cm^2 with a 1-MHz sound head?
   a. Over a recent fracture site
   b. Over noncemented metal implant
   c. Over a recently surgically repaired tendon
   d. Over the quadriceps muscle belly

2. While obtaining the history from a 62-year-old woman weighing 147 pounds, the therapist discovers that the patient has a history of rheumatoid arthritis. The order for outpatient physical therapy includes continuous traction due to an L2 disc protrusion. What is the best course of action for the therapist?
   a. Follow the order.
   b. Consult with the physician because rheumatoid arthritis is a contraindication.
   c. Apply intermittent traction instead of continuous traction.
   d. Use continuous traction with the weight setting at 110 pounds.

3. A 25-year-old woman has been referred to a physical therapist by an orthopedist because of low back pain. The therapist is performing an ultrasound at the L3 level of the posterior back when the patient suddenly informs the therapist that she is looking forward to having her third child. On further investigation, the therapist discovers that the patient is in the first trimester of pregnancy. Which of the following is the best course of action for the therapist?
   a. Change the settings of the ultrasound from continuous to pulsed.
   b. Continue with the continuous setting because first-trimester pregnancy is not a contraindication.
   c. Cease treatment, notify the patient's orthopedic physician, and document the mistake.
   d. Send the patient to the gynecologist for an immediate sonogram.

4. The therapist routinely places ice on the ankle of a patient with an acute ankle sprain. Ice application has many therapeutic benefits. Which of the following is the body's first response to application of ice?
   a. Vasoconstriction of local vessels
   b. Decreased nerve condition velocity
   c. Decreased local sensitivity
   d. Complaints of pain

5. Which of the following theories supports the use of a transcutaneous electrical nerve stimulation (TENS) unit for sensory level pain control?
   a. Gate control theory
   b. Sensory interaction theory
   c. Central summation theory
   d. Sensory integration theory

6. Which of the following tissues absorbs the least amount of an ultrasound beam at 1 MHz?
   a. Bone
   b. Skin
   c. Muscle
   d. Blood

7. The therapist decides to use electrical stimulation to increase a patient's quadriceps strength. Which of the following is the best protocol?
   a. Electrodes placed over the superior/lateral quadriceps and the vastus medialis obliquus; stimulation on for 15 seconds, then off for 15 seconds
   b. Electrodes over the femoral nerve in the proximal quadriceps and the vastus medialis obliquus; stimulation on for 50 seconds, then off for 10 seconds
   c. Electrodes over the vastus medialis obliquus and superior/lateral quadriceps; stimulation frequency set between 50 to 80 hertz, pps
   d. Electrodes over the femoral nerve in the proximal quadriceps and the vastus medialis obliquus; stimulation frequency set between 50 to 80 hertz, pps

8. A therapist should consider using a form of treatment other than moist heat application on the posterior lumbar region of all of the following patients except
   a. Patient with a history of hemophilia
   b. Patient with a history of malignant cancer under the site of heat application
   c. Patient with a history of Raynaud's phenomenon
   d. Patient with a history including many years of steroid therapy

9. A 50-year-old woman has been receiving treatment in the hospital for increased edema in the right upper extremity. The therapist has treated the patient for the past 3 weeks with an intermittent compression pump equipped with a multicompartment compression sleeve. The patient's average blood pressure is 135/80 mm Hg. The daily sessions are 3 hours in duration. The pump is set at 50 mm Hg, 40 mm Hg, and 30 mm Hg (distal to proximal) for 30 seconds, on and off for 15 seconds. The therapist decides to change the parameters. Of the following changes, which is the most likely to increase the efficiency of treatment?
   a. Place the patient in a seated position with the right upper extremity in a dependent position versus supine and elevated.
   b. Increase the maximal pressure from 50 mm Hg to 60 mm Hg.
   c. Change the on/off time to 15 seconds on and 45 seconds off.
   d. Equalize the sleeve compartments versus having greater pressure distally.

10. A therapist chose to work with her patient using fluidotherapy rather than paraffin wax. The patient has a lack of range of motion and also needs to decrease hypersensitivity. There are no open wounds on the hand to be treated. Which of the following would not be an advantage of using fluidotherapy versus paraffin wax in the above scenario?
   a. The therapist can assist range of motion manually while the patient has his hand in the fluidotherapy and not while in the paraffin wax.
   b. The fluidotherapy can be used to assist in desensitzation by adjusting air intensity.
   c. The fluidotherapy can be provided at the same time as dynamic splinting, and this cannot be done while in paraffin wax.
   d. The fingers can be bound, to assist gaining finger flexion, with tape while in fluidotherapy and not in paraffin wax.

11. A therapist is treating a 35-year-old man who has suffered loss of motor control in the right lower extremity due to peripheral neuropathy. The therapist applies biofeedback electrodes to the right quadricep in an effort to increase control and strength of this muscle group. The biofeedback can help achieve this goal in all of the following ways except
   a. Providing visual input for the patient to know how hard he is contracting the right quadricep
   b. Assisting the patient in recruitment of more motor units in the right quadricep
   c. Providing a measure of torque in the right quadricep
   d. Providing the therapist input on the patient's ability and effort in contracting the right quadricep

12. A patient is receiving electrical stimulation for muscle strengthening of the left quadricep. One electrode from one lead wire, 4 × 4 inches in size, is placed on the anterior proximal portion of the left quadricep. Each of two other electrodes from one lead wire are 2 × 2 inches in size. One of the electrodes is placed on the inferior medial side of the left quadricep and one on the inferior lateral side of the left quadricep. This is an example of what type of electrode configuration?
    a. Monopolar
    b. Bipolar
    c. Tripolar
    d. Quadripolar

13. In comparing the use of cold pack and hot pack treatments, which of the following statements is false?
    a. Cold packs penetrate more deeply than hot packs.
    b. Cold increases the viscosity of fluid and heat decreases the viscosity of fluid.
    c. Cold decreases spasm by decreasing sensitivity to muscle spindles and heat decreases spasm by decreasing nerve conduction velocity.
    d. Cold decreases the rate of oxygen uptake, and heat increases the rate of oxygen uptake.

14. A patient is being treated with iontophoresis, driving dexamethasone, for inflammation around the lateral epicondyle of the left elbow. The therapist is careful when setting the parameters and with cleaning the site of electrode application to prevent a possible blister. This possibility is not as strong with some other forms of electrical stimulation, but with iontophoresis using a form of _____, precautions must be taken to ensure that the patient does not receive a mild burn or blister during the treatment session.
    a. Alternating current
    b. Direct current
    c. Pulsed current
    d. Transcutaneous electrical nerve stimulation

15. A physician has ordered a specific type of electrical stimulation that utilizes a frequency of 2500 Hz with a base frequency at 50 Hz to achieve fused tetany. What type of electrical stimulation has the physician ordered?
    a. Iontophoresis
    b. Transcutaneous electrical nerve stimulation
    c. Intermittent flow configuration
    d. Russian stimulation

16. A physical therapist who is pregnant has been studying the use of transcutaneous electrical nerve stimulation during labor and birth to decrease pain perception. Which of the following is the most effective technique in this situation?
    a. Place the electrodes over the upper abdominals during the first stages of labor and over the lower abdominals during the later stages.
    b. Place the electrodes over the paraspinals at the L5 level and S1 level throughout labor and delivery.
    c. Place the electrodes in a V pattern above the pubic region during labor and delivery.
    d. Place electrodes over the paraspinals at the L1 and S1 level initially during labor, and over the pubic region during the latter stages.

17. A patient with chronic back pain is referred to physical therapy for application of a transcutaneous electrical nerve stimulation unit. The parameters chosen by the therapist are set to provide a noxious stimulus described as an acupuncture type of stimulus. Which of the following lists of parameters produces this type of stimulation?
    a. Low intensity, duration of 60 μsec, and a frequency of 50 Hz
    b. High intensity, duration of 150 μsec, and a frequency of 100 Hz
    c. Low intensity, duration of 150 μsec, and a frequency of 100 Hz
    d. High intensity, duration of 150 μsec, and a frequency of 2 Hz

18. A 63-year-old woman presents to physical therapy with a diagnosis of herpes zoster. The physician informs the physical therapist that the L5 dorsal root is involved and that a transcutaneous electrical neuromuscular stimulation (TENS) unit should be used to help control the pain. Where should the TENS unit electrodes be placed?
    a. Posterior thigh
    b. Lateral hip/greater trochanter area
    c. Anterior thigh
    d. Anterior lateral tibia

19. Use of functional electrical stimulation in patients with longstanding spinal cord injury does not improve
    a. Aerobic capacity
    b. Muscle strength
    c. Osteopenia
    d. Muscle mass

20. A physician has ordered electrical stimulation to a 43-year-old male with complaints of sternocleidomastoid spasms. What is the appropriate course of action by the physical therapist?
   a. Begin intervention with low frequency, high phase duration electrical stimulation.
   b. Electrical stimulation in this area is a contraindication. Contact the physician to discuss alternative interventions.
   c. Begin intervention with high frequency, low phase duration electrical stimulation.
   d. Use ultrasound only and do not contact the physician.

21. The physical therapist has decided to use functional electrical stimulation (FES) in order to help a spinal cord injured patient ambulate. What is the lowest spinal injury level that FES would be considered?
   a. T3-T4
   b. T8-T9
   c. T11-T12
   d. L3-L4

22. A physical therapist is using a cold pack to decrease inflammation after a therapeutic exercise session. Which of the following areas needs to be monitored most closely during the ice pack application?
   a. Lateral knee
   b. Lumbar area
   c. Quadriceps area
   d. Acromioclavicular joint

23. In which of the following patient conditions would it be safe to apply spinal traction to help decompress a spinal nerve root?
   a. Acute rheumatoid arthritis
   b. Degenerative joint disease
   c. Osteoporosis
   d. Spinal tumor

24. Which of the following best describes the patient's position when administering positional traction?
   a. Hanging upside down on an inversion table (or with inversion boots)
   b. Hanging by the hands (right side up) from an overhead bar
   c. Side-lying with a pillow placed under one side of the lumbar spine
   d. Sitting with head in a halter that is attached to an over-the-door traction system

25. You plan to administer lumbar traction to a patient who has back pain and nerve root impingement. You determine from your history that this patient has no contraindications to the use of traction. What other piece of information do you need to obtain from this patient in order to determine the appropriate intensity for your traction treatment?
    a. Age
    b. Body weight
    c. Medications currently taken
    d. Pain rating

26. Before a lumbar traction treatment, your patient tells you that his pain is localized in his low back and right buttock. Your examination indicates a medium-sized herniated disk. The day after the traction treatment, he tells you that his back pain has diminished, but he now has deep aching and numbness down the posterior aspect of his right lower extremity. In addition, you are no longer able to elicit his Achilles tendon reflex. Based on these responses, you should
    a. Increase the intensity of the traction during the next treatment session
    b. Reduce the intensity of the traction during the next treatment session
    c. Switch from a static to an intermittent mode of traction application
    d. Discontinue the traction treatments

27. You administer cervical traction to a patient in your clinic to help stretch the tight soft tissues along the posterior aspect of her neck. She responds well to the initial treatment so you arrange for her to lease a home cervical traction unit to continue this treatment on a daily basis. In what position would you instruct her to place the traction unit to produce the optimal effect?
    a. At a downward angle that pulls her neck into slight extension
    b. At an upward angle that slightly flexes her neck
    c. At an upward angle that fully flexes her neck
    d. Lying flat with no angle (no extension or flexion)

28. When the goal of a lumbar traction treatment is to cause distraction of the vertebrae, the magnitude of the traction force should approximate what percent of the patient's body weight?
    a. 10%
    b. 25%
    c. 50%
    d. 75%

29. Which of the following is not a physiologic benefit associated with the use of continuous passive motion (CPM)?
   a. Prevents muscle atrophy by simulating a normal concentric contraction
   b. Prevents adhesions by orienting collagen fibers as they heal
   c. Reduces edema by facilitating the movement of fluid in and out of the joint
   d. Reduces pain via the stimulation of joint mechanoreceptors

30. A patient with venous insufficiency in his lower extremities is referred for instruction on the use of a pneumatic compression pump at home. What inflation pressure and treatment time will you use to initiate this compression treatment?
   a. Continuous pressure equal to the patient's diastolic blood pressure for 20 to 30 minutes
   b. Continuous pressure between 30 and 50 mm Hg for 20 to 30 minutes
   c. Intermittent pressure no higher than 30 mm Hg for one hour
   d. Intermittent pressure between 40 and 80 mm Hg for 2 hours

31. Which of the following conditions would contraindicate the use of an intermittent pneumatic compression pump?
   a. Congestive heart failure
   b. Lymphedema
   c. Recent joint arthroplasty
   d. Venous stasis ulcers

32. You are treating a patient with acute bicipital tendinitis, so your goal is to reduce inflammation. Two of your treatment choices are iontophoresis and phonophoresis. Which of the following comparative statements regarding these two modalities is true?
   a. Both procedures can be performed at home by the patient.
   b. Both procedures require medications to be suspended in a solution.
   c. Iontophoresis can deliver medication to deeper tissues than phonophoresis.
   d. Iontophoresis is more likely to cause skin irritation than phonophoresis.

33. If you are using iontophoresis to deliver dexamethasone (−) to an inflamed tissue, which of the following would be the most appropriate treatment parameters?
   a. (+) Active electrode; intensity = 1.5 mAmps; treatment time = 0 min
   b. (−) Active electrode; intensity = 2 mAmps; treatment time = 20 min
   c. (+) Active electrode; intensity = 4 mAmps; treatment time = 10 min
   d. (−) Active electrode; intensity = 8 mAmps; treatment time = 5 min

34. If you want move ions into the tissue, as in the application of iontophoresis, what type of electrical current will you need to use?
    a. Continuous biphasic
    b. Continuous monophasic
    c. Pulsed biphasic
    d. Pulsed monophasic

35. You have a patient with a diabetic ulcer that has not responded well to conventional treatment, so you think he might be a good candidate for electrical stimulation. Which type of electrical current would most likely facilitate wound healing?
    a. High-volt using a pulsed monophasic waveform
    b. Interferential (medium-frequency)
    c. Iontophoresis using a continuous monophasic waveform
    d. TENS using a pulsed biphasic waveform

36. You are treating a patient who is recovering from a muscle strain and you want to help increase the blood flow to that muscle as well as enhance its extensibility. Which thermal agent is most likely to produce these effects in muscle tissue?
    a. Hot pack
    b. Infrared radiation
    c. Pulsed ultrasound
    d. Shortwave diathermy

37. You are treating an athlete who strained his hamstring muscle. Which of the following modalities would be contraindicated if this patient had a cardiac pacemaker?
    a. Ice massage
    b. Hydrotherapy
    c. Shortwave diathermy
    d. Ultrasound

38. You decide to use sensory-level (i.e., conventional) TENS to provide some relief for incisional pain in your patient who recently underwent knee surgery. The physiological mechanism by which this form of TENS is thought to provide immediate pain relief is known as
    a. Autogenic inhibition
    b. Descending inhibition
    c. Presynaptic inhibition
    d. Reciprocal inhibition

39. When you apply cryotherapy to a patient, you can expect it to _____ that patient's sensory and motor nerve conduction velocity.
    a. Decrease
    b. Increase
    c. Initially increase, then decrease
    d. Not change

40. You want to use neuromuscular electrical stimulation (NMES) to facilitate active range of motion in a patient who is recovering from a fractured wrist. The patient has bony union but is limited by soft tissue tightness in her wrist flexors and extensors because of her immobilization. Which of the following stimulation parameters would you recommend?
    a. Reciprocal stimulation mode using a frequency of 40 Hz and high enough intensity to elicit a full muscle contraction
    b. Reciprocal stimulation mode using a frequency of 2 Hz and high enough intensity to elicit an observable muscle twitch
    c. Synchronous stimulation mode using a frequency of 100 Hz with high enough intensity to elicit a comfortable sensory response
    d. Synchronous stimulation mode using a frequency of Hz with intensity as high as the patient can tolerate

41. You have a patient with subacute rheumatoid arthritis in her hands who also has a history of Raynaud's disease. Which of the following modalities would be contraindicated for this patient?
    a. Cold pack
    b. Fluidotherapy
    c. Paraffin wax bath
    d. Ultraviolet light

42. You plan to administer a combination of ultrasound and electrical stimulation to a patient who is experiencing muscle spasm in her upper trapezius and posterior neck muscles following a recent whiplash injury. To perform this type of treatment, what type of electrode setup would you use?
    a. Bipolar technique using a dispersive pad that is equal to the size of the soundhead
    b. Monopolar technique using a dispersive pad that is much larger than the soundhead
    c. Monopolar technique using a dispersive pad that is much smaller than the soundhead
    d. Quadripolar technique using 2 soundheads and 2 equal-sized dispersive pads

43. You are treating a 12-year-old patient with Osgood Schlatter's disease and want to apply a modality treatment over his tibial tuberosity to help relieve his pain. Which of the following modalities should you probably avoid using in a patient this age?
   a. Ice massage
   b. Iontophoresis
   c. TENS
   d. Ultrasound

44. You have an older patient with balance problems who you think would benefit from walking in a therapeutic pool. However, this patient also has some lower extremity edema associated with venous insufficiency. What effect might the pool therapy have on her edema?
   a. The hydrostatic pressure exerted by the water should reduce her edema.
   b. The relaxing effect of the water is likely to slow her circulation and diminish her edema.
   c. Her edema will probably worsen because therapeutic pools are usually heated to at least 100° F.
   d. It should have no effect on her edema because walking in water is not that strenuous.

45. You are treating a patient who is recovering from Guillain Barre syndrome and is still experiencing considerable weakness and fatigue in her lower extremity muscles. You want to use some electrical stimulation to help facilitate the strength of her muscle contractions. What type of duty cycle would be most appropriate for a patient like this?
   a. 10 seconds ON, 50 seconds OFF
   b. 10 seconds ON, 30 seconds OFF
   c. 15 seconds ON, 15 seconds OFF
   d. 15 seconds ON, 5 seconds OFF

46. You have placed equal-sized electrodes over the dorsal aspect of a patient's proximal and distal forearm as shown in Figure 5-1 in order to stimulate his wrist and finger extensor muscles. However, when you first turn the electrical stimulator on, the response you are getting is finger flexion, rather than extension. How would you correct this problem to get the desired motor response?

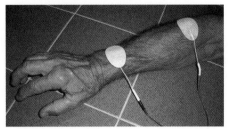

Fig 5-1

a. Increase the pulse duration to maximize the intensity
b. Move the electrodes closer together over the muscle belly
c. Switch from a biphasic current to a monophasic current
d. Use a smaller electrode over the distal forearm

47. You are using electrical stimulation to facilitate the contraction of a muscle that is recovering from a peripheral nerve injury. Because the patient only shows signs of partial innervation at this time, any electrical stimulation treatment will require the use of a stimulator that can produce a
a. High amplitude and long pulse duration
b. High frequency (i.e., >5000 Hz)
c. Monophasic waveform of positive polarity
d. Very low intensity in the microamperage range

48. You are treating a patient with adhesive capsulitis of the glenohumeral joint. You decide to administer some ultrasound in order to increase the extensibility of the patient's joint capsule before you begin joint mobilization procedures. Which ultrasound parameters are most likely to produce the desired results in this particular tissue?
a. 1 MHz continuous ultrasound
b. 1 MHz pulsed ultrasound
c. 3 MHz continuous ultrasound
d. 3 MHz pulsed ultrasound

49. Which of the following patient conditions would contraindicate the use of most thermal, mechanical, and electrical modalities?
a. Diabetic neuropathy
b. Hypertension
c. Metastatic cancer
d. Urinary incontinence

50. Which of the following patients would not be an appropriate candidate for EMG biofeedback training?
   a. Individual with tension headaches
   b. Older adult with Alzheimer's dementia
   c. Poststroke patient who needs balance training
   d. Quadriplegic patient who has had a recent tendon transfer

51. Which of the following physiologic changes would not be associated with the application of superficial heat?
   a. Decreased interstitial fluid
   b. Decreased pain perception
   c. Increased extensibility of collagen tissue
   d. Increased metabolic activity

52. You are preparing to apply cryotherapy to a patient who has never had it before. In your history, which question would help you determine whether your patient might be hypersensitive to cold?
   a. Do your fingers ever go numb when exposed to cold, damp weather?
   b. Have you ever had an allergic response to a cold stimulus (i.e., itchy rash or hives)?
   c. Have you ever been frostbitten?
   d. How often do you wear gloves when you are outside in cold weather?

53. Which of the following modalities produces its thermal effects via evaporation?
   a. Hot pack
   b. Ice massage
   c. Paraffin wax
   d. Vapocoolant spray

54. If you apply a cold pack or ice massage over a patient's biceps muscle for 5 to 10 minutes before a session of resistive exercise, what change would you expect to see in that muscle?
   a. An immediate increase in isometric strength
   b. An immediate decrease in muscle tone and tendon reflex
   c. Elimination of any exercise-induced muscle soreness
   d. Faster recruitment of type II muscle fibers

55. Heat modalities are generally contraindicated in the presence of an infectious lesion because they may
   a. Increase circulation, which can spread the organism to other parts of the body
   b. Increase the rate of cellular mitosis and cause the organism to mutate
   c. Mask the pain associated with the lesion, which may cause further tissue damage
   d. Reduce the effectiveness of the body's immune system

56. In most cases, it is considered safe to apply ultrasound over or near
    a. Cemented and plastic implants
    b. Metal screws, plates, implants
    c. A pacemaker
    d. Reproductive organs

57. When examining an ultrasound machine, you note that it operates at a frequency of 1 MHz and has a Beam Nonuniformity Ratio (BNR) of 8:1. Which of the following statements regarding this machine is true?
    a. Most energy will be absorbed in superficial tissues, and it may produce uneven heating.
    b. Most energy will be absorbed in superficial tissues, and it should produce even heating.
    c. Most energy will be absorbed in deep tissues, and it may produce uneven heating.
    d. Most energy will be absorbed in deep tissues, and it should produce even heating.

58. The most common clinical use of phonophoresis is to
    a. Apply an anti-inflammatory medication to a localized musculoskeletal tissue
    b. Deliver antibiotics to an infected wound
    c. Provide a mechanical stimulus to accelerate repair in bone and cartilage
    d. Slow the conduction velocity of sensory nerves to relieve pain

59. You are administering ultrasound to a localized area around a patient's patellar tendon when she begins to complain of intense pain over her tibial tuberosity. What is the most likely cause of this response?
    a. You are using an ineffective or insufficient amount of coupling medium.
    b. There is a very low attenuation of ultrasound in bony tissue.
    c. You are using an ultrasound unit with a high BNR and/or are moving it too slowly.
    d. The crystal in the soundhead has been damaged.

60. A patient with diabetes is admitted for care of a venous stasis ulcer on the medial aspect of his ankle. You decide to include pulsed ultrasound as part of your treatment plan to take advantage of its nonthermal effects on wound healing. Which of the following is an example of a nonthermal effect produced by ultrasound?
    a. Decreased cell membrane permeability, which reduces edema
    b. Decreased histamine release and macrophage activity
    c. Destruction of surface bacteria and stimulation of antibodies in the wound bed
    d. Increased intracellular calcium and protein synthesis

61. You plan to give a short wave diathermy treatment to a 42-year-old female patient who has low back pain. Which of the following questions would not be necessary or appropriate to ask this patient before giving her this treatment?
    a. Are you currently menstruating?
    b. Could you possibly be pregnant?
    c. Do you know if you might have a urinary infection or a pelvic tumor?
    d. Do you take birth control pills?

62. A college student injures his ankle in an intramural volleyball game. X-rays reveal no evidence of fracture, so he is referred to PT for treatment of an acute ankle sprain. Which of the following modalities would be most appropriate to apply at this time?
    a. Air-activated heat wrap
    b. Cold compression cuff
    c. Fluidotherapy
    d. Short wave diathermy

63. You receive a referral to treat a decubitus ulcer over a patient's sacrum. Following hydrotherapy to clean and debride the ulcer, you decide to irradiate the wound with ultraviolet light. Before administering a UV treatment, you need to ask your patient if he/she
    a. Has a cardiac pacemaker
    b. Has any food allergies
    c. Has ever been severely sunburned
    d. Is currently taking any medications that cause sensitivity to sunlight

64. The intensity of an infrared or ultraviolet lamp is greatest when the lamp is
    a. Positioned closer to the patient at a 45 degree angle
    b. Positioned closer to the patient at a 90 degree angle (perpendicular to skin)
    c. Positioned further from the patient at a 90 degree angle (perpendicular to skin)
    d. Radiating the skin through a sheet or thin towel

65. How does low-powered ("cold") laser light differ from other types of phototherapy?
    a. Laser light has greater divergence from its source.
    b. Laser light is monochromatic (i.e., one wavelength).
    c. Light waves from lasers are transmitted in an asynchronous, noncoherent manner.
    d. Laser light is classified as a form of ionizing radiation.

66. A young woman is referred to you with severe muscle spasm in her back that began shortly after she started working as a ticket agent at the local airport. You think that some deep heat will really help calm down her spasm. When you ask about her past history of back problems she tells you that she had scoliosis as a child but underwent a surgical fusion (with metal rods) to stop the progression of her curve. She thinks her limited spinal mobility may be what triggered her spasm. Based on this history and her current symptoms, which thermal modality would you select?
    a. Diathermy because it selectively heats muscle tissue the best
    b. Ultrasound because diathermy is contraindicated in this patient
    c. Hot pack because both diathermy and ultrasound are contraindicated
    d. None of the above because heat will only make her muscle spasm worse

67. Why must a patient's skin be cleaned and debrided before applying electrodes?
    a. To avoid contaminating your electrodes
    b. To determine whether his or her sensation is intact
    c. To help decrease skin resistance
    d. To reduce current density at the electrode-tissue interface

68. In Figure 5-2, which stimulation parameter is being modulated?

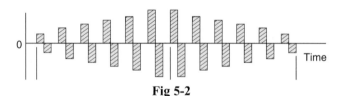

Fig 5-2

    a. Pulse amplitude
    b. Pulse duration/width
    c. Pulse frequency
    d. Pulse waveform

69. For which of the following patient conditions would electrotherapy be an inappropriate treatment modality?
    a. An infected wound
    b. Prior history of seizures
    c. Muscle spasticity
    d. Urinary incontinence

70. A high frequency sinusoidal (i.e., biphasic) waveform that is typically delivered in bursts of approximately 50 per second and used for muscle strengthening is usually referred to as
    a. High-volt galvanic stimulation
    b. Interferential current
    c. Microcurrent
    d. Russian current

71. Why do most neuromuscular electrical stimulation (NMES) protocols recommend frequency settings between 30 and 50 pulses per second?
    a. Frequencies lower than this range cannot produce a muscle contraction.
    b. Higher frequencies usually stimulate the nociceptors and make the patient uncomfortable.
    c. It produces a smooth, tetanic muscle contraction without excessive fatigue.
    d. Most muscle stimulators cannot produce frequencies above or below this range.

72. In which of the following situations would it be appropriate to use a low frequency (i.e., 1 to 5 Hz) to stimulate a muscle?
    a. When the muscle is only partially innervated and very weak
    b. When stimulating the intrinsic muscles of the hand or foot
    c. When you are trying to relax a muscle that is in spasm
    d. When you are trying to stretch a joint contracture

73. When using NMES, when would you want to use a long rise/ramp time (i.e., 2 to 3 seconds)?
    a. When stimulating a completely denervated muscle
    b. When stimulating a hypotonic (i.e., flaccid) muscle
    c. When stimulating a hypertonic (i.e., spastic) muscle
    d. When stimulating the antagonist of a hypertonic (i.e., spastic) muscle

74. Which muscles would you stimulate if you were using NMES to help correct a subluxed glenohumeral joint in a patient who has had a stroke?
    a. Anterior and posterior deltoid
    b. Rhomboids and serratus anterior
    c. Supraspinatus and latissimus dorsi/teres major
    d. Supraspinatus and posterior deltoid

75. The concept of current dosage in iontophoresis refers to the
    a. Current amplitude (intensity) multiplied by treatment time
    b. Current density as determined by the size of the delivery electrode
    c. Current polarity in relation to the medication's polarity
    d. Difference between the phase charge and the treatment time

76. If you are using electrical stimulation to limit edema formation in an acutely injured joint, the amplitude should be adjusted to produce a
   a. Mild muscle contraction (tapping)
   b. Strong muscle contraction (beating)
   c. Sensory response only
   d. Subsensory response

77. Why is a modulated current recommended when using conventional TENS for pain control?
   a. It provides combined effects of sensory and motor level TENS.
   b. It helps prevent sensory adaptation/habituation.
   c. It reduces the placebo effect of TENS.
   d. It selectively activates A-beta fibers.

78. Nerves cannot achieve a continuous state of excitation due to
   a. Threshold
   b. Depolarization Period
   c. Repolarization Period
   d. Refractory Period

79. When utilizing electrical stimulation, what is the pulse frequency range for tetany?
   a. 25 to 50 pps
   b. 0 to 10 pps
   c. 10 to 20 pps
   d. 75 to 100 pps

80. What is the duty cycle for an electrical stimulation program with 6 seconds on time and 18 seconds off time?
   a. 25%
   b. 15%
   c. 33%
   d. 50%

81. When stimulating the wrist extensors, the best current type/electrode configuration is
   a. Symmetric biphasic/monopolar
   b. Symmetric biphasic/bipolar
   c. Asymmetric biphasic/monopolar
   d. Asymmetric biphasic/bipolar

82. When utilizing electrical stimulation, the key element of pulsed current is
   a. A period of electrical silence
   b. The duration of the current
   c. The frequency of the current
   d. The amplitude of the current

83. A 29-year-old woman fractured her right midtibia in a skiing accident 3 months ago. After cast removal, a severe foot drop was noted. The patient wants to try electrical stimulation orthotic substitution. You would set up the functional electrical stimulation to contract the appropriate muscles during
   a. Toe off
   b. Push off
   c. Foot flat
   d. Swing phase

84. A patient has been referred to you following a fracture of the femur six months ago. The cast was removed, but the patient was unable to volitionally contract the quadriceps. You decide to apply electrical stimulation to the quadriceps muscle. Your choice of electrode placement and electrical stimulation duty cycle (on/off) would consist of
   a. Large electrodes, closely spaced (10:10)
   b. Large electrodes, widely spaced (10:30)
   c. Small electrodes, closely spaced (10:30)
   d. Small electrodes, widely spaced (10:10)

85. A 31-year-old patient complains of patellar tendonitis as a result of a mountain climbing accident 3 weeks ago. The patient complains of pain with resisted knee extension, stair climbing, and sit-to-stand movements. You choose to apply iontophoresis using a pain medication with a positive charge. The correct type, polarity, and active electrode placement is
   a. Monophasic current with anode placed on the tendon
   b. Monophasic current with the cathode placed on the tendon
   c. Biphasic current with the cathode placed proximal on the tendon
   d. Low-volt, continuous current with the anode placed distal on the tendon

86. A 28-year-old actor/singer is complaining of TMJ pain. He also complains of headaches and neck tightness. He has been under a lot of stress lately and has noticed an increase in the frequency and magnitude of symptoms. His doctor suggested and you concur that biofeedback might help him relax the neck and shoulder muscles and therefore decrease his symptoms. Initially, the EMG biofeedback protocol should consist of
   a. High detection sensitivity with recording electrodes placed far apart
   b. Low detection sensitivity with recording electrodes placed closely together
   c. Low detection sensitivity with recording electrodes placed far apart
   d. High detection sensitivity with recording electrodes placed closely together

87. A 26-year-old presents with weakness of the knee resulting from an anterior cruciate ligament injury. Your examination reveals moderate pain (5/10) and excessive translation of the tibia during active knee extension. You determine functional stability of the knee should consist of stimulation of the
    a. Hamstrings immediately before the quadriceps to produce co-contraction
    b. Quadriceps only
    c. Hamstrings only
    d. Quadriceps immediately before the hamstrings to produce co-contraction

88. A patient presents with partial- and full-thickness burns on the chest and neck region. You are applying TENS during your debriding procedure to modulate pain. Your TENS treatment of choice would be
    a. Modulated TENS
    b. Conventional (high rate) TENS
    c. Acupuncture-like (low rate) TENS
    d. Brief intense TENS

89. A 73-year-old patient presents with a stage III decubitus ulcer on the plantar surface of the right foot. After a series of conservative treatments with limited success, the therapist chooses to apply electrical stimulation for tissue repair. The electrical current best suited in this case is
    a. Russian current
    b. Asymmetric biphasic pulsed current
    c. Symmetric biphasic pulsed current
    d. Interferential current

90. You are applying pulsed current to the quadriceps to improve patellar tracking during knee extension. Your patient complains that the current is uncomfortable. To make the current more tolerable to the patient, yet maintain a good therapeutic effect, you should consider adjusting the
    a. Current intensity
    b. Pulse rate
    c. Pulse duration
    d. Current polarity

91. Your patient has moderate spasticity of the biceps brachii on the left as a result of a stroke. You choose to use electrical stimulation to temporarily decrease the effects of hypertonicity in order to work on ADL activities. Your objective in applying the current is to
    a. Fatigue the ipsilateral biceps brachii
    b. Stimulate the contralateral biceps brachii
    c. Stimulate the ipsilateral triceps
    d. Stimulate the contralateral triceps

92. A 66-year-old patient with spastic hemiplegia was referred to you for ambulation training. The patient is having difficulty with standing up from a seated position due to co-contraction of the quadriceps and hamstrings during the knee and hip extension phase. You choose EMG biofeedback to assist you in progressively decreasing the motor activity of the hamstrings. You wish to use biofeedback beginning with simple knee extension exercise in the seated position and progressing to sit to stand training. Initially, the biofeedback protocol should consist of
   a. Low detection sensitivity with recording electrodes placed far apart
   b. High detection sensitivity with recording electrodes placed closely together
   c. Low detection sensitivity with recording electrodes placed closely together
   d. High detection sensitivity with recording electrodes placed far apart.

93. A physical therapist is providing intervention for an 11-year-old boy diagnosed with Sever's disease. All are appropriate therapeutic interventions for this patient except
   a. Gastrocnemius/soleus stretches
   b. Tibialis anterior strengthening
   c. Ultrasound
   d. Ice

94. The physical therapist makes recommendations to a patient after hip replacement surgery for positioning in a wheelchair. Which set of instructions would adhere to safety precautions?
   a. Keep the legs abducted with abductor pillow and affected leg in neutral.
   b. Keep the legs together by using an adductor strap to prevent external rotation of legs.
   c. Sit in a regular wheelchair with the feet supported on a footrest.
   d. Sit in regular wheelchair with the affected leg in full extension.

95. The therapist is ambulating a patient with an above-knee amputation. The new prosthesis causes the heel on the involved foot to move laterally at toe-off. Which of the following is the most likely cause of this deviation?
   a. Too much internal rotation of the prosthetic knee
   b. Too much external rotation of the prosthetic knee
   c. Too much outset of prosthetic foot
   d. The prosthetic foot is set in excessive dorsiflexion

96. The therapist in an outpatient physical therapy clinic receives an order to obtain a shoe orthotic for a patient. After examining the patient, the therapist finds a stage I pressure ulcer on the first metatarsal head. Weight-bearing surfaces need to be transferred posteriorly. Which orthotic is the most appropriate for this patient?
    a. Scaphoid pad
    b. Thomas heel
    c. Metatarsal pad
    d. Cushion heel

97. When ordering a customized wheelchair for a patient, the therapist determines that the pelvic belt needs to be positioned so that it allows active anterior pelvic tilt. What is the best position for the pelvic belt in relation to the sitting surface?
    a. 30 degrees
    b. 45 degrees
    c. 60 degrees
    d. 90 degrees

98. The therapist is treating a patient who has suffered a recent stroke. There is a significant lack of dorsiflexion in the involved lower extremity and a significant amount of medial/lateral ankle instability. The therapist believes that an ankle foot orthosis (AFO) would be beneficial. Which of the following is an in appropriate AFO?
    a. Solid AFO
    b. Posterior leaf spring AFO
    c. Hinged solid AFO
    d. Electrical stimulation aided AFO

99. The use of compression stockings on the feet and ankles is contraindicated in which patient population?
    a. Chronic venous disease
    b. Recent total knee replacement
    c. Burn patients
    d. Chronic arterial disease

100. The therapist is examining a 36-year-old woman to fit her with the appropriate wheelchair. Recent injury caused C6 quadriplegia. What is the correct way to measure length of the footrests for the patient's permanent wheelchair?
    a. From the patient's popliteal fossa to the heel and add 1 inch
    b. From the patient's popliteal fossa to the heel and subtract 1 inch
    c. From the patient's popliteal fossa to the first metatarsal head and add 1 inch
    d. From the patient's popliteal fossa to the first metatarsal head and subtract 1 inch

101. The therapist is ambulating a 42-year-old man who has just received an above-knee prosthesis for the left leg. The therapist notices pistoning of the prosthesis as the patient ambulates. Which of the following is the most probable cause of this deviation?
    a. The socket is too small.
    b. The socket is too large.
    c. The foot bumper is too soft.
    d. The foot bumper is too hard.

102. While examining a patient who has just received a new left below-knee prosthesis, the therapist notes that the toe of the prosthesis stays off the floor after heel strike. Which of the following is an unlikely cause of this deviation?
    a. The prosthetic foot is set too far anterior.
    b. The prosthetic foot is set in too much dorsiflexion.
    c. The heel wedge is too stiff.
    d. The prosthetic foot is outset too much.

103. Which of the following is the most appropriate orthotic for a patient with excessive foot pronation during static standing?
    a. Scaphoid pad
    b. Metatarsal pad
    c. Metatarsal bar
    d. Rocker bar

104. A therapist is instructing a patient in the use of a wrist-driven prehension orthotic. What must be done to achieve opening of the involved hand?
    a. Actively extend the wrist
    b. Passively extend the wrist
    c. Actively flex the wrist
    d. Passively flex the wrist

105. The therapist is treating a patient who received an above-elbow amputation 2 years ago. The prosthesis has a split cable that controls the elbow and the terminal device. With this type of prosthesis, the patient must first lock the elbow to allow the cable to activate the terminal device. This is accomplished with what movements?
    a. Extending the humerus and elevating the scapula
    b. Extending the humerus and retracting the scapula
    c. Extending the humerus and protracting the scapula
    d. Extending the humerus and depressing the scapula

106. A 30-year-old man is referred to physical therapy after a recent motor vehicle accident that resulted in total loss of motor control of both legs. Trunk and bilateral upper extremity control allows independent sitting at bedside. The patient is to be discharged from the hospital and will return home a few hours after the physical therapy session. The therapist notices, from the history in the chart, that the patient lives alone and has little or no outside support from family members. The patient also suffers from severe obesity. The therapist decides to practice a transfer from the bed to the wheelchair. Which assistive device should the therapist use for this transfer attempt?
    a. Hoyer lift (pneumatic lift)
    b. Sliding board
    c. Geriatric chair (using a slide sheet transfer)
    d. Trapeze bar

107. The physical therapist has just given the patient a custom wheelchair. The patient has a longstanding history of hamstring contractures resulting in fixation of the knees into 60 degrees of flexion. The patient is also prone to develop decubitus ulcers. Which of the following is incorrect advice to give the family and patient?
    a. Keep the patient's buttocks clean and dry.
    b. Make sure that the wheelchair cushion is always in the wheelchair seat.
    c. Keep the leg rests of the wheelchair fully elevated.
    d. Never transfer using a sliding board from one surface to another.

108. A 27-year-old man with a diagnosis of incomplete spinal cord injury at the L4 level is being examined by a physical therapist. The patient is nearing discharge from the rehabilitation unit. Manual muscle testing reveals the following: right hip flexion = 4/5, right hip adduction = 5/5, right knee flexion = 2/5, right knee extension = 3+/5, right ankle plantar flexion = 1/5, and right ankle dorsiflexion = 2-/5; left hip flexion = 4+/5, left hip adduction = 4+/5, left knee flexion = 2+/5, left knee extension = 3+/5, left ankle plantar flexion = 2-/5, and left ankle dorsiflexion = 2-/5. What is the appropriate orthotic for this patient? What is his most likely functional outcome?
    a. Hip-knee-ankle-foot orthosis (HKAFO) with forearm crutches, household ambulator.
    b. Knee-ankle-foot orthosis (KAFO) with forearm crutches, household ambulator.
    c. KAFO with forearm crutches, functional ambulator.
    d. HKAFO with forearm crutches, functional ambulator.

109. A physical therapist is ordered to provide gait training for an 18-year-old girl who received a partial medial meniscectomy of the right knee one day earlier. The patient was independent in ambulation without an assistive device before surgery and has no cognitive deficits. The patient's weight-bearing status is currently partial weight bearing on the involved lower extremity. Which of the following is the most appropriate assistive device and gait pattern?
    a. Crutches, three-point gait pattern
    b. Standard walker, three-point gait pattern
    c. Standard walker, four-point gait pattern
    d. Crutches, swing-to gait pattern

110. A physical therapist is ordered to provide gait training to a 78-year-old man who received a right cemented total knee replacement 24 hours earlier. The patient also had a traumatic amputation of the left upper extremity 3 inches above the elbow 40 years ago. If the patient lives at home alone, which of the following is an appropriate assistive device?
    a. Rolling walker
    b. Standard walker
    c. Hemi-walker
    d. Wheelchair for 2 weeks

111. Which of the following statements about below-knee amputations is false?
    a. Gel socket inserts should be left in the prosthesis overnight.
    b. The therapist should puncture any blisters that appear on the stump.
    c. Areas of skin irritation on the stump can be covered with a dressing, then a nylon sock, before donning the prosthesis.
    d. When not in use, the prosthesis should be laid on the floor.

112. A therapist is assisting a patient with pre-gait activities who has been fitted with a hip disarticulation prosthesis. To ambulate with the most correct gait pattern, what must be mastered first?
    a. Forward weight shift on to the prosthesis
    b. Swing-through of the prosthesis
    c. Maintain stability while in single limb support on the prosthesis
    d. Posterior pelvic tilt to advance the prosthesis

113. A 68-year-old man is being treated by a physical therapist after a right below-knee amputation. The patient is beginning ambulation with a preparatory prosthesis. In the early stance phase of the involved lower extremity, the therapist notes an increase in knee flexion. Which of the following are possible causes of this gait deviation?
    a. The heel is too stiff.
    b. The foot is set too far anterior in relation to the knee.
    c. The foot is set in too much plantar flexion.
    d. The heel is too soft.

114. Orthotic intervention is usually recommended at _____ for a child
      with idiopathic scoliosis.
      a. 15 degrees
      b. 25 degrees
      c. 40 degrees
      d. 60 degrees

115. An advantage for use of an externally-powered UE prosthetic device
      over a body-powered prosthetic device is
      a. Cost
      b. Ease of use
      c. Improved fit
      d. Weight

116. A patient begins ambulation with axillary crutches for the first time.
      The gait required will be non–weight bearing for the right foot. What
      is the best advice to give them in regard to crutch placement during
      static standing?
      a. Stand with the crutches and weight-bearing foot in a parallel line.
      b. Stand with both crutches under the right arm.
      c. Stand with both crutches under the left arm.
      d. Stand with both crutches approximately 4 inches to the front and
          side of the shoulders.

117. Of the walkers listed below, which is the least stable?
      a. Folding walker
      b. Reciprocal walker
      c. Rolling walker
      d. Nonfolding standard walker

118. The physical therapist is providing intervention for a patient with a
      recent stroke. Gait training with a new ankle foot orthosis (AFO) will
      begin today. What is the most important aspect of the fit of the AFO?
      a. The ankle should be flexed to 90 degrees.
      b. The top of the AFO should be 4 inches below the knee joint.
      c. Any complaints of pain or discomfort are important to AFO fit.
      d. The bottom of the AFO should stop at the metatarsal heads.

119. Which of the following is the most important factor when considering
      using restraints on a patient?
      a. Comfort of application
      b. Consent to apply restraints from patient/family
      c. Current knowledge of staff in securing restraints
      d. Mental status of patient

120. A physician orders gait training for a 16-year-old male with recent open reduction internal fixation of the left femur. The patient is non–weight bearing on the affected leg. Which of the following assistive devices is most appropriate for this patient?
      a. Forearm crutches
      b. Front-wheel walker
      c. Axillary crutches
      d. Quad cane

Answers

1. c.   A therapist can use ultrasound with all of the other choices. Performing an ultrasound over a cemented metal implant is also a contraindication. However, with any ultrasound technique, treatment should be stopped if the patient feels pain.

2. b.   Choices A and C are incorrect because rheumatoid arthritis is a contraindication for continuous or intermittent traction. Choice D is incorrect for the same reason as well as the fact that a 110-pound setting is too great for a 147-pound patient.

3. c.   The therapist should notify the referring physician. The mistake should be documented and the patient informed. The referring physician can determine the need for a consultation with him or her or an obstetrician.

4. a.   Local vasoconstriction is the first response. Nerve conduction velocity decreases after approximately 5 minutes of ice application.

5. a.   This theory supports the use of a TENS unit for sensory level pain control. The activation of the larger fibers decreases the amount of sensory information traveling to the brain.

6. d.   Tissue with a high collagen content absorbs more ultrasound. Bone absorbs the most ultrasound.

7. c.   Correct electrode placement is over the motor points of the involved muscle. On/off cycle time is usually between 1:3 and 1:5. Fused tetany of a muscle usually occurs between 50 to 80 hertz or pps (sources vary).

8. c.   Raynaud's phenomenon is a vasospastic disorder of the vessels of the distal parts of the extremities. Patients with Raynaud's phenomenon do not respond well to cold treatment. Choice B is incorrect because it is believed that moist heat may encourage more rapid growth of cancer. Choice D is incorrect because prolonged use of steroids may cause capillaries to lose their integrity, which compromises the body's ability to dissipate heat. Choice A is incorrect because moist heat may encourage hemorrhaging in patients with hemophilia by causing vasodilation.

9. b. Although the change may be minimal, increasing the maximal pressure to 60 mm Hg is the most likely choice to have a positive effect on edema reduction. The pressure, however, should not exceed the diastolic pressure of the patient. Choice A is not the right choice because placing the extremity in a dependent position causes the pump to work against gravity. Choice C is an incorrect choice because decreasing the on time means that the extremity receives compression for a shorter period. Choice D is an incorrect choice because greater pressure distally is more likely to move fluid than equal pressure throughout the sleeve.

10. d. The fingers can be bound in paraffin wax as well as in fluidotherapy. When using this technique, the hand remains stationary throughout the heating process, which is necessary for paraffin to be most effective (when using the standard method of dipping the hand and wrapping with plastic wrap and a towel).

11. c. The EMG does not record torque. It assists by showing a linear relationship between the EMG and the force produced by the muscle during an isometric contraction.

12. b. This is an example of a bipolar configuration. Another form of bipolar configuration is to have two electrodes of equal size, each from a different lead wire. In a monopolar configuration, one smaller electrode is placed over the intended site and a larger electrode is placed some distance away. The stimulation is perceived by the patient, in this case, only under the smaller electrode. In a quadripolar configuration, two electrodes coming from two different lead wires are placed over the intended area.

13. c. Choice C is correct. Heat decreases spasm by causing the vessels to dilate, which brings more blood (containing oxygen) to the area. Cold decreases spasm by decreasing sensitivity of the muscle spindles.

14. b. Iontophoresis uses direct current to drive medication through the skin by repelling ions. For example, if a medication is positively charged, it can be driven by the anode (the positive electrode); if a medication is negatively charged, it can be driven by the cathode (the negative electrode).

15. d. This is an example of Russian stimulation.

16. d. This is the most common placement suggested by sources used in preparation of this book. Spinal level varies, but the overall consensus is that the electrodes are placed higher and on the back initially. Then they are moved lower and to the anterior pubic region as labor progresses.

17. d. This type of stimulation is usually not well tolerated by patients with acute conditions. Acute conditions are usually treated by TENS with a high frequency, and chronic conditions can be treated with a low frequency (if tolerated by the patient). Treatments providing a noxious stimulus usually have a longer lasting effect.

18. d. Herpes zoster involves a particular dorsal root and its ganglia. TENS unit electrodes should be placed over the involved dermatome (L5 in this case).

19. c. Because functional electrical stimulation involves stimulating the paralyzed muscle groups, the same gains that one can expect from the "well" population can be carried over into the spinal cord injured patient. There has been no research to prove that osteopenia is reversed with electrical stimulation.

20. b. The use of electrical stimulation near the carotid sinus is contraindication. The physical therapist should always contact the physician if there is a change in an order as in choice D.

21. c. A prerequisite for FES is an upper motor neuron lesion. Patients with flaccid paralysis are not suitable candidates for FES. The cauda equina begins below T11-T12.

22. a. The lateral knee would cause the most concern because the common peroneal nerve is superficial in this area. The medial elbow near the ulnar nerve would be another area that would need extra care during ice application.

23. b. Spinal traction is contraindicated for patients with conditions that may cause spinal instability or fracture such as tumors, acute infections, osteoporosis, and rheumatoid arthritis.

24. c. Positional traction is used to alleviate pressure on an entrapped spinal nerve, which is usually a unilateral occurrence; thus, the side-lying position (nonpainful side) is most commonly used.

25. b. Although all pieces of information are important, the body weight is needed to help determine the maximum intensity for a lumbar traction treatment.

26. d. The patient is experiencing peripheralization of his pain, which indicates that his condition has worsened, so the traction treatment should be stopped.

27. b. Pulling the cervical spine into slight flexion is the best way to target your stretch to the posterior cervical musculature. It also reduces tension on the facet joint capsules.

28. c. A force that equals up to 50% of the patient's body weight may be needed to cause distraction of the lumbar vertebra. Much lower forces ($\approx$7%) are needed to distract the cervical vertebrae.

29. a. Because this is passive movement only, CPM can neither cause a muscle contraction nor prevent atrophy.

30. d. The pressure setting should never exceed the patient's diastolic blood pressure. Because venous pressure is usually higher in the lower extremities than in the upper extremities, guidelines suggest a range of 30 to 60 mm Hg for the upper extremity and 40 to 80 mm Hg for the lower extremity. Intermittent compression is usually tolerated better, and recommended treatment times are 2 to 3 hours a day, depending on the severity of the condition

31. a. Congestive heart failure and pulmonary edema are both contraindications for pneumatic compression because the heart and lungs are already overloaded and compression will just further increase that fluid load. This could result in more breathing difficulties or complete heart failure.

32. a. Because iontophoresis is administered with a continuous monophasic (i.e., direct) current, it can cause an acidic or alkaline reaction under the electrode, depending on the polarity used. This can be very irritating to the skin. Home units are available for iontophoresis, but not phonophoresis. Iontophoresis requires medications to be suspended in a solution, whereas phonophoresis requires the medication to be mixed in with a lotion, gel, or cream. Deeper penetration is usually possible with phonophoresis because ultrasound can target tissues several centimeters deep, while iontophoresis only penetrates a few millimeters.

33. b. The active electrode should be the same polarity as the medication. The optimal current dosage (intensity $\times$ treatment time) is 40 to 80 mAmp minutes.

34. b. In order to move ions continuously into the tissue, a continuous monophasic current (i.e., direct current) is needed.

35. a. High-volt stimulation would be the best option because it is a monophasic waveform and can produce polarity effects. These polarity effects have been shown to help stimulate tissue repair and destroy bacteria that may contaminate the wound. Iontophoresis also produces polarity effects but cannot be applied to an open wound because the continuous current will irritate the tissue too much.

36. d. Shortwave diathermy produces deep heat and is best absorbed by muscle tissue. Hot packs and infrared radiation are too superficial to adequately heat the target tissue. Pulsed ultrasound produces little or no thermal effect.

37. c. Diathermy is always contraindicated in patients with pacemakers. Ultrasound is only contraindicated when used to treat a body part in close proximity to the pacemaker. In this case, the patient's thigh is sufficiently distant from the pacemaker.

38. c. Sensory-level TENS is believed to selectively activate the large-diameter A-beta fibers that block (i.e., "close the gait") the slower conduction nociceptive fibers in the dorsal horn of the spinal cord before these neurons can synapse with the second-order neurons in the spinal tracts. Thus, this mechanism is referred to as presynaptic inhibition.

39. a. The application of cold modalities has been shown to reduce nerve conduction velocity.

40. a. A reciprocal mode is used because you want to provide contraction and elongation to both muscle groups (flexors and extensors). In order to simulate a functional muscle contraction, you need to use a frequency in the tetanizing range and enough amplitude to produce a strong muscle contraction that can overcome the force of gravity and move the joint through its full range of motion.

41. a. Raynaud's disease or phenomenon is induced by exposure to a cold stimulus, so the cold pack should be avoided with this patient.

42. b. Because the soundhead is the active electrode in a combination treatment such as this, you want the dispersive pad to be relatively inactive. Thus, a monopolar technique in which a larger dispersive pad is attached adjacent to the targeted treatment area would be most appropriate.

43. d. Although no evidence has supported prior concerns that ultrasound may damage a growing epiphysis, treating over these bony sites with ultrasound is still not generally recommended, particularly when other treatment options exist.

44. a. The hydrostatic pressure exerted by the water at deeper depths (near this patient's legs and feet) will help push fluid up and out of the lower extremities and back into the central circulation.

45. a. Because you are dealing with a very weak, partially innervated muscle, you will need to select a duty cycle that causes the least amount of fatigue. A 1:5 ratio of on/off time is recommended in those cases.

46. b. The illustration shows that these electrodes are spaced pretty far apart. The further apart two electrodes are, the deeper the current will run. Thus, the current is probably running too deep and actually stimulating the flexors, instead of the extensors. Moving both electrodes over the muscle belly should remedy this problem.

47. a. The stimulus threshold for a muscle that is denervated or only partially innervated is much higher than it is for a normal, innervated muscle. The stimulus threshold is reached through a combination of increasing pulse amplitude and duration. Most small stimulators have limited amplitude range and a fixed pulse duration of 150-300 microseconds. This may not be sufficient to reach the stimulus threshold for this patient's muscle.

48. a. To increase the extensibility of collagen tissue, you want some thermal effects from the ultrasound treatment; thus, you need to use the continuous mode. To penetrate to the depth of the shoulder joint capsule, you should use the 1 MHz frequency because ultrasound delivered with higher frequencies tends to be absorbed more in the superficial tissues.

49. c. Most heating, compression, and electrical modalities cause some increase in circulation, which can aggravate a metastatic condition. In addition, the presence of an active cancer in local tissue such as bone can weaken the tissue and cause injury, so traction would also be contraindicated. All of the other conditions are either indications or potential precautions for the use of these modalities.

50. b. EMG biofeedback requires the patient to consciously attend and respond to a visual or auditory stimulus in order to have a learning effect. An individual with dementia is unlikely to have the attention focus or retention needed to benefit from this type of intervention. All of the other conditions are indicated for either facilitating strength or relaxation of the targeted muscle groups.

51. a. Heat tends to cause local vasodilation, so it is more likely to increase the accumulation of fluid in the interstitial spaces than decrease it.

52. b. An allergic response to cold is most likely to present itself as a skin reaction in the form of itching, rash, or hives. Choice A relates to the occurrence of Raynaud's phenomenon. The other two choices are irrelevant.

53. d. Vapocoolant sprays cause a surface cooling when the liquid spray evaporates.

54. a. Studies have shown an increase in muscle strength following a 5-minute application of a cold modality. Long-term cooling may reduce muscle strength as well as muscle tone. Although cold therapy may reduce the amount of delayed onset muscle soreness, the modality would need to be applied immediately after the exercise session, not before it.

55. a. Because heat tends to increase circulation, the greatest danger is that heat applied over an infectious lesion will cause the organism to spread to adjacent tissues or get into the central circulation where it can cause a systemic infection.

56. b. Cement and plastic are rapidly heated by ultrasound, so it should be avoided over tissues with these types of implants. Ultrasound can interfere with a cardiac pacemaker when applied over the chest or upper back. The effects of ultrasound on reproductive organs is not known; thus, it should be avoided over these anatomic areas. Metal tends to reflect ultrasound, so metal implants are not a contraindication.

57. c. A 1MHz ultrasound unit is a relatively low frequency that allows the sound waves to be absorbed deeper into the tissue (higher frequency energy is absorbed more superficially). BNR is the ratio between the spatial peak intensity and the spatial average intensity of the ultrasound beam. The higher the BNR, the less uniform the heating effect will be and the more likely to produce "hot spots" during the treatment. Most units produce a BNR of 5:1 or 6:1 and some are as low as 2:1.

58. a. Phonophoresis is most commonly used to deliver anti-inflammatory medication to soft tissues such as muscles, tendons, and joint capsules.

59. c. Bony tissue has a high attenuation for ultrasound due to both absorption and reflection. Thus, if you are moving the soundhead too slowly or using a unit with a high BNR, the heating effect may be more concentrated over the bone tissue and cause discomfort (i.e., deep aching).

60. d. Nonthermal effects of ultrasound include an increase in intracellular calcium levels, skin and cell membrane permeability, histamine release, rate of protein synthesis, rate of mast cell degeneration, and nitric oxide synthesis, all of which promote wound healing.

61. d. The use of birth control pills does not contraindicate or add precautions to the use of short wave diathermy, so it is an unnecessary question. All of the other questions may have some relevance to the use of this modality over this particular part of the body.

62. b. The combination of cryotherapy and compression is best for reducing edema because the cold will cause vasoconstriction and the compression will prevent the build-up of fluid in the interstitial spaces. The other choices are all heat modalities, which can aggravate the edema formation.

63. d. The use of photosensitive medications can affect the choice of treatment intensity when using ultraviolet treatment. The rest of the questions are not particularly relevant to the use of this modality in terms of precautions or treatment parameters.

64. b. According to the Inverse Square and Cosine Laws, the intensity of the radiation will be most intense when the light source is positioned closer to the object and perpendicular to its surface.

65. b. By definition, a laser emits light of a specific wavelength; thus, it is monochromatic. Cluster diodes used in newer therapeutic lasers usually contain several lasers of differing wavelengths. The other unique characteristics of laser light are that it does not diverge much from its source (i.e., less "scatter" of the light), and the waves travel in a synchronous pattern. Low-powered lasers are nondestructive because they are not in the ionizing range of the electromagnetic spectrum.

66. b. Heat should help reduce this patient's muscle spasm. However, the target tissue in this case is too deep to be effectively heated with superficial modalities such as hot packs. Because she had metal rods in her back, diathermy is contraindicated even though it tends to heat muscle tissue better than ultrasound.

67. c. Rubbing the skin surface with soap or alcohol will remove any dirt, lotions, or skin oils that may create impedance to the electrical current and ensure better conductivity using the least amount of intensity.

68. a. In the illustration provided, the height of each pulse (i.e., amplitude) progressively increases then decreases again. The shape of the pulses, width (i.e., duration) of the pulses, and the space between pulses remain the same.

69. b. Electrotherapy may be used to treat all infected wounds, spasticity, and urinary incontinence (via strengthening of the pelvic floor muscles). However, it is contraindicated in patients with a history of seizures because of the possibility that the stimulus might provoke a seizure.

70. d. This type of current is known as Russian current. The other currents listed have different waveforms and are usually intended for other clinical indications besides muscle strengthening.

71. c. Muscle tetany is usually achieved at a pulse rate between 30 and 50 pulses per second (Hz). Because a smooth contraction is desired for muscle strengthening or range of motion, most NMES protocols include frequency settings in this range. A muscle contraction can be elicited at lower frequency settings (will present as a twitch response), and higher frequency settings may be used, particularly when the treatment goal is to fatigue a muscle that is in spasm.

72. a. A very weak or partially innervated muscle is easily prone to fatigue, so a lower frequency setting is indicated for these patients.

73. d. When using electrical stimulation to help reduce spasticity, many protocols stimulate the antagonist of the spastic muscle because it is usually in a weakened state. However, if the stimulus is brought on too quickly by using a fast rise/ramp time, it may cause a quick stretch to the spastic muscle, thus exacerbating the problem.

74. d. Because the subluxed humerus is displaced anteriorly and inferiorly, the supraspinatus and posterior deltoid muscles are usually stimulated simultaneously to help reverse the subluxed position.

75. a. The important aspect of iontophoresis is to deliver a sufficient amount of medication to the tissues. Thus, it takes a combination of current intensity and treatment time to achieve the desired results. A current dosage of 40 mAmp minutes is usually required for effective results. Thus, if a patient only tolerates 1 mAmp of current, the treatment time would be 40 minutes. If they tolerate more intensity, the treatment time can be reduced accordingly.

76. c. When the injury is acute and edema is still forming, stimulation should be kept at the sensory level to avoid further injury to the tissues. Sensory-level stimulation is all that is needed to affect the cell permeability changes that help reduce the edema formation.

77. b. With sensory-level TENS, the body can quickly adapt, or habituate, to the sensation which diminishes its effects. By modulating the pulse amplitude, frequency, and/or duration, the body does not have the opportunity to get used to the sensation and should continue to respond to it.

78. d. Refractory period is the amount of time it takes for an excitable membrane to be ready for a second stimulus once it returns to its resting state following excitation. In the generation of an action potential, as the membrane potential is increased, both the sodium and potassium ion channels begin to open. This increases both the inward sodium current (which is called depolarization) and the balancing outward potassium current (which is called repolarization). Threshold is the amount of current required for voltage to increase past a critical limit, typically 15 mV higher than the resting value. This results in initiating a process whereby the positive feedback from the sodium current activates even more sodium channels, and this eventually leads to the generation of an action potential.

79. a. Pulse frequency determines the rate of action potential activation. In addition, frequency influences the strength and motor response of a single motor unit. Increasing frequency changes muscle response from twitch to tetany. Tetany is required for most stimulation programs. 25 to 50 pulses per second is the frequency range to achieve tetany in most muscles. Anything less will result in twitch muscle responses. Increases in frequency past 50 pps deplete neurotransmitter supply in neuromuscular junction and depletes muscles energy supplies (ATP).

80. a. Duty cycle is the percentage of time that stimulation is on or active. Duty cycle = {on time/(on + off time)} × 100%. In this case, 6 sec on/(6 on + 18 sec off) = 25% duty cycle (1:3 ratio).

81.   c.   Electrode placement or electrode configuration is dependent on several factors, including the size of electrodes, orientation of electrodes, distance between electrodes, distance from motor points, polarity of electrodes, and type of waveform utilized. A monopolar electrode configuration occurs when one electrode is located over target tissue (active) and a second electrode over a distant site (inactive). A bipolar configuration occurs when both electrodes are over the target area and both electrodes are usually active. Monopolar configurations are often used when current must be kept in a small area. Bipolar is utilized when current is desired in a larger target area. Asymmetrical or monophase configurations refer to a type of electrical waveform. It is utilized when current is desired in greater dosages at a specific electrode site. One active electrode is placed close to the motor point while the other electrode is placed at another point to disperse current. Symmetric or biphasic waveforms are utilized when both electrodes need to be equally active. This is utilized in muscles that are larger or require more current. Wrist extensors are a small muscle mass that requires specific current to a small region. The asymmetric biphasic waveform with monopolar electrode configuration will provide the configuration for this muscle mass.

82.   a.   There are three classes of electrical current. Direct current (DC) is characterized by a continuous or uninterrupted unidirectional flow of charged particles. Alternating current (AC) refers to a continuous or uninterrupted bidirectional flow of charged particles. Pulsed current is a unidirectional or bidirectional flow of charged particles that periodically ceases for a finite period of time. A period of electrical silence is a hallmark characteristic of pulsed current.

83.   d.   While foot drop itself can be the result of numerous pathologies (both neurologic and orthopedic), weakness of the tibialis anterior muscle results in an impaired ability to dorsiflex the foot. This deficit is most apparent during the swing phase of gait in which the foot is required to dorsiflex in order to clear the toes as the foot progresses forward in the air.

84.   b.   Large electrodes should be utilized because the quadriceps are a large muscle group and a wider electrical field will allow for the recruitment of a greater number of motor units. Widely spaced electrodes are needed because electricity will travel the path of least resistance. If the electrodes are placed closely, that pathway will be superficial. By spreading the electrodes out wider, the current will flow deeper to the muscles motor points. The 10:30 duty cycle will provide the muscle with adequate recovery time between contractions as opposed to the 10 second rest cycle of the 10:10 duty cycle.

85.   a.   When ionizable substances such as acids, basis, salts or alkaloids are dissolved in water, the substances dissolve and dissociate into their polar components (ionization). Resulting solutions (electrolytes) can carry an electrical current by virtue of the migration of the dissociated ions. When a direct current (DC) is passed between two electrodes in an electrolytic solution, positive ions will be repelled from the anode (+) and negative ions repelled from the cathode (−). The anode will repel the positively charged ion from the electrode and into the body. Electrostatic repulsion of like charges is the driving force for iontophoresis. Direct current is the continuous or uninterrupted unidirectional flow of charged particles. It allows for continuous transmission of the medication and assures maximum ion transfer per unit of applied current. Pulsed, AC, and interferential currents are less effective in meeting the need of causing a local medication effect.

86.   b.   Biofeedback operates on the theory that we have the innate ability to influence the functions of our bodies through volitional control mechanisms. Biofeedback is the use of electronic instrumentation to provide objective information (feedback) to an individual about physiologic function or response so that the individual becomes aware of his or her response. The individual attempts to alter the feedback signal in order to modify the physiologic response. Biofeedback EMG is the recording of the electrical activity of the muscle membrane in response to the physiologic activation of skeletal muscle. The amplitude of EMG reflects the size and number of active motor units as well as the distance of the active muscle fibers from the recording electrodes. Therefore, distance between the electrodes is critical in determining the activity of a muscle group. Electrodes placed close together will require the patient to contract the muscle hard in order to register a response in the biofeedback unit. Electrodes placed far apart will make it easier to register a response. Progression of the use of biofeedback to decrease muscle recruitment would involve placing electrodes close together initially and progressing to moving them farther apart as the patient is able to recruit the muscle more effectively. Detection sensitivity is utilized to monitor how much muscle recruitment is being generated. High detection sensitivity refers to the biofeedback unit's ability to detect small muscle contractions. The setting allows for a high ability to detect muscle contractions. Low detection sensitivity will require a larger muscle contraction for the biofeedback unit to detect the muscle activation. In this patient case, the activity of the masseter muscle is high and you wish to decrease that activity. Placing the electrodes close with a low detection sensitivity is the best arrangement.

87. a. The hamstring muscles function to reduce or prevent anterior translation of the tibia during terminal knee extension. The ACL plays a similar role. In an ACL deficient knee, rehabilitation should be geared towards recruiting the hamstring during functional activities. The hamstring should be recruited before the quadriceps to provide for joint stability.

88. d. Brief intense pain TENS is also known as Motor Level TENS or Counter Irritation TENS. Physiologically, it utilizes the concept that if someone's hand hurts, causing pain in the leg will result in the person feeling less pain in the hand. Physiologically, the mechanism is still unclear, but it is hypothesized that changes occur cortically as the CNS shifts its focus away from the painful area to the new area of pain. Because of the nature of the pain involved with wound debridement, a very noxious stimulant should be utilized to counter the pain generated from the procedure. Brief intense TENS is the best setting to achieve the noxious stimulant.

89. b. Results from animal and human studies support electrical stimulation as a means of promoting faster healing rate (epithelization) and enhanced wound (dermal) strength. The proposed physiologic effects include improved epidermal cell proliferation and migration, increased dermal fibroblastic activity, diminished edema, improved blood flow, increased oxygen, increased nutrients, decreased waste products, inhibited bacterial growth, enhanced phagocytosis, and changes in the "skin battery." The skin, like cell membranes, separates charge across its membrane. This separation of charge creates an electrical potential difference across the membrane. With wounds, electrical charge escapes the wound and the potential difference decreases. With healing wounds, there is a current flow across the wound and with nonhealing wounds there is no current flow. This is called the skin battery. Electrical stimulation has been postulated to create this current flow and therefore promote wound healing. The current has been hypothesized to promote epithelial cell migration, increased capillary permeability, and increased macrophages. Asymmetric waveforms have been shown to be more effective then symmetric waveforms indicating that polarity may play a role in healing. Biphasic waveforms appear to be more effective than monophasic.

90. a. The quadriceps are a large muscle group and as a result require a relatively significant amount of current to effectively recruit enough motor units to strengthen the muscle. Studies on the quadriceps indicate that it is difficult to selectively recruit one of the quadricep muscles individually during functional activities. The focus of treatment is not to improve strength of the muscle but rather to improve the muscle's motor control. Maximal muscle recruitment is

not required to improve muscle motor control. Therefore, the clinician could decrease the amount of current (current intensity). This would make the treatment more comfortable for the patient, but the patient should be encouraged to actively recruit the muscle in conjunction with the stimulation. Modifying the pulse rate and pulse duration would affect the ability to recruit muscle fibers and therefore should not be changed. With a muscle group as large as the quadriceps, a biphasic waveform is probably preferable to monophasic; therefore, changing polarity will not affect the comfort of the intervention because a biphasic waveform will have equal current at each electrode.

91. c. While stimulation of any of the mentioned muscles could potential lead to an inhibition of the biceps muscle, the best results would be accomplished through stimulation of the ipsilateral triceps. Physiologically, the stimulation of the ipsilateral triceps would result in reciprocal inhibition of the biceps muscle via the Ia inhibitory pathway.

92. c. Biofeedback operates on the theory that we have the innate ability to influence the functions of our bodies through volitional control mechanisms. Biofeedback is the use of electronic instrumentation to provide objective information (feedback) to an individual about a physiologic function or response so that the individual becomes aware of his or her response. The individual attempts to alter the feedback signal in order to modify the physiologic response. Biofeedback EMG is the recording of the electrical activity of the muscle membrane in response to the physiologic activation of skeletal muscle. The amplitude of EMG reflects the size and number of active motor units as well as the distance of the active muscle fibers from the recording electrodes. Therefore, distance between the electrodes is critical in determining the activity of a muscle group. Electrodes placed close together will require the patient to contract the muscle hard in order to register a response in the biofeedback unit. Electrodes placed far apart will make it easier to register a response. Progression of the use of biofeedback to decrease muscle recruitment would involve placing electrodes close together initially and progressing to moving them farther apart as the patient is able to recruit the muscle more effectively. Detection sensitivity is utilized to monitor how much muscle recruitment is being generated. High detection sensitivity refers to the biofeedback unit's ability to detect small muscle contractions. The setting allows for a high ability to detect muscle contractions. Low detection sensitivity will require a larger muscle contraction for the biofeedback unit to detect the muscle activation. In this patient case, the activity of the hamstring muscle is high and you wish to decrease that activity. Placing the electrodes close with a low detection sensitivity is the best arrangement.

93. c. All are appropriate interventions except ultrasound. It is contraindicated to apply ultrasound directly over active epiphyseal regions (growth plates) in children.

94. a. Following hip precautions, it is essential to avoid hyperextension or flexion of the hip past 90 degrees. In a wheelchair, a cushion or pillow should be placed in the seat to reduce the angle of the hip while seated, and the legs should be positioned in neutral to prevent internal or external rotation with the use of an abductor pillow.

95. a. This deviation is commonly referred to as a lateral heel whip. Excessive internal rotation of the prosthetic knee is one of the causes of this deviation. Excessive external rotation of the knee causes a medial heel whip.

96. c. Metatarsal pads successfully transfer weight onto the metatarsal shafts of this patient. A Thomas heel and a scaphoid pad are for patients with excessive pronation. A cushion heel absorbs shock at contact.

97. d. A belt that is angled at 90 degrees with the sitting surface limits the patient's involuntary efforts to extend the trunk because of increased tone. This angle also allows the patient to actively tilt the pelvis anteriorly, which is a functional movement that does not need to be restricted.

98. b. Choices A and C provide the most medial/lateral ankle support. A posterior leaf-spring ankle-foot orthosis only provides assistance with dorsiflexion. Electrical stimulation aided AFOs also only assist with dorsiflexion and do not address the ankle instability.

99. d. Compression stockings (e.g., Jobst, TED hose) are used in patients with poor venous return. A patient with chronic arterial disease already has difficulty with getting blood to the lower extremities; there is no need to further inhibit the flow.

100. b. The correct procedure is choice B. Subtracting 1 inch allows correct pressure distribution over the patient's buttocks and thighs.

101. b. A socket that is too large may cause the prosthetic limb to "drop" during ambulation.

102. d. If the foot is outset too much, it is likely to cause the prosthetic knee to bow inward during standing.

103. a. Metatarsal pads, metatarsal bars, and rocker bars transfer weight onto the metatarsal shaft. A scaphoid pad is for patients with excessive pronation.

104. d. This type of orthotic uses tenodesis to achieve opening and closing of the hand. To close the hand, the patient actively extends the wrist. To open the hand, the patient passively flexes the wrist.

105. d. To lock the elbow with this type of prosthesis, the patient must extend the humerus and depress the scapula.

106. b. Use of a sliding board is the most functional transfer for this patient. The pneumatic lift requires assistance from another person, on which this patient cannot rely because he lives alone and has poor outside family support. A fully reclined geriatric chair is often used to transfer obese patients with a slide sheet transfer, which requires two or more people. A trapeze bar may be useful, but transferring wheelchair to bed with a sliding board teaches the patient the skill needed to transfer from the wheelchair to many other surfaces (that may not have a trapeze bar to assist).

107. c. Fully elevating the leg rests of the patient's chair increases hip flexion. The already tight hamstrings (secondary to contracture) would tilt the pelvis posterior. This maneuver would increase weight on the ischial tuberosity, risking a decubitus ulcer. Choice D is correct advice because sliding board transfers can lead to abrasions. Choices A and B are also correct measures to decrease the chance of developing ulcers.

108. c. Because the hip flexors are strong, there is no need for the hip component of an orthotic.

109. a. A patient of this age usually can begin with crutches instead of a standard walker. If the patient has no cognitive deficits and was independent in ambulation without an assistive device before surgery, she most likely will have the balance and coordination necessary to ambulate with crutches. A three-point gait pattern is necessary because of the current partial weight-bearing status. A swing-to pattern also can be used, but a three-point pattern assists more quickly in returning a more normal gait pattern.

110. c. Although the patient will have to use the hemi-walker with the right upper extremity, answer C is still the best choice for this patient. Choices A and B are unsafe with one upper extremity. Choice D does not encourage weight-bearing and is not the most functional choice. A person with a cemented prosthesis can bear weight as tolerated on the involved lower extremity in early rehabilitation.

111. b. Blisters should be allowed to subside naturally. Gel inserts lose their shape if not left in the prosthesis overnight. The prosthesis should be propped up in a corner or laid on the floor to prevent it from falling and cracking.

112. d. All of the above are important skills for a patient with a hip disarticulation prosthesis to master, but posterior pelvic tilt should be mastered first to advance the prosthesis.

113. a. A heel that is too stiff causes excessive knee flexion. Choices B and C cause excessive knee extension during this stage of the gait cycle.

114. b. The type of orthosis used depends on the degree of curve, location, and curve type. Skeletally immature patients with a curve of 25 to 45 degrees have shown good results with orthotics.

115. a. An externally powered prosthesis uses muscle contractions by the child that activates an electrode in the prosthesis. A body-powered prosthesis uses a cable and harness system.

116. d. Choice A provides a very small base of support, while choice D widens the base of support. Crutches should never be placed under the same arm.

117. b. The reciprocal walker has hinges that allow each side of the walker to move with the lower extremity being advanced. This walker is unsafe. The order of most to least stable is nonfolding standard walker, folding, rolling, and reciprocal.

118. c. Any complaints should be investigated immediately. Pain could be a sign of possible pressure areas or a compartment syndrome. The fit of the brace should be examined after there are no complaints.

119. b. Without legal consent for restraints, none of the other choices are a concern. Legal documentation is imperative with any medical procedure.

120. c. Axillary crutches are the most appropriate device based on the patient's age and diagnosis.

CHAPTER 6

Safety and Professional

1. The BEST example of a statement that would be documented in the assessment portion of a subjective, objective, assessment, and plan (SOAP) note is
   a. Client and spouse participated in a discussion about planning activities of interest for the patient
   b. Client complains of difficulty donning night-time splint and requests that the splint be re-examined by the therapist
   c. Family was referred to social services for consideration of alternative placement
   d. Client demonstrates good understanding of the home program but requires supervision to perform independently

2. Which is the BEST means for documenting a goal statement?
   a. Therapist will instruct the patient in overhead dressing techniques.
   b. Patient will participate in meal preparation for 15 minutes without breaks.
   c. Patient will perform 10 repetitions of active assistive shoulder ladder exercises.
   d. Patient will show increased endurance for performing ADLs.

3. Which statement would be the MOST appropriate for the PT to document in the plan section of the SOAP note?
   a. Client given educational materials to practice correcting posture and trunk balance during daily routine.
   b. Client able to respond to verbal instructions and questions with correct responses 3 out of 3 times.
   c. Client indicates that the long-term goal is to return to work on a full-time basis.
   d. Client assessed for use of compensatory techniques while cooking in the clinic kitchen.

4. During a treatment session, a patient with a C5 spinal cord injury complains of dizziness and a severe headache and is noticed by the PT to be flushed and sweating profusely. The best course of action for the PT to take is to
   a. Lie the patient down to rest for about 30 minutes or until symptoms subside
   b. Contact the physician and report signs of autonomic dysreflexia
   c. Take the blood pressure because of the suspected signs of orthostatic hypotension
   d. Assist the patient in taking medication for the symptoms

5. A client being treated in outpatient therapy for extensor tendon repair missed three appointments while sick with the flu. When writing the monthly report, the therapist explained why the client did not achieve her short-term goals in the time frame specified. Which is the MOST appropriate section of the subjective, objective, assessment, and plan (SOAP) note for this documentation?
   a. S
   b. O
   c. A
   d. P

6. After talking to nursing, the inpatient rehab PT treated the patient in the room for instruction in safety and adaptive equipment for toileting, along with dressing and grooming activities. The patient was motivated and worked hard throughout the treatment session. Which is the BEST choice for the subjective portion of the daily SOAP note?
   a. Patient was cooperative and engaged in social conversation throughout the treatment session.
   b. Patient reports that the patient feels good today.
   c. Patient is unable to move her right upper extremity as well today as yesterday, although it doesn't really hurt but feels "tight."
   d. Nursing staff reports that patient is unsafe to toilet independently.

7. After a stroke, a patient had difficulty picking up pills from the table; difficulty buttoning; and difficulty completing jigsaw puzzles, which was a favorite leisure activity. During part of the treatment session, the patient worked on putting in and removing pieces from a jigsaw puzzle and practiced manipulating different sized coins from a flat table surface. When documenting the treatment, the BEST choice for an objective statement is
   a. Patient worked for 15 minutes placing and removing jigsaw puzzle pieces.
   b. Patient worked on tripod grasp using various coins and jigsaw puzzle pieces.
   c. Patient worked for 15 minutes on tripod grasp in order to be able to grasp objects used for leisure activities and ADLs.
   d. Patient worked on tripod grasp to be able to perform leisure activities and ADLs.

8. Which statement would be documented in the "plan" portion of a SOAP note?
   a. Problems include decreased coordination, strength, sensation, and proprioception in left upper extremity.
   b. In order to return to work, patient will demonstrate increase of 10# of grasp in left hand, in 3 weeks.
   c. Patient would benefit from further instruction in total hip precautions for lower extremity dressing, bathing, and hygiene.
   d. Patient attended job skills group with prompting by nursing and OT staff.

9. The BEST example of a statement that would document the patient's prognosis is
   a. The patient may require prolonged time to perform transfers because of poor motor planning ability.
   b. The patient received a home program on energy conservation and work simplification.
   c. Compared to the norm, grip strength is within normal limits and age appropriate.
   d. The patient performed a stand pivot transfer to and from the wheelchair to bathtub.

10. When discharging a patient with Alzheimer's to a skilled nursing facility, what is the most important information to share?
    a. Summary of cognitive performance
    b. Recommendations to a support group
    c. Summary of the patient progress
    d. Results of the initial examination

11. A PT walks into a patient's room and finds the patient lying on the floor next to the bed. The PT has been previously reprimanded for forgetting to put the bed rails up after treatment. After checking to be sure the patient has no broken bones and is not in severe pain, the therapist helps the patient back into bed, and then leaves the room without reporting the incident. Which terms best describe the PT's conduct?
    a. Legal and ethical
    b. Legal but unethical
    c. Ethical but illegal
    d. Illegal and unethical

12. A PT suspects physical abuse after noticing bruises on the face and back of a child during the treatment session. The appropriate action to take is
    a. To ask the child questions about the bruises
    b. To confront the parents about the cause for the inflictions
    c. To make a report to the appropriate authorities
    d. To ignore the bruises because proof of suspicion is difficult

13. To facilitate effective communication between a physical therapy supervisor and employee, the supervisor should
    a. Communicate what is expected of the employee
    b. Express disappointment regarding the employee's behavior
    c. Offer criticism to stimulate discussion
    d. Meet with the employee away from the workplace to facilitate a conversation

14. The term that refers to the process of providing information to individuals to assist them in the decision-making process about their own health care is
    a. Beneficence
    b. Fidelity
    c. Autonomy
    d. Informed consent

15. A patient tells the PT how much the services provided have helped in coping with his/her depression. The patient then offers a gift of appreciation to the therapist. The PT's best response is to say
    a. "I love the gift, but I need to report it to my administrator in order to follow regulations."
    b. "Thank you, that's great. What is it?"
    c. "Just knowing that you appreciate my help is reward enough. I appreciate the gesture, but I cannot accept the gift."
    d. "Please mail it to my house. I cannot accept the gift on the hospital premises."

16. The single most important measure to prevent the spread of infectious diseases is
    a. Hand washing
    b. Proper cooking
    c. Canning
    d. Pasteurization

17. A 30-year-old female patient presents with right calf pain and may have a deep vein thrombosis (DVT). What would be the MOST appropriate initial course of action?
    a. Prescribe rest and inactivity until symptoms subside
    b. Treat with RICE protocols until symptoms subside
    c. Treat with massage, muscle stripping, and stretching procedures
    d. Refer for medical evaluation

18. The most important step to take upon involvement in an emergency is to
    a. Let the patient know that you have arrived
    b. Assess the scene and environment
    c. Make sure that you have plenty of gloves
    d. Immediately care for the patient

19. What is the BEST method for controlling bleeding and should be attempted first?
    a. Elevation
    b. Direct pressure
    c. Trauma dressing
    d. Tourniquet

20. When caring for a fractured, dislocated, or sprained extremity, when is it important to check for pulses, sensation, and motor function?
    a. After the splint has been removed at the hospital
    b. Before applying a splint
    c. Before and after applying a splint
    d. During the detailed physical examination of the patient, usually en route to the hospital

21. A therapist is treating a 35-year-old man diagnosed, with lumbar disc degeneration, in an outpatient clinic. Through conversation with the patient, the therapist learns that he is also being treated by a chiropractor for cervical dysfunction. What is the best course of action by the therapist?
    a. Continue with the current treatment plan and ignore the chiropractor's treatment.
    b. Ask the patient what the chiropractor is doing and try the same approach.
    c. Stop physical therapy at once and consult with the referring physician.
    d. Contact the chiropractor to coordinate his or her plan of care with the physical therapy plan of care.

22. Which of the following duties cannot be legally performed by a physical therapist assistant?
    a. Confer with a doctor about a patient's status
    b. Add 5 pounds to a patient's current exercise protocol
    c. Allow a patient to increase in frequency from 2 times/week to 3 times/week
    d. Perform joint mobilization

23.   The therapist is treating a patient in an outpatient facility for strengthening of bilateral lower extremities. During the initial assessment, the patient reveals that he has a form of cancer but is reluctant to offer any other information about his medical history. After 1 week of treatment, the therapist is informed by the physician that the patient has Kaposi's sarcoma and AIDS. Which of the following is the best course of action for the therapist?
    a.   Cease treatment of the patient, and inform him that an outpatient facility is not the appropriate environment for a person with his particular medical condition.
    b.   Continue treatment of the patient in the gym, avoiding close contact with other patients and taking appropriate universal precautions.
    c.   Continue treatment of the patient in the gym as before, taking appropriate universal precautions.
    d.   Cease treatment, but do not confront the patient with the knowledge of his HIV status.

24.   A patient's lawyer calls the therapist requesting his or her client's clinical records. The lawyer states that he or she needs the records to pay the patient's bill. What is the best course of action?
    a.   Tell the lawyer either to have the patient request a copy of the records or to have the patient sign a medical release.
    b.   Fax the needed chart to the lawyer.
    c.   Mail a copy of the chart to the patient.
    d.   Call the patient and tell him or her of the recent development.

25.   A 12-year-old male has been referred to physical therapy after recently being involved in a car accident. The patient's mother has signed all the necessary paperwork for admission to the clinic, including a form allowing release of her son's records to the parties listed. The patient's mother included herself, doctors involved in the patient's care, and their attorney on the list. The patient's stepfather comes to the clinic after the patient is discharged and requests a copy of the stepson's record. Which of the following would be the correct response from the office staff?
    a.   Give the stepfather a copy of the records.
    b.   Give the stepfather a copy of the records after he has signed a release form.
    c.   Inform the patient's stepfather that he is not on the list that authorizes the records to be released to him.
    d.   Call the patient's mother and get verbal permission to release the records to the stepfather.

26. The home health physical therapist arrives late at the home of a patient for a treatment session just as the occupational therapist has finished. The patient is angry because the sessions are so close together. The patient becomes verbally abusive toward the physical therapist. The most appropriate response to the patient is
    a. "I'm sorry I'm late, but you must try to understand that I am extremely busy."
    b. "I know you are aggravated. It is inconvenient when someone does not show up when expected. Let's just do our best this session and I will make an effort to see that we do not have PT and OT scheduled so close together from now on."
    c. "You have to expect visits at any time of the day with home health."
    d. "The OT and I did not purposefully arrive so close together. I apologize, please let's now begin therapy."

27. When should a physical therapist begin discharge planning for a patient admitted to a rehabilitation unit with a diagnosis of a recent stroke?
    a. At the first team meeting
    b. At the last team meeting
    c. Two weeks before discharge
    d. After the initial examination by the physical therapist

28. A therapist is performing a chart review and discovers that lab results reveal that the patient has malignant cancer. When examining the patient, the therapist is asked by the patient, "Did my lab results come back and is the cancer malignant?" The appropriate response for the therapist is
    a. To tell the patient the truth and contact the social worker to assist in consultation of the family.
    b. "It is inappropriate for me to comment on your diagnosis before the doctor has assessed the lab results and spoken to you first."
    c. "The results are positive for malignant cancer, but I do not have the training to determine your prognosis."
    d. To tell the patient the results are in, but physical therapists are not allowed to speak on this matter.

29. A physical therapy technician calls the therapist immediately to the other side of the outpatient clinic. The therapist discovers a 37-year-old female lying face down on the floor. Which of the following sequence of events is most appropriate for this situation?
    a. Have someone call 911, determine unresponsiveness, establish an airway, and assess breathing (look/listen/feel)
    b. Determine unresponsiveness, have someone call 911, establish an airway, and assess breathing (look/listen/feel)
    c. Have someone call 911, determine unresponsiveness, assess breathing (look/listen/feel), establish an airway
    d. Determine unresponsiveness, have someone call 911, assess breathing (look/listen/feel), and establish an airway

30. Which of the following acts forced all federally supported facilities to increase corridor width to a minimum of 54 inches to accommodate wheelchairs?
    a. Americans with Disabilities Act
    b. National Healthcare and Resource Development Act
    c. Civil Rights Act
    d. Older Americans Act (Title III)

31. A patient at an outpatient facility experiences the onset of a grand mal seizure. Which of the following is the most appropriate course of action by the therapist?
    a. Assist the patient to a lying position, move away close furniture, loosen tight clothing, and prop the patient's mouth open.
    b. Assist the patient to a lying position, move away close furniture, and loosen tight clothing.
    c. Assist the patient to a seated position, move away close furniture, and loosen tight clothing.
    d. Assist the patient to a seated position, move away close furniture, loosen tight clothing, and prop the patient's mouth open

32. A therapist is instructing a physical therapy student in writing a SOAP note. The student has misplaced the following phrase: Patient reports a functional goal of returning to playing baseball in 5 weeks. Where should this phrase be placed in a SOAP note?
    a. Subjective
    b. Objective
    c. Assessment
    d. Plan

33. An acute-care physical therapist is ordered to examine and treat a patient who has suffered a right hip fracture in a recent fall. During the examination, the family informs the therapist that the patient suffered a stroke approximately 1 week before the fall. The patient's chart has no record of the recent stroke. What should the physical therapist do first?
    a. Immediately call the referring physician and request a magnetic resonance scan.
    b. Examine and treat the patient as ordered.
    c. Immediately call the referring physician and request a computed tomography scan.
    d. Immediately call the referring physician for an occupational therapy referral.

34. A physical therapist in an outpatient clinic is urgently called into a room to assist an infant who is unconscious and not breathing. The therapist opens the airway of the infant and attempts ventilation. The breaths do not make the chest rise. After the infant's head is repositioned, the breaths still do not cause the chest to move. What should the therapist do next?
    a. Give five back blows.
    b. Look into the throat for a foreign body.
    c. Have someone call 911.
    d. Perform a blind finger sweep of the throat.

35. A physical therapist is setting up a portable whirlpool unit in the room of a severely immobile patient. What is the most important task of the physical therapist before the patient is placed in the whirlpool?
    a. Check for a ground fault circuit interruption outlet.
    b. Check to make sure the water temperature is below 110° F.
    c. Make sure the whirlpool agitator is immersed in the water.
    d. Obtain the appropriate assistance to perform a transfer.

36. A 37-year-old man fell and struck his left temple area on the corner of a mat table. He begins to bleed profusely but remains conscious and alert. Attempts to stop blood flow with direct pressure to the area of the injury are unsuccessful. Of the following, which is an additional area to which pressure should be applied to stop bleeding?
    a. Left parietal bone one inch posterior to the ear
    b. Left temporal bone just anterior to the ear
    c. Zygomatic arch of the frontal bone
    d. Zygomatic arch superior to the mastoid process

37. A physical therapist is beginning the examination of a patient with AIDS. The patient was admitted to the acute floor of the hospital on the previous night after receiving a right total hip replacement. The physician has ordered gait training and a dressing change of the surgical site. Of the following precautions, which is the least necessary?
    a. Mask
    b. Gloves
    c. Hand washing
    d. Gown

38. A physical therapist is treating a 17-year-old boy with an incomplete T11 spinal cord injury. The patient was treated for 2 months in the rehabilitation unit of the hospital before beginning outpatient physical therapy. He is currently ambulating with a standard walker with maximal assist of two. The therapist sets an initial long-term goal of "ambulation with a standard walker with minimum assist of 1 for a distance of 50 feet, with no loss of balance, on a level surface—in 8 weeks." If the patient achieves the long-term goal in 4 weeks, which of the following courses of action should be taken by the therapist?
   a. Discharge the patient secondary to completion of goals.
   b. Set another long-term goal regarding ambulation and continue treatment.
   c. Return the patient to the rehabilitation unit of the hospital for more intensive treatment.
   d. Call the patient's physician and ask for further instructions.

39. A physical therapist is ordered to examine a 74-year-old man who has suffered a recent stroke. The therapist performs a chart review before performing the examination. Which of the following is of the least importance to the physical therapist in assessing the patient's chart?
   a. Nursing assessment
   b. Physician's orders/notes
   c. Respiratory assessment
   d. Dietary assessment

40. Each of the following choices consists of a list of two summaries of some of the principles in the code of ethics of the American Physical Therapy Association. Which of the answers below is a false summary?
   a. (1) Obey regulations governing physical therapists, and (2) maintain high standards when providing therapy.
   b. (1) Respect the rights of patients, and (2) inform people appropriately of the services provided.
   c. (1) Maintain high standards when providing therapy, and (2) provide services for the length of time ordered.
   d. (1) Assist the public when there are public health needs, and (2) accept fair monetary compensation for services.

41. A physical therapist is scheduled to examine the shoulder of a patient with hepatitis B. The therapist notices no open wounds or abrasions and also notices that the patient has good hygiene. The physician has ordered passive range of motion to the right shoulder because of adhesive capsulitis. Which of the following precautions is absolutely necessary to prevent the therapist from being infected?
   a. The therapist must wear a gown.
   b. The therapist must wear a mask.
   c. The therapist must wear gloves.
   d. There is no need for any personal protective equipment.

42. A contraindicated activity for a child with osteogenesis imperfecta would be
    a. Spontaneous active extremity movement
    b. Pull-to-sit maneuver
    c. Prone scooter activity
    d. Light weights attached close to joints

43. The best recommendation for strength training in prepubescent children is
    a. No strength training recommended
    b. Strength training programs should be the same as adolescents
    c. Strength training should be done only for the lower extremities
    d. Strength training should be closely supervised, correctly taught, and involve low load/high repetition tasks

44. You are working with a 2-year-old child who has a tumor in the posterior fossa. She demonstrates a significant right torticollis. Which intervention is most likely contraindicated?
    a. Facilitated active range of motion
    b. Gentle anterior-posterior glides in the upper cervical region
    c. Home positioning program
    d. Upper trapezius strengthening

45. A patient with an acute infection of the left knee has been admitted to the hospital. A chart review shows that the patient currently has a body temperature of 102.5° F. The physician has ordered for therapy to begin intervention with this patient immediately.
    What is the most appropriate course of action by the physical therapist?
    a. Begin examination of the patient.
    b. Begin intervention with ROM first.
    c. Begin intervention with ambulation first.
    d. Contact the physician as an acute infection is a contraindication to exercise.

46. During documentation after an intervention a mistake is made in the note. Which of the below is NOT an appropriate step to make in correcting the mistake?
    a. Strike one line through the error so that it is still legible.
    b. Write your initials in the margin near the mistake.
    c. Write "mistaken entry" or "error" near the mistake.
    d. Use liquid correction fluid or an eraser over the mistake.

47. A physical therapist has determined that hamstring stretching should be incorporated in the intervention of 75-year-old female with complaints of low back pain. Which of the following conditions is a contraindication to stretching of the hamstring muscle group?
    a. Soreness lasting approximately 2 to 3 hours after therapy
    b. Hemophilia
    c. Patient's age
    d. Minimal complaints of pain in the lumbar area

48. A physical therapist is about to begin intervention of a patient with recent total hip replacement using an anterior approach. Which of the following are contraindicated motions of the hip during early rehabilitation?
    a. Hip flexion above 90 degrees
    b. Hip hyperextension
    c. Hip adduction past neutral
    d. Hip internal rotation

49. Which of the following conditions would be a contraindication to performing manual lymphatic drainage techniques performed over the abdomen?
    a. Menstrual period
    b. Undiagnosed abdominal pain
    c. Crohn's disease
    d. Diverticulitis

50. Which of the following is proper placement of a catheter bag?
    a. In the patient's lap while in a wheelchair
    b. On the patient's stomach while in a supine position on a hospital bed
    c. Hooked onto the therapist's pocket during ambulation
    d. Below the waist of the patient

51. The physical therapist is beginning a program of functional electrical stimulation (FES) for a patient with T4 paraplegia in order to promote cardiovascular fitness. At what systolic blood pressure should the exercise be terminated?
    a. 140 mm Hg
    b. 160 mm Hg
    c. 180 mm Hg
    d. 220 mm Hg

52. A physical therapist decides to use cervical traction for a patient with complaints of cervical pain. Which of the following conditions is a contraindication for cervical traction?
    a. Hyperthyroidism
    b. Hypertension
    c. Diabetes
    d. Down's syndrome

53. Which of the following positions should be avoided in postpartum patients?
    a. Left side-lying
    b. Right side-lying
    c. Supine with a pillow under the knees
    d. Prone with the knees pulled to the chest

54. When disrobing and draping a patient to prepare for intervention, which of the following is the most important advice?
    a. Avoid wrinkles in the draping garment.
    b. Do not use the patient's clothing for draping.
    c. Obtain the patient's consent before disrobing him or her.
    d. Ask for appropriate assistance in situations where the gender of the patient could be concern.

55. At which stage of scar tissue formation can maximal load be placed on the scar tissue without risk of failure?
    a. Inflammatory phase
    b. Granulation phase
    c. Fibroplastic phase
    d. Maturation phase

56. What motions should not be stretched early in rehabilitation after an open rotator cuff repair?
    a. Horizontal abduction, extension, and internal rotation
    b. Horizontal adduction, extension, and internal rotation
    c. Horizontal abduction, flexion, and internal rotation
    d. Horizontal abduction, extension, and external rotation

57. A young patient just starting antidepressant medication is telling you that "life is not worth living." You should tell the patient not to worry since this is
    a. experienced by most patients at the beginning of drug therapy
    b. only a transient reaction to the medication and of no consequence
    c. a good sign because the medication has a period of up to 4 weeks before it can take effect
    d. passing but inform the psychiatrist immediately about your conversation

58. A patient who just returned from abroad is being treated for a worm infection. What precautions do you have to take?
    a. Reschedule appointment until the patient has stopped taking the worm medication.
    b. Wear a mask and change work cloth after therapy.
    c. Disinfect toilet after the patient has used it.
    d. Do not take special precautions because the drug kills the worms and the eggs.

59. Your patient is on antipsychotic drug therapy. During your therapy session you notice a number of adverse reactions. The most severe one requiring immediate attention by a physician is
    a. Increased body temperature with some muscle rigidity
    b. Dizziness with almost fainting when getting up quickly
    c. A sudden but short-lasting tachycardia
    d. Appearance of a yellow skin and eyes

60. A patient on clopidogrel therapy is at increased risk of experiencing
    a. Internal bleeding episodes
    b. Sudden fainting spells
    c. Orthostatic hypotension
    d. Intermittent tachycardia

61. Smoking involves the inhalation of many compounds that can cause all of the following health problems except
    a. Korsakoff-Wernicke syndrome
    b. Emphysema
    c. Bladder cancer
    d. Hypertension

62. A patient receiving drug therapy experiences a slight fever and sore throat with some mouth ulcerations. The physician has to be notified since this could present a/an
    a. Agranulocytosis
    b. Thrombotic thrombocytic purpura
    c. Exfoliate dermatitis
    d. Churg Strauss syndrome

63. A patient receiving drug therapy experiences a cough, fever, and rash across the face spreading to the body. The physician has to be notified since this could present a
    a. Phototoxic reaction
    b. Epidermal necrosis
    c. Stevens-Johnson syndrome
    d. Lupus syndrome

64. A 78-year-old patient with COPD uses oxygen at all times. At rest, the pulse oximeter reads 91%. During a walk with the physical therapist, the pulse oximeter indicates the O_2 saturation is 86%, and the patient indicates fatigue. What is the appropriate action of the physical therapist?
    a. Stop walking and turn the oxygen up until the patient recovers.
    b. Turn the oxygen up and keep walking.
    c. Stop walking and monitor the patient closely.
    d. Keep walking and monitor the patient closely.

65. Which of the following vital sign issues should cause concern?
    a. The systolic blood pressure falls during exercise.
    b. The pulse rate increased by 15 beats/min with activity and recovered within 2 minutes.
    c. The patient reported the activity was rated a 13 on the Rate of Perceived Exertion Scale (RPE).
    d. The 6-year-old child had a resting pulse rate of 90 beats/min.

66. Patients with hyperlaxity always
    a. Have flat feet
    b. Can protect their joints with muscle strength
    c. Will develop patellar instability
    d. Must avoid the butterfly stroke in swimming

67. Postoperative knee braces have been associated with all the following complications except
    a. Deep vein thrombosis
    b. Peroneal nerve injury
    c. Avascular necrosis
    d. Ankle edema

68. Prophylactic bracing
    a. Prevents all injury
    b. Can protect ankles and medial collateral knee ligaments
    c. Has been shown to decrease ACL injuries
    d. Provides psychological benefits only

69. According to the APTA Guide for Physical Therapist Practice, the following are elements of patient management (in order of process during an initial session)
    a. Examination, assessment, impairment, treatment
    b. Evaluation, treatment, documentation, assessment
    c. Examination, evaluation, diagnosis, prognosis
    d. Interview, evaluation, tests and measures, diagnosis

70. You are working as part of an interdisciplinary team of an inpatient rehabilitation unit. Your patient suffered a spinal cord injury 3 weeks earlier. She was making progress in functional mobility, but lately has been behaving erratically: missing therapy, falling out of bed twice, and skipping medications. You suspect these may be self-destructive behaviors related to her recent injury. What is the BEST course of action?

    a. The patient needs encouragement from PT as she is clearly depressed.
    b. Wait for the next weekly conference, and then discuss with the team, as this is not your area of expertise.
    c. You consider self-destructive behaviors as serious, and notify the team with a request for immediate psychiatric assistance.
    d. The patient is at risk for suicide; warn the family to monitor her constantly and recommend they speak to the physician regarding appropriate medications.

71. Which of the following pieces of legislation guarantees patients the right to make autonomous decisions about their health care?

    a. The Americans with Disabilities Act (ADA)
    b. The Emergency Medical Treatment and Active Labor Act (EMTALA)
    c. The Health Insurance Portability and Accountability Act (HIPPA)
    d. The Patient Self-Determination Act (PSDA)

72. A physical therapist owns a private practice in a small community located 40 miles from the nearest hospital or outpatient clinic. Her spouse is offered a great job opportunity in another city so they decide to make the move at the end of the month. The therapist informs her office staff that she will be closing the practice in 2 weeks and asks her secretary to call all her patients and cancel their appointments. When she does this, several patients ask where they are supposed to go to finish their therapy sessions. The secretary replies, "Anywhere you can find another PT!" Given the situation just described, this therapist's patients could file a complaint based on

    a. Breach of confidentiality
    b. Failure to provide informed consent
    c. Fraudulent billing
    d. Patient abandonment

73. Which bioethical principle addresses a physical therapist's duty to provide honest information to his or her patients?

    a. Beneficience
    b. Fidelity
    c. Justice
    d. Veracity

74. You are treating an older adult who recently fell at home. The patient sustained no major injuries from the fall; however, your examination indicates that she is at high risk for falling again and your cognitive screening suggests that she probably has mild dementia. The patient lives alone and desperately wants to stay in her own home. However, you do not believe that she can live safely in this environment by herself and think it is in her best interests to investigate an alternative living arrangement. What ethical duty does this exemplify?
    a. Autonomy
    b. Beneficience
    c. Disclosure
    d. Nonmaleficence

75. You are ambulating a post-op patient up in the hospital corridor using a gait belt and appropriate guarding techniques. Suddenly the patient slips on an unnoticed wet spot on the floor and falls down. Although not seriously injured, the patient is in a lot of pain, has to spend extra days in the hospital, and requires additional rehab services. The patient's family sues the hospital and receives a financial settlement to cover the costs of additional hospitalization and home care. This settlement is an example of
    a. Comparative justice
    b. Compensatory justice
    c. Distributive justice
    d. Fiduciary justice

76. You are treating a patient who recently underwent total hip arthroplasty when she tells you that she urgently needs to use the bathroom. You immediately take her to the bathroom and, observing all positional precautions, assist her on and off the toilet using her walker, a gait belt, and a raised toilet seat. However, as the patient sits back down in her wheelchair, she states that she felt a "funny sensation" in her hip. You check out her hip position and movements but don't find anything unusual. Before returning to her room, the patient is transported to radiology for a previously scheduled x-ray. The next day one of the nurses informs you that the patient is back in surgery because she "dislocated her hip the previous day in physical therapy." You do not believe you were responsible for this patient's injury. What is your best defense against liability in this situation?
    a. The patient was confused and did not follow instructions well.
    b. You followed standard protocol and safety precautions during your treatment session.
    c. One of your transporters reported that the radiology techs frequently "mishandle" patients.
    d. It was an emergency situation so you are protected from liability by "Good Samaritan" laws.

77. A male therapist is performing an initial prosthetic check-out on a female patient with a transfemoral amputation. She is complaining of "pinching" from her prosthesis when she bears weight on it or sits down. To determine whether or not the socket is too tight, the therapist takes the patient into a private treatment room and asks her to undress so he can better palpate the tissues in her groin region. The patient doesn't say anything at that time, but later files a complaint against the therapist for sexual misconduct. What other action could this therapist have taken to protect him from this type of accusation?
    a. Ask the patient to sign a specific written consent form for palpation procedures.
    b. Distract the patient with some casual conversation to make her feel more comfortable.
    c. Request the presence of a female chaperone during the patient's examination.
    d. Wear gloves while performing the examination.

78. You are examining a 9-year-old child with cerebral palsy who appears to have an unusually large number of painful bruises around his wrists and ankles. His mother sees you examining these bruises and tells you that he falls down a lot due to his spasticity and poor balance. However, during your examination the child demonstrates a safe, independent gait using a reverse walker. When you reviewed his medical record you notice two prior emergency room visits to treat limb fractures. Given your observations and the patient's prior history of injuries, what are you obligated to do?
    a. Call 911 and request immediate assistance from a law enforcement officer.
    b. Continue to treat the child and observe for future signs of abuse.
    c. Report your suspicion of abuse to the appropriate child protective service agency.
    d. Request a consult from a medical social worker.

79. You are treating an elderly patient who is about to be discharged from the hospital following a recent stroke. The patient has some residual hemiparesis but he is oriented, communicates appropriately, and follows safety precautions when performing transfers and walking. You tell the patient that you want to arrange for continued therapy at home or on an outpatient basis to help him regain more strength and motor control. The patient agrees to this discharge plan; however, his son is present and tells you that his father has already had plenty of therapy and just needs to go home and rest. Under what circumstances is this patient's son able to act as his father's surrogate decision maker?
    a. The son may act as a surrogate decision maker if his father experienced a temporary or permanent loss for consciousness during his hospitalization.
    b. The son may act as a surrogate decision maker if his father has exceeded his Medicare benefits and cannot afford to pay for additional health care services on his own.
    c. The son may act as a surrogate decision maker if his father has been declared legally incompetent and has appointed the son to act on his behalf via a durable power of attorney.
    d. The son may act as a surrogate decision maker if his father is over 65 and has no spouse or advance directives.

80. According to the Americans with Disabilities Act, what circumstances would legally preclude an employer from having to hire, or provide accommodations for, a disabled worker?
    a. If the employer suspects that the worker's disability is not legitimate
    b. If the employer has to spend more than $500 on accommodations
    c. If the worker is not qualified to perform the essential job functions
    d. If the employment setting is privately owned and employs less than 100 people

81. Your patient presents with dizziness, lip paresthesias, nystagmus, lower extremity paresthesias, and drop attacks. This would be most indicative of
    a. A concussion
    b. Vertebral basilar insufficiency
    c. A labyrinthine syndrome
    d. Carotid artery tear

82. A physical therapist measures the knee range of motion of a patient status after anterior cruciate ligament reconstruction or repair using a goniometer. After completing the measurement, the therapist concludes that the patient lacks 20 degrees of knee extension and can flex the knee to 95 degrees. Knee flexion range of motion should be documented in the patients chart as
    a. 20 to 95 degrees
    b. 95 to 20 degrees
    c. 20-0-95 degrees
    d. −20-0-95 degrees

83. A physical therapist has been asked to determine whether a ramp to enter a local shopping mall meets the minimum accessibility standards required by law. The maximum grade for wheelchair ramps is best identified as for every inch of rise there should be _____ inches of length.
    a. 3
    b. 6
    c. 9
    d. 12

84. A physical therapist is educating a patient with low back pain about appropriate body mechanics. The patient's symptoms were reproduced with forward bending and sitting. Which instructions below are most appropriate for that patient?
    a. Use of a lumbar roll will eliminate your risk of aggravating your back pain during sitting.
    b. Bend the hips and knees when reaching down, and try to keep the spine neutral to avoid aggravation.
    c. Lifting light weights is not likely to cause any problems, but lifting heavier items should be avoided.
    d. Consider placing items you reach for frequently overhead to reduce forward bending.

85. A physician orders gait training for a 14-year-old male with recent open reduction internal fixation of the left femur. Which of the following is not the responsibility of the physical therapist?
    a. Determining weight-bearing status
    b. Assessing balance
    c. Choosing assistive device
    d. Assessing endurance

86. A 3-year-old male sustains a femur fracture after falling off his bike. He received an open reduction internal fixation (ORIF) yesterday. The MD writes an order for PT examination and treatment. He is cleared to ambulate non–weight bearing (NWB) on the affected extremity. The patient's insurance, however, will only authorize one piece of equipment. What is the most appropriate assistive device for this patient?
    a. Front wheeled walker
    b. Axillary crutches
    c. Wheelchair
    d. Posterior walker

87. You are a physical therapist that is performing an examination on a 10-week-old infant with a brachial plexus injury. The patient cannot flex his elbow and has residual signs of Horner's syndrome. The appropriate plan of care is
    a. Begin passive ROM of the upper extremity immediately
    b. Utilize electrical stimulation to regain biceps function
    c. Surgical management
    d. Refer to a brachial plexus specialty center

88. An appropriate physical therapy program for a 2-week old infant with a brachial plexus injury would include teaching the parents how to support the arm while dressing and moving the infant to prevent further injury, and
    a. Functional strengthening
    b. Daily PROM exercises including full shoulder abduction and elevation
    c. Daily PROM exercises with shoulder abduction and elevation to only 90 degrees
    d. Serial sensory testing

89. A 13-year-old male is referred to physical therapy for left knee pain. During the objective examination, the left hip is found to be limited in flexion, abduction, and internal rotation. Observation also reveals that the left hip is positioned in external rotation in supine and in standing positions. The appropriate plan of care is
    a. Stretching of the hip extensors and external rotators
    b. Referral to an orthopedic surgeon
    c. TENS and cold pack to the left knee for pain management
    d. Strengthening of the quadriceps and gluteus medius

90. Deep vein thrombosis (DVT)
    a. Can break off and cause a pulmonary embolism (PE)
    b. Usually occurs in people who are highly mobile
    c. Is usually prevented by daily administration of a thrombolytic
    d. Is a clot that develops in a superficial vein

91. Which of the following is an incorrect direction for proper inhaler usage?
    a. Tilt the head back, open the mouth wide, and inhale a puff from the inhaler.
    b. Place the inhaler in the mouth with the lips sealed securely around mouthpiece.
    c. Press down on the inhaler (actuate) and inhale at the same time.
    d. Hold the breath for approximately 10 seconds.

92. Which is NOT a sign of preeclampsia?
    a. Increased HR
    b. BP > 140/90
    c. Edema
    d. Proteinuria

93. A football athlete with an incomplete C7 spinal cord injury seeks the PT's opinion about the ability to live independently. The BEST response from the PT would be
    a. "You will be able to live independently with modifications such as adapted devices for activities of daily living (ADLs), a wheelchair, and sliding board."
    b. "You can live alone most of the time, but will require a caregiver for such tasks as driving, cooking, and ADLs."
    c. "Persons with this level of spinal cord lesion will require an attendant."
    d. "Persons with this level of injury can live independently with a manual wheelchair for mobility."

94. During an interview with a new patient on the psychiatric unit, the patient asks if they should divorce their spouse. Your best response would be
    a. "That's not a decision that I can make. I don't know what it is like to be in your situation, but we can talk about it and see if it helps you to make a good decision for yourself."
    b. "Why don't you ask your doctor?"
    c. "Yes. Your spouse seems to be no good from what you have told me. Go ahead and divorce."
    d. "If it were me, I'd dump your spouse."

95. During the examination of a patient, the patient says that things are hopeless and "I might as well be dead," In this case you would
    a. Ask some questions to find out more.
    b. Tell the patient that those thoughts are stupid.
    c. Ignore it and change the subject to something brighter.
    d. Tell the patient that you have thought about suicide too and that it is normal.

96.	In an attempt to establish a home exercise program, the therapist gives a patient written exercises. After 1 week, the patient returns and has not performed any of the exercises. After further questioning, the therapist determines that the patient is illiterate. What is an inappropriate course of action?
	a.	Go over the exercises in a one-on-one review session.
	b.	Give the patient a picture of the exercises.
	c.	Give a copy of the exercises to a literate family member.
	d.	Contact the physician for a social services consult.

97.	A supervisor in a physical therapy clinic observes a new graduate performing incorrect exercises on a patient. The exercises are not life threatening but are incorrect. What is the best way to handle this situation?
	a.	The supervisor should immediately tell the new therapist to stop exercising the patient and instruct the patient and therapist in the correct procedure.
	b.	The supervisor should tactfully tell the new therapist to come into his or her office and discuss the situation in private.
	c.	The supervisor should put a note on the new therapist's desk to meet with him/her after work.
	d.	The supervisor should give the new therapist research articles about the correct options.

98.	The therapist has just returned from an in-service training offering new treatment techniques in wound care. The therapist would like to share the information with interested members of the hospital staff. What is the best way to share this information?
	a.	Prepare a handout on the new treatment techniques and give it to the members of the hospital staff.
	b.	Schedule a mandatory in-service training during lunch for the entire hospital staff who participate in some form of wound care.
	c.	Post bulletins in view of all hospital staff and send memos to the department heads inviting everyone to attend an in-service training during lunch.
	d.	Call each department head and invite him or her and their staff to an in-service training during lunch.

99.	A patient is scheduled to undergo extremely risky heart surgery. The patient seems really worried. During the treatment session, the patient and family look to the therapist for comfort. Which of the following is an appropriate response from the therapist to the patient?
	a.	"Don't worry, everything will be okay."
	b.	"Your physician is the best, and he will take care of you."
	c.	"I know it must be upsetting to face such a difficult situation. Your family and friends are here to support you."
	d.	"Try not to worry. Worrying increases your blood pressure and heart rate, which are two factors that need to be stabilized before surgery."

100. A physical therapist instructs a physical therapy assistant to teach a patient how to ascend and descend the front steps of her home. After first exercising the patient at her home, the assistant realizes that, because of her increased size and severe dynamic balance deficits, training on the steps is unsafe at this time. The assistant contacts the therapist by telephone. Which of the following is the best course of action by the therapist?
    a. The therapist should instruct the assistant to attempt step training cautiously.
    b. The therapist should instruct the assistant to recruit the family members to assist with step training.
    c. The therapist should instruct the assistant to discontinue step training until both of them can be present.
    d. The therapist should contact the physician and seek further instructions.

101. A physical therapist is performing an isokinetic test on a 16-year-old boy's shoulder. This particular test compares the right shoulder with the left shoulder. The patient's father asks the physical therapist, "What is the purpose of this test?" How should the therapist respond?
    a. "This isokinetic test will show changes in concentric and eccentric strength."
    b. "This test will show strength differences between the injured arm and the noninjured arm."
    c. "This test shows differences in external rotation strength at specific ranges in the arc of motion."
    d. "This test will provide muscular torque data, which will help us to determine when to discontinue therapy."

102. A physical therapist in the rehabilitation unit is ordered to examine and treat a 3-year-old girl with cerebral palsy. The patient's supportive family is present during the examination. When should the physical therapist explain the treatment plan and possible functional outcomes to the family?
    a. During the examination
    b. After the examination
    c. After the first full treatment session
    d. After the first rehabilitation team conference meeting

103. During the history portion of an examination of a geriatric gentleman, the physical therapist is concerned about lapses in medication dosage. What is the most appropriate way to ask the patient about his medications?
    a. "Do you take your medications?"
    b. "Does someone help you with your medications?"
    c. "How do you take your medications?"
    d. "How long have you been taking your medications?"

104.   The physical therapist is speaking to a group of nurses on proper
        body mechanics. Which of the following is inappropriate advice to
        give to this population regarding body mechanics?
        a.   Carry heavy objects in your dominant arm only.
        b.   Keep your back straight during lifting.
        c.   Maintain a wide base of support.
        d.   Push rather than pull when there is an option of either.

105.   A physical therapist is working with a patient on gait training.
        Verbal cues that are provided only when the patient's performance lies
        outside what the physical therapist considers safe and acceptable, is
        an example of _____ feedback.
        a.   Concurrent
        b.   Delayed
        c.   Bandwidth
        d.   Immediate

106.   A physical therapist is teaching a 72-year-old patient who has had a
        knee replacement to walk using a straight cane. Verbal feedback
        _____ is most beneficial for long-term motor skill acquisition.
        a.   When provided after every practice trial
        b.   That is delayed until several trials of the task have been completed
        c.   That is provided concurrently during the performance of the task
        d.   When provided at the beginning of every practice trial

107.   What is the BEST strategy to communicate with a patient diagnosed
        with Wernicke's aphasia?
        a.   Use a writing board for communication.
        b.   Attend to nonverbal behaviors and the emotional content of the
              message.
        c.   Correct patient errors frequently to assist in his learning strategies.
        d.   Use easier "who/what/when" questions.

108.   The PT administered a visual perceptual assessment tool to a patient
        with Bell's palsy degeneration at the beginning of therapy and before
        the family-rehab team meeting. Administering an assessment tool in
        this fashion measures
        a.   Interrater reliability
        b.   Test-retest reliability
        c.   Standard error of measurement
        d.   Central tendency

109.   Evidence-based practice is the determination of intervention strategies based on
   a.   Extant research findings
   b.   Research findings, the PT's own experiences, and family priorities
   c.   A PT's expert opinion
   d.   Other disciplines' practice

110.   Which is MOST likely to be found in quantitative research?
   a.   Lengthy, descriptive, narrative text
   b.   Open-ended interviewing
   c.   Small samples chosen according to the goals of the study
   d.   Standardized tests and scales

111.   A local plant asks a therapy team to perform a study of its workers. The study needs to determine the frequency of lung cancer in workers who insulate the inside area of an electrical oven appliance. Using company files, the therapy team studies all past employees with this job description. The employees were initially free of lung cancer, as determined by a routine physician's examination required by the plant. From these files, the team records the frequency with which each one of the employees developed lung cancer. What type of study is the therapy team performing?
   a.   Historical prospective or historical cohort
   b.   Retrospective
   c.   Case control
   d.   Matched pairs design

112.   A study of the local population was necessary to determine the need for a new fitness center in the area. The therapists performing the study divided the population by sex and selected a random sample from each group. This is an example of what type of random sample?
   a.   Systematic random sample
   b.   Random cluster sample
   c.   Two stage cluster sample
   d.   Stratified random sample

113.   A therapist is preparing a poster that will clarify some of the data in an in-service presentation. The poster reflects the mode, median, and mean of a set of data. The data consist of the numbers 2, 2, 4, 9, and 13. If presented in the above order (mode, median, mean), which of the following is the correct list of answers calculated from the data?
   a.   4, 2, 6
   b.   2, 4, 6
   c.   6, 2, 4
   d.   6, 4, 2

114. An outpatient physical therapist notices that a large number of patients with impingement of the rotator cuff have been treated in the past 6 months. The clinic finds that most patients are employed at a new auto manufacturing plant. The therapist is invited to the plant to perform an ergonomic assessment and finds that a certain number of the employees must work with their shoulders at 120 degrees of flexion 6 to 8 hours/day. Which of the following recommendations would decrease the frequency of injury?
    a. Provide the employees with a step stool to perform their tasks.
    b. Raise the employees' work surface.
    c. Adjust their tasks so that overhead activities are performed with the palm of the hand downward.
    d. Adjust the task so heavier tools are used.

115. When conducting clinical research, external validity refers to your ability to
    a. Apply the results of your study to a different population of patients
    b. Compare your results to those from similar intervention studies
    c. Generalize the results of your study to similar patients who were not in your study
    d. Verify that the instruments used are measuring what they are supposed to measure

116. If you wanted to determine how well the items on a test or survey related to each other, you would be analyzing that instrument's
    a. Content validity
    b. Internal consistency
    c. Intrarater reliability
    d. Stability

117. Why is a random sample more desirable than other methods of sampling when designing an experimental study?
    a. Confidence intervals tend to be wider.
    b. Data are more likely to be normally distributed.
    c. Group variances will always be homogenous.
    d. Maturation effects of subjects can be avoided.

118. Which of the following factors is inversely related to statistical power in a research study?
    a. Alpha level that has been set for the study
    b. Amount of variance in the outcome measure(s)
    c. Magnitude of the effect size (of the outcome measure)
    d. Sample size

119. What does the term "alpha level" refer to?
    a. Amount of variance in the first sample
    b. Extent to which a statistical conclusion can be generalized
    c. Level of significance when testing a hypothesis
    d. Power of a statistical analysis

120. If you are comparing two or more groups of subjects and accept a null hypothesis when group differences really do exist, you have
    a. Committed a type I statistical error
    b. Committed a type II statistical error
    c. Committed a random error
    d. Drawn an appropriate conclusion

121. A test or instrument that has high specificity is able to accurately identify
    a. False negatives
    b. False positives
    c. True negatives
    d. True positives

122. In order for an instrument to have good predictive validity, the scores must be highly correlated with
    a. Another measure that is considered to be the gold standard
    b. Occurrence of some type of clinical condition or outcome
    c. Scores from the same instrument administered by at least one other tester
    d. Scores from the same instrument repeated at a later time

123. Which of the following clinical measures exemplifies an ordinal level of measurement?
    a. Gait speed
    b. Heart rate
    c. Joint range-of-motion
    d. Visual analog pain rating

124. If you wanted to compare balance measures in older adults who do and do not have a history of falling, which statistical test would be most appropriate to use?
    a. Square dependent (paired) t-test
    b. Independent (unpaired) t-test
    c. One-way analysis of variance
    d. Pearson product moment coefficient

125. If you wanted to classify a group of women as having normal bone density, low bone density, or osteoporosis, based on measures of their age, height loss, and activity level, what type of statistical analysis would you use?
    a. Analysis of variance
    b. Chi square analysis
    c. Discriminant analysis
    d. Factor analysis

126. A sampling technique in which you send a research survey to a small group of subjects who meet your criteria and ask them to share it with others who also meet that criteria is known as
    a. Quota sampling
    b. Random sampling
    c. Snowball sampling
    d. Stratified sampling

127. What is the purpose for doing a power analysis when you are planning an experimental study?
    a. To assess the number of dependent variables you can analyze in a single study
    b. To decide whether to pose a directional or non-directional research hypothesis
    c. To estimate the amount of time you will need to collect sufficient data
    d. To help you determine an appropriate sample size

128. A portion of your patient satisfaction survey asks patients to rate the level of importance of various factors when selecting a health care provider. They are asked to use the scale below to rate their responses
    1 = not important at all
    2 = somewhat important
    3 = very important
    4 = critically important
    This type of scale is best described as a
    a. Guttman scale
    b. Likert scale
    c. Semantic differential scale
    d. Visual analog scale

129. When might you use a coefficient of variation (CV) to describe the variability of a set of measurements?
   a. Any time your data are measured at the nominal or ordinal level
   b. When you want to compare the variability in multiple variables that have different units of measure
   c. When your data have been converted to percentages
   d. Whenever your standard deviations are very large

130. What do statistical measures of "central tendency" represent?
   a. The amount of variance in a distribution of numbers
   b. The average value in a distribution of numbers
   c. The range of a distribution when outliers are removed
   d. The shape of a distribution of numbers

131. You create a box plot like the one in shown in Figure 6-1 to illustrate the distribution of GPAs. What does the line in the middle of the box represent?

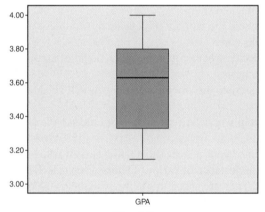

Fig 6-1

   a. Mean of the distribution
   b. Mode of the distribution
   c. 50th percentile of the distribution
   d. An outlier

132. You want to know the average amount of joint contracture that your patients who have had knee surgery demonstrate at the time of discharge. When you graph your results with a histogram it looks like Figure 6-2. How would you describe this distribution?

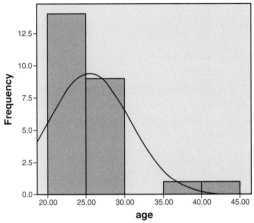

Fig 6-2

   a. Bimodal
   b. Normal (bell-shaped curve)
   c. Skewed to the right
   d. Skewed to the left

133. To meet the definition of "reliable," a test must be both consistent and
   a. Cost-effective
   b. Efficient to use in a clinical setting
   c. Free from error
   d. Highly specific

134. If you wanted to graphically illustrate the relationship of two variables, which type of graph would you select?
   a. Bar graph
   b. Line graph
   c. Pie chart
   d. Scatter plot

135. If you wanted to examine the test-retest reliability of a grip dynamometer, which correlational statistic would be most appropriate to analyze this relationship?
   a. Cronbach's alpha
   b. Intraclass correlation coefficient
   c. Phi coefficient
   d. Pearson product moment correlation

136.   What does the scatter plot in Figure 6-3 illustrate about the nature of the relationship between the GPAs of a group of recent graduates and their scores on the national licensure exam?

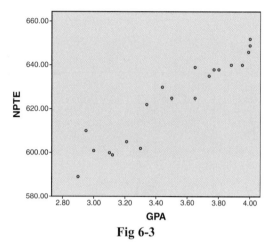

Fig 6-3

 a. There is a moderate, curvilinear relationship between these variables.
 b. There is a strong, positive, linear relationship between these variables.
 c. There is a weak, inverse, linear relationship between these variables.
 d. There is no relationship between these variables.

137.   What is the diagnostic advantage of having a highly sensitive test?
 a. When the test is negative, you can confidently rule in that diagnosis.
 b. When the test is negative, you can confidently rule out that diagnosis.
 c. When the test is positive, you can confidently rule in that diagnosis.
 d. When the test is positive, you can confidently rule out that diagnosis.

138.   A study that follows the same group of subjects over an extended period of time to determine the extent to which exposure to certain risk factors actually results in the incidence of a disease/health condition is known as a
 a. Case series
 b. Cohort study
 c. Cross-sectional study
 d. Quasi-experimental study

139.   When comparing the means between two groups of subjects, you discover that there is a significant difference between the variances of your outcome measure in those groups. What does this result tell you?
 a. You are more likely to have committed a type I statistical error.
 b. You are more likely to have committed a type II statistical error.
 c. You need to run some additional post hoc tests.
 d. You should use a nonparametric statistical test to analyze your data.

140. A therapist who is conducting a back school gives the participants a pretest at the beginning of the first class to determine their baseline knowledge of body mechanics and injury risk factors. She then compares those scores to the score on a quiz she gives during the last class session. What could you conclude from the statistical output displayed in Figure 6-4?

Paired Samples Statistics

	Mean	N	Std. Deviation	Std. Error Mean
Pair 1 Pretest	64.4500	20	11.03332	2.46713
Posttest	85.8500	20	6.71428	1.50136

Paired Samples Test

| | Paired Differences | | | | | | | |
| | | | | 95% Confidence Interval of the Difference | | | | |
	Mean	Std. Deviation	Std. Error Mean	Lower	Upper	t	df	p
Pair 1 Pretest-Posttest	-21.40000	7.14069	1.59671	-24.74195	-18.05805	-13.403	19	.000

Fig 6-4

a. Although the p value was very low, the confidence intervals suggest that there was not really a significant difference in the two test scores.
b. On average, there was a significant improvement of 21.4 points between the pretest and posttest scores.
c. On average, there was a negative change of 21.4 points in the students' pretest and posttest scores, but it was not significant.
d. There was greater variability in the posttest scores than there was in the pretest scores.

141. A surgeon wants to compare functional outcomes among his total knee arthroplasty patients, some of whom received physical therapy after their hospital discharge and some who did not receive therapy. He wants to measure their knee range of motion, gait speed, and pain ratings before surgery and at 2 months postoperatively. What type of data analysis procedures would be most appropriate to use in this situation?
a. Chi square analysis
b. Multiple linear regression
c. Repeated measures multivariate analysis of variance
d. Three-way analysis of variance

142. You are comparing the balance scores of older adults who live in the community versus assisted living facilities versus nursing homes. Your analysis of variance produced a p value of .033. To fully analyze the group differences, what would be your next step?
   a. Analyze the descriptive statistics and compare the variances of each group.
   b. Rerun the ANOVA and enter age as a covariate.
   c. Run a logistic regression to determine the predictive value of the balance scores.
   d. Run a post hoc comparison test to determine which groups differed from each other.

143. A study that statistically analyzes and integrates the results of several studies in order to make a clinical recommendation regarding the overall efficacy of a particular type of treatment would be described as a(an)
   a. Delphi study
   b. Epidemiologic study
   c. Factor analysis
   d. Meta-analysis

144. A therapist conducted a study to compare the effects of real versus placebo laser radiation on the joint pain and mobility of patients with arthritic knee joints. Subjects' pain and mobility were measured before and after 2 weeks of daily laser treatments. The dependent variable(s) in this study was/were
   a. Laser intensity
   b. Pain and functional ratings
   c. Treatment duration (2 weeks)
   d. Type of laser treatment received (real versus placebo)

145. Using a regression analysis, a physical therapy instructor analyzes the effects of multiple predictors of academic success on the students' final GPA. The analysis produces an R^2 (coefficient of determination) value of 0.36. How should the instructor interpret this statistic?
   a. The correlation between the predictor variables and GPA is not statistically significant.
   b. The correlation between the predictor variables and GPA is very strong.
   c. The predictor variables account for 36% of the variance in the students' GPAs.
   d. The predictor variables are inversely related to students' GPAs.

146. When conducting a qualitative research study, data validity is usually established by
    a. Analyzing data at a lower alpha level
    b. Increasing the sample size to include a broader variety of subjects
    c. Repeating the observations or interviews multiple times
    d. Triangulating data from multiple sources

147. Which of the following graphic methods is commonly used to analyze the data in a single-subject research study?
    a. Forest plot
    b. Limits of agreement graph
    c. Receiver operating curve
    d. Two standard-deviation band method

148. The combined effect of two or more independent variables on one or more dependent variable is known as the _____ effect.
    a. Additive
    b. Interaction
    c. Integrative
    d. Regression

149. One threat to internal validity may occur in a research study where subjects know they are being studied, so they perform differently than usual, producing biased results. This phenomenon is known as the _____ effect.
    a. Hawthorne
    b. Maturation
    c. Placebo
    d. Selection

150. You have performed a study investigating the influence of gender on cutting mechanics. Your dependent variable is peak knee valgus moment (a continuous variable) and your independent variable is gender (a nominal variable). What is the most appropriate statistic to evaluate your data?
    a. Two-factorial ANOVA with repeated measures
    b. Independent samples t-test
    c. Multiple regression
    d. Spearman's rank test

Answers

1. d. Assessment is the PT's judgment of clients' progress, limitations, and expected benefit from therapy.

2. b. Goals should be objective, functional, measurable, and action-oriented statements.

3. a. The plan relates to information presented in the "O" and "A" section of the SOAP note and is a description of the interventions, methods, or approaches used to achieve the goals.

4. b. Persons with spinal cord lesions at T6 and above are at risk for autonomic dysreflexia, which can occur as a result of the individual being overheated, stressed, in pain, or having urinary and bowel complications. Autonomic dysreflexia is considered a medical emergency, and symptoms include hypertension, pounding headache, sweating, flushing, pupil constriction, and nasal congestion.

5. c. In the assessment portion of the SOAP note, the therapist indicates progress in treatment or explains the failure to progress as quickly as anticipated.

6. c. The patient's observations about the right upper extremity are most pertinent to this treatment session because it relates to the entire session. Nursing's comments are important but do not belong in the S section. The S section is usually reserved for the patient's comments.

7. c. The emphasis is on the performance component and the functional application, not the specific media used in the treatment. Many third-party payers also want to see the amount of time per Current Procedural Terminology code charged.

8. b. Choice A is the problem list, which goes in the "A" section; choice C is a justification for further treatment, which goes in the "A" section; choice D is what occurred in treatment, which goes in section "O."

9. a. Prognosis is determined when the PT considers the severity of the patient's functional limitations and impairments and predicts the possible level of expected improvement or outcome.

10. a. An update on the patient's cognitive performance is essential in identifying the performance deficits of someone with a diagnosis of Alzheimer's.

11. b. The behavior was legal because there was no crime and it brought no harm to the patient. It was unethical because the therapist was more concerned about the therapist's needs than the patient's needs. It also violated the principle of veracity.

12. c. Most states mandate that all health care professionals report suspected abuse and neglect of vulnerable individuals.

13. a. Effective communication by supervisors/managers involves communicating expectations, offering constructive criticism, and expressing interest in an employee's professional growth.

14. d. Informed consent refers to providing and sharing health care information to individuals so that they can make the best decisions about their treatment or health care.

15. c. It is crucial to take the patient's feelings into consideration when you have to let them know that it is unethical to accept gifts. By explaining the situation and acknowledging the gesture you are more likely to avoid offending the patient.

16. a. While cooking, canning, and pasteurization can reduce the chances of food-borne infections, hand washing is acknowledged as the single most important measure to prevent spread of infectious diseases. Hand washing with plain soap aids in the mechanical removal of dirt and microbes present on the hands, including potential pathogens, thus preventing the spread of many infectious diseases.

17. d. Deep vein thrombosis (DVT) is a potentially serious condition that requires special studies to be properly identified and possible anticoagulant therapy for treatment. Medical referral is indicated as soon as DVT is suspected.

18. b. It is imperative for a rescuer to ensure that the scene is safe to enter before providing emergency rescue. This ensures that the rescuer does not become an additional victim.

19. b. Direct pressure is the first line of defense for external hemorrhage. If it is unsuccessful, then elevation and pressure applied to pulse pressure points are added sequentially. Tourniquets are used as a last resort.

20. c. Pulse, sensation, and motor function are assessed before splinting to assess the integrity of extremity neurovascular function. They are checked again after splinting to ensure that the splint is not applied too tightly.

21. d. In the ideal situation, the therapist should coordinate his or her plan of care with the chiropractor in case the problems are related.

22. c. A physical therapist assistant (PTA) can do all of the listed options except change the frequency or duration as prescribed by a therapist or physician. Choice B allows the PTA to work within the protocol established by the physical therapist.

23. b. The patient can be successfully treated by using universal precautions. The patient should be treated in a relatively isolated area because of his weakened immune system. The diagnosis of AIDS with Kaposi's sarcoma is an indication that the patient's immune system is weak. Gloves should be used if the patient's sarcomas are open; otherwise, hand washing before and after patient contact is appropriate.

24. a. A patient can obtain his or her medical records simply by signing a release form. Charts and records should never be given or faxed to an attorney unless the patient has signed a release.

25. c. The patient's biological father would have the right to access the records whether or not he is on the list, but not the stepfather. Choice B is incorrect because unless he is on the original list, he cannot simply sign a form and receive the records. Choice D is incorrect because you cannot verify that you are speaking to the mother.

26. b. Choice B is the most empathetic response. It also lets the patient know that the therapists will make an effort to prevent the problem from recurring.

27. d. After the therapist assesses the patient for the first time, he or she needs to begin discharge planning. This is true for an assessment of any patient, not just in the inpatient rehabilitation setting.

28. b. A therapist should never comment on such a serious prognosis before the physician has assessed the lab results and consulted with the patient first.

29. b. According to the American Heart Association, a person is determined unresponsive before emergency medical service is activated.

30. a. The ADA allowed structural modifications of federal buildings and protection from discrimination based on disability.

31. b. The person should lie down to prevent head injury. Tight clothing is loosened to make sure that nothing is too constricting. Close furniture is moved away for the patient's safety. Nothing should be placed in the patient's mouth because of the danger of obstructing the airway.

32. a. Any phrase stated by the patient that is relevant information goes into the subjective portion of the note.

33. b. Although a stroke may have occurred, the physical therapist can first examine the patient. After the examination has been performed, the therapist will be more informed about the patient's condition and can then contact the physician if necessary.

34. a. Back blows should be followed by chest thrusts with complete airway obstruction when CPR is performed on an infant. The therapist then should check for a foreign body in the airway. A blind finger sweep of the throat should not be performed on an infant.

35. a. A ground fault interruption circuit protects the patient from a potentially life-threatening situation. The other choices are valid concerns, but choice A is the most important.

36. b. Pressure on the left temporal bone just anterior to the ear helps to occlude blood flow from the temporal artery.

37. a. AIDS is transmitted by blood or bodily fluids. Masks are usually used with airborne precautions. Hand washing should be done between all wound care patients. Gloves are also indicated with all open wounds. Gowns may not be a necessity but should be used if there is a chance of soiling the clothing with infected fluids.

38. b. Because the goals were not completed in a short amount of time, a new long-term goal should be set. Because of the significant progress made in outpatient therapy, there is no need to return to the rehabilitation unit.

39. d. All of the choices are important, but the dietary assessment contains the least amount of critical information at this stage of the physical therapy examination.

40. c. "Provide services for the length of time ordered" is not a summary of one of the principles of the code of ethics. If a physician orders an inappropriate frequency and/or duration, it is the responsibility of the therapist to resolve the dilemma to ensure that the patient is treated with an appropriate frequency and duration.

41. d. The therapist does not need to wear a gown, gloves, or mask. These precautions are necessary only if there is a chance that the therapist or his clothing can become contaminated with blood, serum, or feces.

42. b. A pull-to-sit maneuver would put undue stress on the upper extremities. Rather, the child should be facilitated by supporting the child around the shoulders as he attempts to sit up.

43. d. Strength training in this group should be closely monitored because of skeletal immaturity. Proper technique should be taught and reinforced.

44. b. With an ongoing tumor in this area, any passive ROM or mobilization is contraindicated.

45. d. Exercise during acute infections can affect performance and may make the current condition worse. It could also compromise the cardiovascular and immune systems and exacerbate dehydration.

46. d. Choices A, B, and C should all be performed each time a documentation error is made. One should never use erasers or liquid correction.

47. b. Although soreness lasting 24 hours or more is a concern, and care should be taken because of the age of the patient, it is not a contraindication to stretching. Excessive complaints of pain should be a contraindication. Hemophiliacs should not be stretched in any joint because of the possibility of effusion.

48. b. Hyperextension is contraindicated because of the anterior approach. This motion would put undue stress on the anterior portion of the hip capsule. Choices A, C, and D are all contraindications for the posterior approach.

49. a. The menstrual cycle is a concern, but not a direct contraindication. The other conditions involve the digestive tract, and could be worsened with any manual therapy technique.

50. d. The catheter bag should always be below the level of the waist. This will keep urine in the catheter line from moving back to the patient's urinary tract. Infections can result if urine is allowed to reenter the urinary tract.

51. c. Exercise should be terminated when systolic blood pressure is
         180 mm Hg or above because of the risk of autonomic dysreflexia.
         Systolic blood pressure should be between 180 mm Hg and 80 mm
         Hg, diastolic between 120 mm Hg and 50 mm Hg, and heart rate
         between 160 beats/min and 50 beats/min.

52. d. Studies have shown that 15% percent of individuals with Down's
         syndrome have atlantoaxial (C1-C2) instability. Instability in that
         region is a contraindication to cervical traction.

53. d. The uterus moves superiorly in this position. This could cause
         an air embolism to enter the vagina and uterus. Eventually the
         embolism could enter the circulatory system through the placental
         wound.

54. c. All of the above are good advice that needs to be followed, but
         consent to disrobe is the first and most important choice. Wrinkles
         can cause areas of pressure, and the patient's clothing could be
         soiled. Gender situations could obviously be a cause for concern.

55. d. The order of scar tissue formation consists of the following:
         inflammatory phase, granulation phase, fibroplastic phase, and
         maturation phase.

56. b. Horizontal adduction, extension, and internal rotation would
         stretch the tissues that are early in the healing process. Care must
         be taken not to damage these structures in the anterior capsule.

57. d. Antidepressants work slowly (it takes about 4 weeks before
         antidepressant effects become apparent) but can somewhat
         "energize" patients early on in drug therapy so that they are more
         likely to commit suicide. Such suicidal ideas must be mentioned to
         the treating psychiatrist as soon as possible.

58. c. Antihelminthics kill the worms but do not kill the eggs, which
         can leave the patient during a bowel movement and remain on
         the toilet or hands to be spread to others. Disinfection of the toilet
         and always informing the individual to wash hands thoroughly is
         recommended.

59. a. This could be the beginning of a malignant hyperthermia, which
         requires immediate drug treatment since it could be fatal. The
         other signs and symptoms are of importance but do not require
         immediate attention.

60. a. Clopidogrel interferes with ADP-induced platelet aggregation and can lead to bleeding episodes while the other reactions are unlikely.

61. a. Nicotine can cause increases in blood pressure and gastritis; tar can cause cancers and emphysema; and CO interferes with oxygen transport in the blood, but alcohol abuse can cause the Korsakoff-Wernicke syndrome (psychosis, memory losses).

62. a. Agranulocytosis manifests itself with a slight fever and a sore throat possibly with ulcerations caused by a deficiency of granulocytes. Thrombotic thrombocytic purpura exhibits bizarre behavior, hemolytic anemia (dark urine) and jaundice (yellowing of eyes and skin) caused by microthrombi. Exfoliate dermatitis is characterized by redness, scaling, and shedding of the skin. Churg-Strauss syndrome is manifested by rashes and nodules under the skin, later on damaging internal organs caused by vasculitis.

63. c. Stevens-Johnson syndrome starts with a nonspecific upper respiratory infection, cough, aching, headaches, feverishness followed by a red rash across the face and the trunk of the body spreading later to other parts. Finally the top layer of the skin or epidermis starts to peel off. Epidermal necrolysis manifests itself with fever followed by a rash, redness, blisters, pain and the peeling of the skin from the underlying dermis. Lupus syndrome manifests itself as an inflammation of the joints, mostly fingers, hands and wrists, caused by an autoimmune reaction.

64. c. Normal O_2 values are 96% to 100%. Oxygen flow rates are prescribed by the physician and should not be altered by the physical therapist. Exercise should be stopped if O_2 saturation falls 5% below resting value.

65. a. Systolic blood pressure should always rise as workload increases. The other values are within normal limits for rest or exercise response.

66. b. Hyperlaxity patients may or may not have symptoms from their laxity. One certainty is that muscle strength around joints helps stabilize and protect those joints.

67. c. Braces can cause many problems from direct pressure or constriction. Avascular necrosis has not been found with bracing.

68. b. Prophylactic bracing has been extensively studied. Only in prevention of ankle sprains and MCL tears has effectiveness been shown.

69. c. Examination, evaluation, diagnosis, prognosis is the correct order according to the APTA.

70.   c.   You consider self-destructive behaviors as serious, and notify the team with a request for immediate psychiatric assistance. Choice C is the best for managing an urgent issue and functioning as a member of the interdisciplinary team. A physical therapist cannot diagnose depression. Treatment is outside the scope of PT practice. Waiting a week is a very bad idea as patient behavior is escalating and likely to cause serious harm. This is an urgent issue. Do not warn family members as you are not qualified to diagnose the condition. Plus this choice puts the problem inappropriately into the family's hands. The PT should communicate with the physician.

71.   d.   Autonomy means "self-governance" and refers to an individual's right to make his/her own decisions. The term "self-determination" is synonymous with autonomy. In patient care, this right is protected by a federal statute known as the Patient Self-Determination Act of 1990. The PSDA codifies the rights of hospitalized patients and long-term care residents to participate in treatment decision making and to control the use of extraordinary treatment measures including artificial life support.

72.   d.   Patient abandonment occurs when the health care professional unilaterally terminates his or her relationship with a patient improperly or prematurely. By failing to refer her patients to another physical therapist, this therapist has breached her duty to provide care for her patients and could be charged with professional negligence.

73.   d.   *Veracity* refers to telling the truth. *Fidelity* refers to faithfulness, *justice* refers to fairness, and *beneficence* refers to doing what's best for someone else.

74.   b.   Beneficence is the ethical principle of acting in a way that reflects the best interests of the patient. In this case, the therapist was attempting to do what he/she thought was best in terms of protecting the patient from future risk of physical harm resulting from another fall.

75.   b.   This is an example of ordinary negligence that is incident to health care delivery. Premises liability provides for monetary damages on the part of premise owners for injuries incurred by patrons. The concept of justice refers to fair treatment, or equity. Compensatory justice is one type of justice that compensates individuals fairly for injuries or wrongdoings that they have suffered. The other types of justice listed deal more with fair allocation of health care resources at the societal or individual level.

76.   b.   Liability for professional negligence occurs when health care professionals fail to care for patients in a manner that complies with legal and professional standards of care. To allege negligence on the part of this therapist, the patient would have to provide evidence that the therapist did not follow standard policies and procedures related to patient safety during transfers and that this action was the direct cause for the injury. Thus, the therapist's best defense is not to place the blame elsewhere, but rather emphasize that appropriate standard of care was rendered. The Good Samaritan Laws do not apply to this case because the situation did not place the patient in eminent or serious peril.

77.   c.   To protect oneself against allegations of sexual misconduct, health care providers should implement some risk management strategies including: (1) providing same-sex chaperones when conducting intimate, hands-on procedures or upon patient request; (2) implementing a "knock-and-enter" clinic policy; (3) implementing a general informed consent policy that ensures that patients understand the nature of questions they will be asked and types of therapeutic procedures they may experience; and (4) providing ongoing continuing education to health care professionals and support staff on how to prevent sexual abuse and harassment.

78.   c.   All states have statutes that mandate health care professionals to report cases of actual or suspected child abuse or neglect to a child/family protective agency that is designated to investigate these types of cases. Suspicions of abuse may be based on objective, credible evidence of possible child, spousal, and/or elder abuse.

79.   c.   One purpose of The Patient Self-Determination Act of 1990 was to educate patients about their rights to formulate advance directives for their health care. One type of advance directive is a durable power of attorney for health care decisions. This legal document, signed by the patient, delegates health care decisions to an agent, or surrogate, of the patient's choice. The power only becomes operative when the patient is no longer competent to make his or her own decisions (i.e., must be declared legally incompetent in a court of law). In the scenario posed, the therapist would have no reason to believe that this patient was incompetent unless the son provided some evidence to the contrary.

80. c. The ADA legislation applies to public and private businesses
         employing 25 or more people on July 26, 1992, or those with 15
         or more people on July 26, 1994. Title I of the ADA prohibits
         employment discrimination of "a qualified individual with a
         disability," which means that the job applicant or employee can
         perform the essential job functions, with or without reasonable
         accommodations. The employer determines what the essential job
         functions are and the ADA defines what a disability is. The Equal
         Employment Opportunity Commission (EEOC) provides definitions
         for "reasonable accommodations."

81. b. The cardinal signs described in this question are classic signs of
         vertebral basilar instability. With a labyrinthine involvement you
         will mostly get dizziness but not all of the cardinal signs. With a
         carotid artery tear you may lose consciousness because it supplies
         the higher centers of the brain. A concussion may cause a variety
         of symptoms to include loss of consciousness but not drop attacks,
         lip paresthesias, and lower extremity paresthesias.

82. a. Goniometric texts recommend recording the starting and ending
         values for passive range of motion. The patient's starting point and
         ending points during the examination is most accurately represented
         by 20 to 95 degrees of flexion.

83. d. According to code, 12 inches of length is necessary for each 1
         inch of rise when making an area accessible.

84. b. Good body mechanics cannot guarantee pain control, but the use
         of good body mechanics is critical regardless of the load (light
         versus heavy) being lifted. Heavier items should be placed at waist
         level not below the waist or overhead.

85. a. Weight-bearing status is the physician's responsibility.

86. c. Due to the patient's age and diagnosis, he will have difficulty
         maintaining NWB status. Balancing on a single limb and
         coordinating and using an assistive device safely will be difficult.
         Therefore, to reduce the risk of falling and re-injuring the affected
         extremity, a wheelchair is the safest device for mobility for this
         patient.

87. d. If complete return of biceps function has not returned by 2 months
         of age, the infant should be referred to a brachial plexus specialty
         center. More urgent referrals are needed for a patient with Horner's
         syndrome and complete paralysis.

88. c. The physical therapist can teach parents to perform ROM exercises. Passive ROM is initiated around week 1, and no later than 3 weeks of age, when soft tissue swelling subsides. Shoulder abduction and elevation is limited to 90 degrees for the first 3 weeks.

89. b. The patient has a suspected left slipped capital femoral epiphysis and should be referred to an orthopedic surgeon. The patient typically presents with an antalgic gait and pain in the groin, often referred to the anteromedial aspect of the thigh and knee, but may have pain only in the thigh or knee. The involved extremity is usually held in external rotation in supine and standing positions and there is decreased flexion, abduction, and internal rotation ROM.

90. a. DVT usually occurs in sedentary or immobilized people due to a decrease in blood flow from inactivity. A serious complication of DVT is pulmonary embolism (PE), which is when a clot travels to the pulmonary system, and blocks blood flow. It is a major cause of death in many hospitals.

91. a. The mouth and lips should close around the inhaler (the mouth should not be open wide).

92. a. Usually occurring later in second and third trimesters, preeclampsia is a dangerous condition that can affect both mother and baby. It has an incidence rate of 5% to 8%. Preeclampsia is characterized by protein in the urine and high blood pressure. Other symptoms include headaches, swelling, or changes in vision.

93. a. Functional outcomes of a C7 spinal cord lesion are independence in mobility with a manual or powered wheelchair, independence in transfers with adapted devices or a sliding board, and independence in ADLs with adapted equipment.

94. a. Giving advice or sending the patient to her doctor to get the decision made is not appropriate therapeutic behavior. The PT's role is to help the patient to review her options and encourage her to make the best decision she can for herself.

95. a. Ethically, it is not appropriate to ignore the comment or judge the patient. Suicidal thoughts are not normal, and sharing such personal information about yourself would create a boundary issue. It is important to find out more about these feelings to determine what action should be taken to keep the patient safe.

96. d. This answer is correct because patients need a written home program with diagrams and instructions. One-on-one teaching is also necessary to ensure that the patient understands the program. Bringing in another family member is also definitely advisable to assist the patient with the program at home. Although a social services consult maybe necessary in the long run, it will not help the patient to perform the exercises over the next several days.

97. b. The supervisor can best handle this situation by discussing the exercise program away from the patient. Correcting the new graduate in front of the patient probably would decrease the confidence of the patient in the treatment and the therapist.

98. c. Posting the in-service training date on the bulletin board and sending a memo to the department heads is the most effective way to invite everyone interested. Scheduling during lunch often makes it easier for people to attend.

99. c. This answer is the most appropriate. The therapist cannot guarantee everything will be okay (choice A) or that the physician is the best (choice B). Choice D is too insensitive.

100. c. The physical therapist should tell the assistant to wait until they can both work together with the patient. The family is not qualified to help the assistant during the first attempt at ambulation in this situation.

101. b. This is the most appropriate response to a person who has not indicated that he or she has a medical background. If the patient's father inquires further, the therapist can be more detailed.

102. b. The physical therapist can give his or her ideas about the treatment plan and possible functional outcomes after the evaluation. These ideas may change after treatment sessions and team meetings. The family should be continually informed of the patient's progress and expected level of function after discharge.

103. c. The physical therapist should always use open ended questions as in choice C. If the patient only responds in short answers, some important information may be left out.

104. a. Choices B, C, and D are all correct suggestions. Heavy objects that cannot be supported with two hands should be alternated between hands to avoid excessive lumbar rotation.

105. c. Bandwidth is a type of feedback that is used during intervention to provide cues or feedback only when the patient's performance lies outside of an acceptable range of safety. Bandwidth feedback has been shown to be an effective method to enhance skill acquisition.

106. b. Feedback to promote long-term skill acquisition is most beneficial when it is not provided before or after every trial. Providing feedback as the activity is being performed may enhance immediate performance but has been shown to be less valuable than delayed feedback. Providing feedback less frequently is reported to enhance long-term learning.

107. b. Attend to nonverbal behaviors and the emotional content of the message. Wernicke's aphasia is a receptive aphasia. Use of a writing board or simpler questions will not be successful as that requires receptive communication. Frequent correction is not ideal as the patient cannot process receptive feedback.

108. b. Test-retest reliability is a measurement of the stability of a test over time. Test-retest reliability is proven by giving the test to the same individual on two different occasions.

109. b. Evidence-based practice includes deciding on an intervention strategy based on research findings, the PT's own experiences, and family priorities. Basing a decision about how to approach intervention solely on research findings without considering one's own experience and the family's priorities does not allow for consideration of all of the unique characteristics and needs of the child and family.

110. d. Quantitative research answers questions that require standardized measures. Qualitative methods lend themselves to the study of small groups with research questions that may be broad and evolve throughout the study process.

111. a. In cohort studies, records are taken at a specific time, and then the subjects are followed over time. The records of the factory are used to determine the frequency of disease. In a case-control study, the people are selected based on whether or not they have a disease; then the frequency of the possible cause of the disease in the past is studied. A retrospective study looks for causes of disease between two groups regardless of time. A matched pair design means that one control is matched to one case study.

112. d. A stratified random sample is taken by dividing the test population into two groups or strata (in this case, male and female) and taking a random sample from each group.

113. b. The mean is the average of the set of numbers. The mode is the number that appears most often in the set of data. The median is the middlemost value.

114. a. A step stool decreases the overall shoulder elevation required. Choice B increases shoulder elevation, and choice C maintains internal rotation with increased elevation. External rotation with elevation decreases the impingement to the rotator cuff muscles. Heavier tools would cause more fatigue of the rotator cuff and increase impingement.

115. c. The study usually only includes a representative sample of the population from which it was drawn. Thus, to have external validity, the study results should be able to be applied to the general population from which that sample was drawn. Thus, if the investigator uses sampling techniques that create bias, this can adversely affect the external validity of the study.

116. b. Internal consistency is a form of reliability that assesses the degree to which a set of items in an instrument measure a similar trait.

117. b. Random sampling is more likely to result in a representative sample; thus, the data from that sample are more likely to be normally distributed and not skewed. This is important because one of the underlying assumptions for the use of parametric statistics is normal distribution of data.

118. b. Statistical power increases with larger sample sizes, higher alpha levels, and greater effect sizes; it tends to be lower when data variances are higher.

119. c. *Alpha level* refers to the level of significance used when testing a hypothesis. This is represented by the p value provided in the data analysis.

120. b. A type I error occurs when one incorrectly rejects the null hypothesis, and a type II error occurs when one incorrectly accepts a null hypothesis.

121. c. Specificity is that characteristic of a diagnostic test that indicates the likelihood that a person who does not have a disease or condition will test negative (i.e., true negative).

122. b. Predictive validity and concurrent validity are both forms of criterion validity. Predictive validity is the ability of a test to predict some future performance or occurrence. Concurrent validity is the degree to which one test measure correlates with another measure, usually the "gold standard." The last two responses refer to the definitions for interrater reliability and test-retest reliability.

123. d. Most rating scales represent ordinal levels of measures in that they have scores that are rank ordered but do not represent equally spaced measures as in an interval or ratio level measurement.

124. b. You are comparing two independent groups on a single, ratio level measure. Thus, a parametric test is appropriate. In this case, that would be an independent t-test.

125. c. Regression techniques are used to assess the combined relationship of several independent, or predictor, variables on a single, dependent variable. When that predictor variable is a category or classification, discriminant analysis is the best type of regression analysis to use. Logistic regression techniques may also be used when the classification contains only two categories.

126. c. Snowball sampling is a method in which a target group of subjects successively recruit additional subjects who meet the same criteria. In random sampling, every individual within a population has an equal chance of being selected to participate in the study. Stratified samples represent subgroups of a population, from which subjects are randomly recruited. In quota sampling, an equal proportion of subjects are recruited from each subgroup.

127. d. During the planning stage of a study, a power analysis is used to help determine the optimal number of subjects to recruit in order to avoid the possibility of committing a type II statistical error. The investigator has little control over any of the other factors that affect power (i.e., group variance, effect size of outcome measure, and alpha level), with the exception of the alpha level, which is usually set at .05 to reduce the risk of committing a type I error.

128. b. This is a classic example of a Likert scale in which participants are asked to rate their level of agreement with a set of statements. A Guttman scale is a cumulative scale in which a higher rating assumes all levels of measure below it. A semantic differential scale asks respondents to rate perceptions of a concept or characteristic on a 7-point scale that includes opposite descriptors at each end of the scale. A visual analog scale asks respondents to rate perceptions of a phenomenon, such as pain intensity, on a numeric scale, usually from 0 to 10.

129. b. A coefficient of variation (CV) is a standardized measure of variation that is based on the standard deviation of a measure, divided by its mean, and multiplied times 100. Thus, it can be used to compare variability in a set of variables, or outcomes, that have different units of measure.

130. b. Measures of central tendency are descriptive statistics that represent average values in a distribution of scores. These measures include the mean, median, and mode.

131. c. A box plot is a graphic representation of a distribution of scores that illustrates the high, low, and median scores, as well as the boundaries for the 25th and 75th percentiles. The 50th percentile is indicated by the horizontal line within the box.

132. c. When one tail in a curve is longer than the other, the distribution is said to be skewed. The direction of skewness is determined by the longer tail; in this case, the longer tail is to the right of the curve.

133. c. In addition to being consistent, a measurement must reduce the amount of error in order to be considered reliable. Sources of error may be systematic (e.g., due to poor calibration of an instrument) or random (e.g., changes in subject performance). Statistical tests such as ICCs take into account these multiple sources of error when estimating the reliability of a measure.

134. d. Scatter plots illustrate the relationship of two variables, one plotted on the x-axis and the other plotted on the y-axis. A line of fit for the data points may also be illustrated. A perfect relationship is illustrated by a diagonal line from one corner of the graph to the opposite corner.

135. b. An intraclass correlation coefficient (ICC) is best for determining inter- or intrarater reliability of a numeric measure. A phi coefficient is used to correlate two dichotomous (i.e., categorical) measures. Cronbach's alpha is used to establish the internal consistency of a multi-itemed instrument. A Pearson correlation coefficient is sometimes used to analyze test-retest reliability, but it cannot account for systematic measurement errors.

136. b. Because these dots align themselves well along a diagonal from the bottom left-hand side of the graph to the upper right-hand side of the graph, they indicate a strong, positive correlation. An inverse relationship would be illustrated if the points aligned themselves from the upper left-hand side of the graph to the bottom right-hand side. In a weak or moderate relationship, the dots would not fit well along a diagonal line, but would be more scattered.

137. b.   According the rules of SpPin and SnNout, a test with high specificity (Sp) that is positive (P) will help rule in (in) a diagnosis, and a test with high sensitivity (Sn) that is negative (N) will help rule out (out) a diagnosis.

138. b.   A cohort is a group of subjects that are observed or studied over a period of time to determine their risk for developing a certain health condition. A case series follows a few subjects with similar diagnoses to determine how they respond to a certain treatment. A cross-sectional study measures certain traits in a population at one specific point in time. A quasi-experimental study is one that compares two or more groups of subjects that cannot be randomly assigned to their groups because those groups are based on pre-existing characteristics such as age, gender, diagnosis, etc.

139. d.   Homogeneity of variance is one of the underlying assumptions of parametric statistics. When group variances are significantly different, then this assumption has been violated and you should run the nonparametric version of that statistical test, if that option is available.

140. b.   The p value is less than .001 indicating a significant difference between the pretest and posttest scores. Because the mean of the posttest scores was 21.4 points higher than the mean of the pretest scores, subjects demonstrated significant improvements on the posttest.

141. c.   A multivariate analysis incorporates tests for more than one dependent variable within the same statistical model. This guards against the risk of committing a type I error when running multiple univariate analyses such as multiple t-tests. The repeated measures design is appropriate because there is only one group of subjects whose measures are being compared at different points in time. The repeated measures model takes into account the fact that each pair of measures will probably be highly correlated.

142. d.   The ANOVA resulted in a significant p value ($< .05$), so it tells you that there is a significant difference in the balance scores among these 3 groups of older adults. However, in order to determine which groups differ from each other, you must then run some post hoc comparisons (post hoc indicates tests run after the main analysis). Examples of post hoc comparisons include Scheffe's comparison, Bonferroni t-test, Tukey's honestly significant difference, Newman-Keuls test, Duncan's multiple range test, and Fisher's least significant difference.

143. d. A meta-analysis is a statistical procedure used in a systematic review to calculate an overall effect size of the outcomes produced by several studies that included similar dependent variables. A factor analysis is an exploratory method for identifying the constructs reflected in a large set of variables. A Delphi study is a survey method in which decisions on items are based on a consensus of the respondents. An epidemiologic study involves an assessment of the incidence or risk of certain health conditions within a population.

144. b. The outcomes being measured are the dependent variables in a study. The treatment groups would represent the independent variable.

145. c. The multiple correlation coefficient (R) reflects the combined relationship of these predictor variables to GPA. When squared, the coefficient of determination (R2) reflects the percentage of variance in the dependent variable (in this case, GPA) that is accounted for by the predictor variables (in this case, 36%). No p values are provided to assess the significance of this regression model. Likewise no R is provided, although this can be determined by taking the square root of R2, which would be .60, a correlation of only moderate strength.

146. d. No statistical tests are used to analyze qualitative data. Instead, the investigator uses multiple methods to document the same phenomena and looks for similar themes to emerge from these data sources.

147. d. The two standard deviation band method is one way of analyzing the significance of changes that occur in a single subject study. The mean and standard deviation of an outcome measure is calculated from multiple baseline measures. Additional measures taken during and/or after the treatment phase are then compared to these baseline measures. Those measures that fall outside the range of normal variance (i.e., two standard deviations) are attributed to the treatment effect. A forest plot is a graphic method used to illustrate the results of meta-analysis studies. Limits of agreement graphs are an alternate method used to illustrate test reliability. Receiver operating curves are used to help determine optimal cut-off scores in studies that establish test validity.

148. b. The interaction effect is identified in an ANOVA table using an "X"; for example, the interaction between group and treatment effect would be indicated as "Group X Treatment."

149.   a.   The Hawthorne effect was named for an experiment conducted at the Hawthorne plant of the Western Electric Company back in the 1920s in which workers' productivity improved no matter what the researchers did to change the work environment. This outcome was attributed to the special attention the workers received from the researchers as opposed to the variables that were introduced into the work setting.

150.   b.   Independent samples t-test is the most appropriate evaluation. Given the data described, a t-test is the best test. Because the groups are not matched (males and females), an independent samples t-test is best.

Selected Bibliography and Suggested Readings

Adams G, Beam W: *Exercise physiology laboratory manual*, ed 5, New York, 2007, McGraw-Hill.

Afifi AK, Bergman RA: *Functional neuroanatomy*, ed 2, New York, 2005, McGraw-Hill.

American College of Sports Medicine (editor), Durstine LJ, Moore G, Painter P, Roberts S: *ACSM's exercise management for persons with chronic diseases and disabilities*, ed 3, Champaign, 2009, Human Kinetics.

American College of Sports Medicine (editor): *ACSM's health-related physical fitness assessment manual*, ed 3, Philadelphia, 2009, Lippincott Williams & Wilkins.

American College of Sports Medicine (editor): *ACSM's resource manual for guidelines for exercise testing and prescription*, ed 6, Philadelphia, 2009, Lippincott Williams & Wilkins.

American College of Sports Medicine (editor): *ACSM's resources for clinical exercise physiology: musculoskeletal, neuromuscular, neoplastic, immunologic and hematologic conditions*, ed 2, Philadelphia, 2009, Lippincott Williams & Wilkins.

American Physical Therapy Association: *Guide to physical therapist practice*, Alexandria, 2003, American Physical Therapy Association.

American Physical Therapy Association: *Guidelines for pulmonary rehabilitation programs*, ed 3, Champaign, 2004, Human Kinetics.

Andreoli TE, Carpenter CCJ, Griggs RC, Benjamin I: *Cecil essentials of medicine*, ed 7, Philadelphia, 2007, Saunders.

Andrews JR, Harrelson GL, Wilk KE: *Physical rehabilitation of the injured athlete*, ed 3, Philadelphia, 2004, Saunders.

Baldry P: *Acupuncture, trigger points and musculoskeletal pain*, ed 3, New York, 2005, Churchill Livingstone.

Bandy WD, Sanders B: *Therapeutic exercise: techniques for intervention*, Philadelphia, 2001, Lippincott Williams & Wilkins.

Baranoski S, Ayello EA: *Wound care essentials: practice principles*, ed 2, Philadelphia, 2007, Lippincott Williams & Wilkins.

Batavia M: *Clinical research for health professionals*, ed 2, Philadelphia, 2003, Butterworth-Heinemann.

Batavia M: *Contraindications in physical rehabilitaion:doing no harm,* Philadelphia, 2006, Saunders.

Baxter RE: *Pocket guide to musculoskeletal assessment,* ed 2, Philadelphia, 2003, Saunders.

Bear MF, Connors BW, Paradiso MA: *Neuroscience: exploring the brain*, ed 3, Philadelphia, 2006, Lippincott Williams & Wilkins.

Belanger AY: *Evidence-based guide to therapeutic physical agents*, Philadelphia, 2002, Lippincott Williams & Wilkins.

Benjamin PJ, Tappan FM: *Handbook of healing massage techniques: classic, hollistic, and emerging*, ed 4, Stamford, 2004, Prentice Hall.

Berg KE, Latin RW: *Essentials of research methods in health, physical education, exercise science, and recreation*, ed 3, Philadelphia, 2007, Lippincott Williams & Wilkins.

Berk LE: *Development through the lifespan*, ed 4, Boston, 2006, Allyn & Bacon.

Berman J: *Color atlas of basic histology*, ed 3, New York, 2003, McGraw-Hill.

Bickley LS, Szilagyi PG: *Bates' guide to physical examination and history taking*, ed 10, Philadelphia, 2008, Lippincott Williams & Wilkins.

Bogduk N: *Clinical anatomy of the lumbar spine and sacrum*, ed 4, New York, 2005, Churchill Livingstone.

Boissonnault WG: *Primary care for the physical therapist: examination and triage*, Philadelphia, 2004, Saunders.

Borcherding S: *Documentation manual for writing soap notes in occupational therapy*, ed 2, Thorofare, 2005, Slack Incorporated.

Bottomley JM: *Essentials of geriatric physical therapy*, 2e, Stamford, 2010, Prentice Hall.

Brotzman SB, Wilk KE: *Clinical orthopaedic rehabilitation*, ed 2, St Louis, 2003, Mosby.

Brown SP, Miller WC, Eason JM: *Exercise physiology: basis of human movement in health and disease*, Philadelphia, 2006, Lippincott Williams & Wilkins.

Brukner P, Khan K: *Clinical sports medicine,* ed 3, New York, 2010, McGraw-Hill.

Bryant DP, Bryant BR: *Assistive technology for people with disabilities*, Boston, 2002, Allyn & Bacon.

Bryant R, Nix D: *Acute and chronic wounds: current management concepts*, ed 3, St Louis, 2006, Mosby.

Cameron MH: *Electrical stimulation, ultrasound and laser light handbook*, Philadelphia, 2006, Saunders.

Cameron MH: *Physical agents in rehabilitation handbook: ultrasound, electrical stimulation & laser light*, ed 2, Philadelphia, 2006, Saunders.

Campbell SK, Vander Linden DW, Palisano RJ: *Physical therapy for children*, ed 3, Philadelphia, 2006, Saunders.

Cantu RI, Grodin AJ: *Myofascial manipulation: theory and clinical application*, ed 2, Gaithersburg, 2001, Aspen Publishers.

Carr JH, Shepherd RB: *Neurological rehabilitation: optimizing motor performance*, Philadelphia, 2000, Butterworth-Heinemann.

Carr JH, Shepherd RB: *Stroke rehabilitation-guidelines for exercise and training to optimize motor skill*, Philadelphia, 2003, Butterworth-Heinemann.

Case-Smith J: *Occupational therapy for children*, ed 6, St Louis, 2004, Mosby.

Cech D, Martin S: *Functional movement: development across the life span*, ed 2, Philadelphia, 2002, Saunders.

Cerny FJ, Burton HW: *Exercise physiology for health care professionals*, Champaign, 2001, Human Kinetics.

Ciccone CD: *Pharmacology in rehabilitation*, ed 4, Philadelphia, 2007, FA Davis.

Cleland J: *Orthopaedic clinical examination: an evidence-based approach for physical therapists*, Philadelphia, 2005, Saunders.

Cole MB: *Group dynamics in occupational therapy*, ed 3, Thorofare, 2005, Slack Incorporated.

Cook AM, Polgar J: *Assistive technologies: principles and practice*, ed 3, St Louis, 2007, Mosby.

Cottrell RR, Girvan JT, McKenzie JF: *Principles and foundations of health promotion and education*, ed 4, San Francisco, 2008, Benjamin Cummings.

Crossman AR, Neary D: *Neuroanatomy: an illustrated colour text with student consult access*, New York, 2006, Churchill Livingstone.

Cuppett M, Walsh K: *General medical conditions in the athlete,* St Louis, 2005, Mosby.

Dandy DJ, Edwards DJ: *Essential orthopaedics and trauma*, ed 5, New York, 2009, Churchill Livingstone.

DeDomenico G: *Beard's massage: principles and practice of soft tissue manipulation*, ed 5, Philadelphia, 2007, Saunders.

DePoy E, Gitlin LN: *Introduction to research*, 3e, St Louis, 2005, Mosby.

Dittmar SS, Gresham GE: *Functional assessment and outcome measures for the rehabilitation health professional*, Dallas, 2005, Pro-Ed.

Domholdt E: *Rehabilitation Research,* ed 3, Philadelphia, 2004, Saunders.

Donatelli R: *Biomechanics of the foot and ankle*, ed 2, Philadelphia, 1995, FA Davis.

Donatelli RA, Wooden MJ: *Orthopaedic physical therapy*, ed 4, New York, 2001, Churchill Livingstone.

Donatelli RA: *Physical therapy of the shoulder*, ed 4, New York, 2004, Churchill Livingstone.

Dorland: *Dorland's illustrated medical dictionary*, ed 31, Philadelphia, 2007, Saunders.

Drake RL, Vogl W, Mitchell AWM: *Gray's anatomy for students*, ed 2, New York, 2009, Churchill Livingstone.

Drench ME, et al: *Psychosocial aspects of healthcare*, ed 2, Stamford, 2003, Prentice Hall.

Dutton M: *Orthopaedic examination, evaluation, and intervention*, ed 2, New York, 2004, McGraw-Hill.

Echternach J: *Introduction to electromyography & nerve conduction testing*, Thorofare, ed 2, 2002, Slack Incorporated.

Edelman CL, Mandle CL: *Health promotion throughout the lifespan*, St Louis, 2009, Mosby.

Edmond SL: *Joint mobilization manipulation: extremity and spinal techniques*, ed 2, St Louis 2006, Mosby.

Edmunds MW, Mayhew MS: *Pharmacology for the primary care provider*, ed 3, St Louis, 2008, Mosby.

Effgen SK: *Meeting the physical therapy needs of children*, Philadelphia, 2005, FA Davis.

Esterson SH: *Starting and managing your own physical therapy practice,* 2004, Jones and Bartlett Publishers.

Felton DL, Jozefowicz R: *Netter's atlas of human neuroscience*, Philadelphia, 2003, Saunders.

Field D, Owen-Hutchinson J: *Anatomy, palpation and surface markings: palpation and surface markings*, ed 4, Philadelphia, 2006, Butterworth-Heinemann.

Foley M, et al: *Cardiopulmonary rehabilitation: basic theory and application*, ed 3, Philadelphia, 1997, FA Davis.

Fritz S: *Mosby's fundamentals of therapeutic massage, enhanced reprint*, ed 3, St Louis, 2004, Mosby.

Frontera WR, Slovik DM: *Exercise in rehabilitation medicine*, ed 2, Champaign, 2006, Human Kinetics.

Frownfelter D, Dean E: *Cardiovascular and pulmonary physical therapy: evidence and practice*, ed 4, St Louis, 2005, Mosby.

Gann N: *Orthopaedic case studies*, Gaithersburg, 1998, Aspen Publishers.

Ganong WF: *Ganong's review of medical physiology*, ed 23, New York, 2009, McGraw-Hill Medical.

Gelb D: *Introduction to clinical neurology*, ed 3, Philadelphia, 2005, Butterworth Heinemann.

Gillen: *Stroke rehabilitation: a function-based approach*, ed 2, St Louis, 2004, Mosby.

Gladson B: *Pharmacology for physical therapists*, Philadelphia, 2005, Saunders.

Goodman CC, Fuller K : *Pathology: implications for the physical therapist*, ed 3, Philadelphia, 2009, Saunders.

Goodman CC, Snyder TEK: *Differential diagnosis for physical therapists: screening for referral,* ed 4, Philadelphia, 2006, Saunders.

Greene D, Roberts SL: *Kinesiology: movement in the context of activity*, ed 2, St Louis, 2004, Mosby.

Greenspan A, Chapman MW: *Orthopedic imaging: a practical approach*, ed 4, Philadelphia, 2004, Lippincott Williams & Wilkins.

Guccione A: *Geriatric physical therapy*, ed 2, St Louis, 2000, Mosby.

Gulick D: *Ortho notes: a clinical examination pocket guide*, ed 2, Philadelphia, 2009, FA Davis.

Gutman SA: *Quick reference neuroscience for rehabilitation professionals*, ed 2, Thorofare, 2001, Slack Incorporated.

Guyton AC, Hall JE: *Textbook of medical physiology*, ed 11, Philadelphia, 2005, Saunders.

Guyton AC, Hall JE: *The pocket companion to the textbook of medical physiology*, ed 10, Philadelphia, 2000, Saunders.

Haines DE: *Fundamental neuroscience for basic and clinical applications,* New York, 2005, Churchill Livingstone.

Haines DE: *Neuroanatomy: an atlas of structures, sections, and systems*, ed 7, Philadelphia, 2003, Lippincott Williams & Wilkins.

Hall SJ: *Basic biomechanics*, ed 5, Boston, 2006, McGraw Hill.

Hamill J, Knutzen KM: *Biomechanical basis of human movement*, ed 3, Philadelphia, 2008, Lippincott Williams & Wilkins.

Hansen JT: *Essential anatomy dissector: following Grant's method*, ed 2, Philadelphia, 2002, Lippincott Williams & Wilkins.

Hay WW, Levin MJ, Sondheimer JM, Deterding RR: *Current pediatric diagnosis & treatment*, ed 18, New York, 2006, McGraw-Hill Medical.

Henderson G, Bryan WV: *Psychosocial aspects of disability*, ed 3, Springfield, 2004, Charles C. Thomas Publisher.

Hertling D: *Management of common musculoskeletal disorders: physical therapy principles and methods,* ed 4, Philadelphia, 2005, Lippincott Williams & Wilkins.

Hiatt JL, Gartner LP: *Color atlas of histology*, ed 4, Philadelphia, 2005, Lippincott Williams & Wilkins.

Hicks CM, Hicks C: *Research methods for clinical therapists: applied project design and analysis,* ed 4, New York, 2004, Churchill Livingstone.

Hillegrass EA, Sadowsky HS: *Essentials of cardiopulmonary physical therapy*, ed 2, Philadelphia, 2001, Saunders.

Hillman SK: *Interactive functional anatomy*, ed 2, Champaign, 2005.

Hislop HJ, Montgomery J: *Daniels and Worthingham's muscle testing: techniques of manual examination*, ed 8, Philadelphia, 2007, Saunders.

Huber & Wells: *Therapeutic exercise: treatment planning for progression*, Philadelphia, 2006, Saunders.

Irion G: *Comprehensive wound management*, ed 2, Thorofare, 2009, Slack Incorporated.

Irwin S, Tecklin JA: *Cardiopulmonary physical therapy: a guide to practice*, ed 4, St Louis, 2004, Mosby.

Jacobs MA, Austin NM: *Splinting the hand and upper extremity: principles and process*, Philadelphia, 2002, Lippincott Williams & Wilkins.

Jenkins DB, Hollinshead WH: *Hollinshead's functional anatomy of the limbs and back,* ed 9, Philadelphia, Saunders.

Jones MA, Rivett DA: *Clinical reasoning for manual therapists*, Philadelphia, 2003, Butterworth-Heinemann.

Kaltenborn FM, et al: *Manual mobilization of the joints: the spine*, ed 5, Minneapolis, 2009, Orthopedic Physical Therapy Products.

Kandel ER, Schwartz JH, Jessell TM: *Principles of neural science*, ed 4, New York, 2000, McGraw-Hill Medical.

Katzung BG, Masters S, Trevor A: *Basic and clinical pharmacology*, ed 11, Boston, 2009, McGraw Hill.

Kauffman TL, Barr JO, Moran ML: *Geriatric rehabilitation manual*, ed 2, New York, 2007, Churchill Livingstone.

Kendall FP, et al: *Muscles: testing and function, with posture and pain*, ed 4, Philadelphia, 2005, Lippincott Williams & Wilkins.

Kisner C, Colby LA: *Therapeutic exercise: foundations and techniques*, ed 5, Philadelphia, 2007, FA Davis.

Konin JG, et al: *Special tests for orthopedic examination*, Thorofare, 2006, Slack Incorporated.

Kumar V, et al: *Robbins and Cotran pathologic basis of disease*, ed 8, Philadelphia, 2004, Saunders.

Lattanzi JB, Purnell LD: *Developing cultural competence in physical therapy practice*, Philadelphia, 2005, FA Davis.

Leonard PC: *Building a medical vocabulary: with Spanish translations*, ed 7, Philadelphia, 2008, Saunders.

Leonard CT: *The neuroscience of human movement*, St Louis, 1997, Mosby.

Levangie PK, Norkin CC: *Joint structure and function: a comprehensive analysis,* ed 4, Philadelphia, 2005, FA Davis.

Lewis C, Bottomley J: *Geriatric rehabilitation: a clinical approach*, ed 3, Stamford, 2007, Prentice Hall.

Lewis CB: *Aging: the health care challenge*, ed 4, Philadelphia, 2002, FA Davis.

Lippert LS: *Clinical kinesiology for physical therapist assistants*, ed 4, Philadelphia, 2006, FA Davis.

Long T, Toscano K: *Handbook of pediatric physical therapy*, ed 2, Philadelphia, 2001, Lippincott Williams & Wilkins.

Los Amigos Research and Education: *Observational gait analysis*, Downey, 2001, Los Amigos Research and Education.

Lowe W, Chaitow L: *Orthopedic massage*, ed 2, New York, 2003, Churchill Livingstone.

Lundy-Ekman L: *Neuroscience: fundamentals for rehabilitation*, ed 3, Philadelphia, 2002, Saunders.

Magee DJ, Quillen WS, Zachazewski JE: *Athletic injuries and rehabilitation*, Philadelphia, 1996, Saunders.

Magee DJ, Zachazewski JE, Quillen WS: *Scientific Foundations and Principles of Practice of Musculoskeletal Rehabilitation*, Philadelphia, 2007, Saunders.

Magee DJ: *Orthopedic physical assessment,* ed 5, Philadelphia, 2005, Saunders.

Magill RA: *Motor learning: concepts and applications with powerweb: health and human performance*, ed 6, New York, 2000, McGraw-Hill.

Maitland GD, Hengeveld E, Banks K, English K: *Maitland's vertebral manipulation*, ed 7, Philadelphia, 2005, Butterworth-Heinemann.

Martin S, Kessler M: *Neurologic intervention for physical therapist assistants*, ed 2, Philadelphia, 2000, Saunders.

Maxey L, Magnusson J: *Rehabilitation for the post surgical orthopedic patient*, ed 2, St Louis, 2006, Mosby.

McArdle WD, Katch FI, Katch VL: *Essentials of Exercise Physiology*, ed 3, Philadelphia, 2006, Lippincott Williams & Wilkins.

McArdle WD, Katch FL, Katch VL: *Essentials of exercise physiology and student study guide and workbook for essentials of exercise physiology*, ed 2, Philadelphia, 2004, Lippincott Williams & Wilkins.

McCance KL, Huether SE: *Pathophysiology: the biologic basis for diseases in adults and children*, ed 4, St Louis, 2005, Mosby.

McGill S: *Low back disorders,* ed 2, Champaign, 2007, Human Kinetics.

McKinnis LN: *Fundamentals of musculoskeletal imaging*, ed 2, Philadelphia, 2005, FA Davis.

McPhee SJ, Papadakis MA: *Current medical diagnosis and treatment 2010*, ed 49, New York, 2010, McGraw-Hill Medical.

Mettler FA: *Essentials of radiology*, ed 2, Philadelphia, 2004, Saunders.

Moore AP, Petty NJ: *Neuromusculoskeletal examination and assessment: a handbook for therapists*, ed 3, New York, 2001, Churchill Livingstone.

Moore K, Persaud TVN: *Before we are born: essentials of embryology and birth defects*, ed 7, Philadelphia, 2007, Saunders.

Moore KL, Dalley AF, Agur AMR: *Clinically oriented anatomy*, ed 6, Philadelphia, 2009, Lippincott Williams & Wilkins.

Mosby: *Mosby's medical, nursing & allied health dictionary*, ed 5, St Louis, 2002, Mosby.

Myers BA: *Wound management: principles and practice*, ed 2, Stamford, 2007, Prentice Hall.

Netter FH: *Atlas of human anatomy,* ed 4, Philadelphia, 2006, Saunders.

Neumann DA: *Kinesiology of the musculoskeletal system: foundations for physical rehabilitation*, St Louis, 2009, Mosby.

Nieman DS: *Exercise testing and prescription*, ed 5, New York, 2002, McGraw-Hill.

Nolte: *The human brain: an introduction to its functional analysis*, ed 6, St Louis, 2008, Mosby.

Nordin M, Frankel VH: *Basic biomechanics of the musculoskeletal system*, ed 3, Philadelphia, 2001, Lippincott Williams & Wilkins.

Norkin CC, White DJ: *Measurement of joint motion: a guide to goniometry*, Philadelphia, 2003, FA Davis.

Nosse: *Managerial and supervisory principles for physical therapists*, ed 3, Philadelphia, 2009, Lippincott Williams & Wilkins.

Nowak TJ, Handford AG: *Pathophysiology: concepts and applications for health care professionals*, ed 3, New York, 2004, McGraw Hill.

Oatis CA: *Kinesiology: the mechanics & pathomechanics of human movement*, ed 2, Philadelphia, 2004, Lippincott Williams & Wilkins.

Oschman JL: *Energy medicine in therapeutics and human performance*, Philadelphia, 2003, Butterworth-Heinemann.

O'Sullivan SB, Schmitz TJ: *Physical rehabilitation*, ed 5, Philadelphia, 2006, FA Davis.

Oyelowo T: *Mosby's guide to women's health: a handbook for health professionals*, St Louis, 2007, Mosby.

Pagana KD, Pagana TJ: *Mosby's diagnostic and laboratory test reference,* ed 9, St Louis, 2004, Mosby.

Pagliarulo MA: *Introduction to physical therapy*, ed 3, St Louis, 2001, Mosby.

Palastanga N, Soames R, Field D: *Anatomy & human movement: structure and function*, ed 5, Philadelphia, 2006, Butterworth-Heinemann.

Palisano RJ: *Movement sciences: transfer of knowledge into pediatric practice*, London, 2004, Routlege.

Payne VG, Isaacs LD, Isaacs L: *Human motor development: a lifespan approach,* New York, 2007, McGraw-Hill.

Paz JC, West MP: *Acute care handbook for physical therapists*, ed 2, Philadelphia, 2008, Saunders.

Peckenpaugh NJ, Poleman CM: *Nutrition essentials and diet therapy*, 11 ed, Philadelphia, 2009, Saunders.

Pierson FM, Fairchild SL: *Principles and techniques of patient care*, ed 4, Philadelphia, 2004, Saunders.

Porterfield JA, DeRosa C: *Mechanical low back pain: perspectives in functional anatomy* 1998

Porterfield JA, DeRosa C: *Mechanical neck pain: perspectives in functional anatomy*, ed 2, Philadephia, 1998, Saunders.

Portney LG, Watkins MP: *Foundations of clinical research: applications to practice*, ed 3, Stamford, 2008, Prentice Hall.

Powers SK, Howley ET: *Exercise physiology: theory and application to fitness and performance*, ed 7, New York, 2008, McGraw-Hill.

Prentice WE, Voight ML: *Techniques in musculoskeletal rehabilitation*, Philadelphia, 2001, McGraw-Hill Medical.

Purtilo R: *Ethical dimensions in the health professions*, ed 4, Philadelphia, 2004, Saunders.

Purtilo RB, Haddad AM: *Health professional and patient interaction*, ed 7, Phildelphia, 2007, Saunders.

Quinn L, Gordon J: *Functional outcomes: documentation for rehabilitation*, Philadelphia, 2003, Saunders.

Ratliffe KT: *Clinical pediatric physical therapy*, St Louis, 1997, Mosby.

Reese NB, Bandy WD: *Joint range of motion and muscle length testing*, ed 2, Philadelphia. 2010, Saunders.

Reese NB: *Muscle and sensory testing*, ed 2, Philadelphia, 2005, Saunders.

Reynolds F: *Communication and clinical effectiveness in rehabilitation,* Philadelphia, 2005, Butterworth-Heinemann.

Richmond T, Powers D: *Business fundamentals for the rehabilitation professional*, ed 2, Thorofare, 2009, Slack Incorporated.

Royeen M, Crabtree JL: *Culture in rehabilitation: from competency to proficiency,* Stamford, 2005, Prentice Hall.

Sahrmann S: *Diagnosis and treatment of movement impairment syndromes*, St Louis, 2001, Mosby.

Saidoff DC, McDonough AL, Duprey LP: *Critical pathways in therapeutic intervention: extremities and spine*, St Louis, 2002, Mosby.

Saunders HD: *Evaluation treatment & prevention of musculoskeletal disorders (volume 1 - the spine)*, ed 4, Philadelphia, 2004, Saunders.

Schmidt R, Lee TD: *Motor control and learning: a behavioral emphasis*, ed 4, Champaign, 2005, Human Kinetics.

Scott & Petrosino: *Physical therapy management*, St Louis, 2007, Mosby.

Scott R: *Foundations of physical therapy: a 21st century-focused view*, New York, 2001, McGraw-Hill.

Scott RW: *Legal aspects of documenting patient care*, ed 3, Sudbury, 2000, Jones & Bartlett Publishers.

Scott RW: *Promoting legal awareness in physical and occupational therapy*, St Louis, 1997, Mosby.

Shamus E, Stern DF: *Effective documentation for physical therapy professionals*, New York, 2004, McGraw-Hill.

Shepard KF, Jensen GM: *Handbook of teaching for physical therapists*, ed 2, Philadelphia, 2002, Butterworth Heinemann.

Sherpherd CJ, Carr JH: *Movement science: foundations for physical therapy in rehabilitation*, ed 2, Dallas, 2000, Pro-Ed.

Shiland BJ: *Mastering healthcare terminology*, ed 3, St Louis, 2003, Mosby.

Shumway-Cook A, Woollacott MH: *Motor control: translating research into clinical practice*, ed 3, Philadelphia, 2006, Lippincott Williams & Wilkins.

Sine R, Liss SE, Roush RE: *Basic rehabilitation techniques: a self-instructional guide*, ed 4, Gaithersburg, 2000, Aspen Publishers.

Sisto SA, Durin E, Sliwinski MM: *Spinal cord injuries: management and rehabilitation*, St Louis, 2008, Mosby.

Skinner HB: *Current diagnosis and treatment in orthopedics*, ed 4, New York, 2006, McGraw-Hill.

Skinner JS: *Exercise testing and exercise prescription for special cases: theoretical basis and clinical application*, ed 3, Philadelphia, 2005, Lippincott Williams & Wilkins.

Smith L, Weiss E, Lehmkuhl LD: *Brunnstrom's clinical kinesiology*, Philadelphia, 1996, FA Davis.

Snell RS: *Clinical anatomy for medical students*, ed 6, Philadelphia, 2000, Lippincott Williams & Wilkins.

Snell RS: *Essential clinical anatomy*, ed 3, Philadelphia, 2006, Lippincott Williams & Wilkins.

Somers MF: *Spinal cord injury: functional rehabilitation*, ed 3, Stamford, 2001, Prentice Hall.

Spencer JW, Jacobs JJ: *Complementary and alternative medicine: an evidence-based approach*, St Louis, 2003, Mosby.

Spring H, et al: *Stretching and strengthening exercises*, New York, 1991, Thieme Medical Publishers.

Springhouse (editor): *Clinical pharmacology made incredibly easy*, ed 3, Philadelphia, 2008, Lippincott Williams & Wilkins.

Staheli LT: *Fundamentals of pediatric orthopedics*, ed 4, Philadelphia, 2007, Lippincott Williams & Wilkins.

Standring S: *Gray's anatomy: the anatomical basis of clinical practice*, ed 40, New York, 2008, Churchill Livingstone.

Stone RJ, Stone JA: *Atlas of skeletal muscles*, ed 6, Boston, 2008, McGraw Hill.

Straus SE, et al: *Evidence-based medicine*, ed 3, New York, 2005, Churchill Livingstone.

Sullivan SB, Markos PD: *Clinical procedures in therapeutic exercise*, ed 2, Stamford, 1996, Prentice Hall.

Swisher LL, Page CG: *Professionalism in physical therapy: history, practice, and development*, Philadelphia, 2005, Saunders.

Tortora GJ, Grabowski SR: *Principles of anatomy and physiology*, ed 10, New York, 2002, Wiley & Sons Publishing.

Trevor AJ, Katzung BG, Masters SB: *Katzung and Trevor's pharmacology examination and board review*, ed 8, New York, 2007, McGraw-Hill.

Umphred DA: *Neurological rehabilitation*, ed 5, St Louis, 2006, Mosby.

Watchie J: *Cardiopulmonary physical therapy: a clinical manual*, ed 2, Philadelphia, 2009, Saunders.

Watson T: *Electrotherapy: evidence-based practice*, ed 12, New York, 2002, Churchill Livingstone.

Weir J, Abrahams PH: *Imaging atlas of human anatomy*, ed 3, St Louis, 2003, Mosby.

West JB: *Respiratory physiology: the essentials*, ed 8, Philadelphia, 2004, Lippincott Williams & Wilkins.

White AA, Panjabi MM: *Clinical biomechanics of the spine*, ed 2, Philadelphia, 1990, Lippincott Williams & Wilkins.

Whitmore I, et al: *Human anatomy: color atlas and text*, ed 4, St Louis, 2002, Mosby.

Whittle MW: *An introduction to gait analysis,* ed 4, Philadelphia, 2001, Butterworth-Heinemann.

Wilkins R, Sheldon R: *Clinical assessment in respiratory care*, ed 6, St Louis, 2009, Mosby.

Index